Unravel the Thread

Applying the ancient wisdom of yoga to live a happy life

Rubén Vásquez

Unravel the Thread

Library of Congress Control Number: 2021915034

ISBN 978-1-7376482-0-8

Contact information: https://simple-yoga.org/

Simple Yoga Publications, Saint Petersburg, Florida

Printed in USA

'Unravel the Thread' by Rubén Vásquez is an excellent book that gives a practical and down-to-earth review and interpretation of the Yoga Sutras of Patanjali. The writing style is coherent and easy to read. The author has made a text that is generally very difficult to read, let alone understand or use, very accessible for the general public. By using modern day-to-day examples, the author has made it very easy for the reader to relate to the subject matter. If you are in any way interested in yoga, then I wholeheartedly recommend this book.

Simon Borg-Olivier MSc BAppSc (Physiotherapy) APAM c-IAYT

Reading Unravel the Thread may transform your life! But only if you put it into daily regular practice.

What you will find in this beautiful new book by Rubén Vásquez is a friendly, compassionate and joyful map toward establishing a workable, daily practice that reflects the essence of Yoga as codified and understood through the ancient text of Patanjali Yoga Sutras. Rubén helps to de-mystify these ancient writings and offers suggestions for designing a life practice that is simply defined, practical and inherently joyful to implement. His writing voice is kind, down-to-earth, and evocative.

Keep this book by your bedside. It will inspire you to rise in the morning, curious about how you will show up in your own life, and eager to continue the process of bringing your best Self forward into this present moment.

Peentz Dubble, Certified Iyengar Yoga Teacher (CIYT), IYNAUS Teacher Trainer and Assessor, IAYT accredited Yoga Therapist

Rubén Vásquez has taken the time to make the Yoga Sutra's of Patanjali accessible to all, his examples and use of practical questions for the reader to answer, make it accessible to all. I highly recommend this book!

Bianca Machliss BSc BAppSc (Physiotherapy) YA-ERYT 500

Today is forever, still.

Antonio Machado

CONTENTS

PREFACE

From its origins in India thousands of years ago, yoga has now become many things to many people. While many people see yoga as stretching and physical exercise, others find in yoga a remedy for stress and other ailments. And a growing number of thoughtful practitioners seek in yoga the traditional complete system for deep personal transformation and spiritual freedom used for thousands of years in India. That may explain why the classic yoga text, Patañjali's Yoga Sutra, has become the most popular it has ever been (White xvi). In the last century, many scholars have continued the tradition that began around the fifth century CE by offering commentaries on Patañjali's 196 aphorisms. As scholar Edwin Bryant has pointed out, the Yoga Sutra can be approached from an academic perspective by emphasizing its historic context. Alternatively, a practitioner's point of view on the Yoga Sutra emphasizes instead the practical application of the text. This book takes the practitioner's approach by using the Yoga Sutra as a practical guide for liberating ourselves from the limitations keeping us from experiencing inner freedom, peace of mind, and awareness of the deep interconnectedness between everything that exists.

How this book developed

In 1995, a few years after my introduction to yoga and Zen meditation, I started practicing yoga every day. Since then, I have been on a journey of self-discovery using yoga as the guide for my exploration. Feeling the benefits of yoga in my body, mind, and emotions compelled me to learn more about the foundations of yoga. This led me to the Yoga Sutra. In 2003 I started studying the Yoga Sutra and today I continue to feel grateful for the breadth and depth of wisdom in Patañjali's work.

Over the last fifteen years I have studied the Yoga Sutras to answer a simple question: *How can I use the Yoga Sutra as a framework for my yoga practice and for my life?* Exploring the Yoga Sutra has led me on a journey of learning and transformation. Since I am not a Sanskrit scholar, I have studied over a dozen translations and interpretations of the Yoga Sutra. I have also studied how to chant the Yoga Sutra in Sanskrit by listening and chanting for hundreds of hours. I have also taught myself the Devanagari script to be able to read and hand copy the complete text. This added one more way to experience the Yoga Sutra directly. I also benefited from a course with Dr. Rajan Narayanan where we studied the Yoga Sutra one aphorism at a time. Contemplating the meaning of the Yoga Sutra for daily application has been motivating and inspiring. I feel grateful to Patañjali and to the many authors, yoga scholars, and teachers who have shared their insights for more than a thousand years.

The major criteria I have used in my interpretation of the Yoga Sutras are:

- To honor the wisdom that Patanjali, his predecessors and his commentators have generously shared over centuries.

- To offer an easy-to-understand interpretation of the Yoga Sutra focused on daily application at this moment in history.

- To use common sense explanations and suggestions that invite readers to explore, question, and ultimately make their own intelligent choices.

I acknowledge that the interpretation of any text is deeply influenced by the perspectives, attitudes, and personal history of the person reading that text. Certainly, that is the case with my own interpretations of the Yoga Sutra, which have been evolving over the last fifteen years. Patañjali lists in the Yoga Sutra various forms of knowledge, indicating that the major source of correct knowledge is direct experience (*pratyaksha*) [Yoga Sutra 1.6-1.7]. As a practitioner's manual, this book is an invitation to embark on the journey of self-discovery in order to live in wisdom and free from suffering. The journey requires reflection and application.

In the following pages, I present simple, practical, yet powerful ways of integrating the various aspects of yoga into contemporary life – your life – at a gradual and sustainable pace. I invite you to approach the Yoga Sutra as a set of guidelines to be reflected upon in order to better understand yourself and the interpenetrating systems you are made of. Knowing yourself thoroughly enables you to choose the best way of putting these ideas into practice. You can test if your exploration is working by noticing if you are growing in inner harmony and inner wisdom. This wisdom will guide you to participate in your life with an open mind and an open heart. My desire is to assist you in unraveling the thread of worldly distractions and to instead recognize the common thread of living presence which we all inherently share.

This journey of exploration and application begins from the most concise summary of the whole Yoga Sutra, a single word from the original text. This handbook, filled with questions to guide you as you take charge of your own personal inquiry, beckons you toward a gradual but deep immersion into the fountain of wisdom offered by Patañjali. True wisdom is tested in its usefulness through application. It is up to you to decide which techniques and practices will ultimately enhance your actions and interactions.

May your path be filled with joy, health and clarity,

Rubén

THIS JOURNEY IS NOT FOR YOU IF…

You are truly free from obstructions, distractions and suffering.

You already have satiated your curiosity about the great mysteries of life.

You already are unconditionally accepting, forgiving and loving.

You already fully know yourself intimately.

You already feel ever-expanding enthusiasm about being alive.

You already feel that your life is meaningful, filled with abundance and with a deep sense of connection to yourself and to the people

ACKNOWLEDGMENTS

No human endeavor is accomplished by a single person alone – it's our ability to learn from and cooperate with each other that enables us to expand the boundaries of our specific knowledge and individual limitations. I am grateful to Patañjali, as well as to the many nameless authors whose work inspired Patañjali. My passion for the message of the Yoga Sutra has been fueled by the many authors who have added to Patañjali's work through the centuries. I have often thought that writing a book on Patañjali's Yoga Sutra requires a combination of naiveté and arrogance: it is arrogance to think one can add something new and meaningful to a 1,500-year-long conversation, and naiveté to think that there will be people interested and willing to listen. I am indebted to the many students who have shown me there is growing interest in living the wisdom of the Yoga Sutra not just in contemporary yoga practice, but also in life.

Although most of my exploration of the Yoga Sutra has been a process of trying to make sense of the different texts by testing them out in my own personal practice and life, I have found many teachers along the way. One of the teachers who has influenced my perspective and practice greatly is Erich Schiffmann. Erich has inspired me to make my own practice and teaching clear and effective. I am also grateful to Rajan Narayanan for his patient guidance through the Yoga Sutras one aphorism at a time. My understanding of yoga has also been greatly enriched by the teachings of Simon Borg-Olivier and Bianca Machliss that combine anatomy, physiology, and yoga into a logical, safe, and very effective practice. I also appreciate the common-sense perspective on anatomy offered by Amy Matthews and Leslie Kaminoff. In addition, I would be remiss if I did not mention how much I have benefited from the work of Gregor Maehle, Andrey Lappa, Michael Singer, Michael Brown, Adyashanti, Don Miguel Ruíz, and Yogani, I am thankful to live in a time when so much wisdom is available.

All of life is an opportunity to learn and grow, and everything and everyone we encounter offer countless lessons. My heartfelt thanks to the many students who have attended my workshops on the Yoga Sutras and the teacher training sessions I've led over the last decade: your questions and comments have helped me expand my understanding and have guided me to try to communicate my message effectively. Special thanks to Andrea, Christa, Carol, Carole, Candace, Diane, Jennifer Rose, Johanna, Kristal, Liz B, Liz G, Michele, Michelle, Sandy, Susan, Suzanne, and Tachi for their dedication and interest. I am deeply grateful for the encouragement and support of my friend and colleague Cindy Mastry, who has offered feedback on many versions of this manuscript and who is always willing to geek out about all things yoga and especially about yoga philosophy. I am extremely fortunate that students like Chris Chen and Chris Davis generously provided excellent feedback and suggestions on an earlier draft of this book. I also feel gratitude for dear friends like Sharen Lock and LeGrand Jones who are fellow explorers on the yogic path. There are not enough words to thank LeGrand for his kindness and generosity in offering detailed and insightful feedback on the complete manuscript. The Yoga Sutra study group has been a wonderful venue for exploring many different perspectives on the Yoga Sutra, so thank you Bill, Denise, Peentz, Tricia and all who have attended. I am greatly indebted to Lisa Maier for her generosity and support and for guiding me in the process of making my message more widely accessible. I am deeply grateful for my friend Enee, for her kindness, thoughtfulness, and generosity. Thanks also to Jim for always offering useful insights and suggestions about writing and publishing. To Rusty, you are amazing! Thank you for editing the book with so much care, mindfulness, and clarity. I am fortunate to know dear friends like Amanda, CF, Doug, Julie, Michael, and Yannick. My gratitude goes also to my family Rubén, Ladys, Claudia, Luz Victoria, Adolf, Adri, Carlos, Luca, Jitka, and Zdenek for their love, kindness, and support. My greatest source of inspiration, motivation and support is my beloved Camilla, who has shown me her unwavering unconditional love and support every day of our life together: I love you and thank you with all that I am.

This book represents my best at this time. And even with all the support and help I have received, there are many things that I may have overlooked, places where my understanding has fallen short and where my message might be improved. All errors and mistakes are, of course, my own.

Let's begin our journey, imperfect beings experiencing the one perfect moment – which is the *now* – together.

INTRODUCTION

In the most authoritative Sanskrit-English dictionary, meanings of *sutra* include thread, yarn, string, line, cord, and wire (Monier-Williams). The word *sutra* is related to the English word suture, in the sense of stitches or a seam which joins. In the Indian tradition, a sutra is a compilation of condensed texts on a specific topic such as ritual, philosophy, or grammar. *Sutra* also refers to each one of the concise sentences that make up a complete text. There are *sutras* for topics other than yoga, each one following a coherent line of thinking on a specific subject. Since some of these *sutra* texts were memorized and/or transmitted from teacher to student directly, they were reduced to the minimum number of words possible, both for ease of memorization and for succinctness of messaging.

Traditionally in India, *sutra* study is a dialogue between teacher and student, wherein the teacher elaborates on the meaning and application of each sutra. From the perspective of the teacher, the collection of aphorisms is a teaching aid containing the complete system of yoga. The teacher uses the *sutra* as a starting point for instruction, to be complemented by knowledge the teacher has gathered through direct experience. From the student's point of view, the complete Yoga Sutra is a tool for contemplating the yogic teachings and their import on his or her individual life.

About the Yoga Sutra

The Yoga Sutra of Patañjali offers the first complete handbook of yoga theory and practice (Feuerstein, 2001, p. 214) . Although there is consensus on the idea that the Yoga Sutra is a compilation of ideas and practices that has been around for many centuries, there is no unanimous agreement on the date when the sutras were actually compiled by Patañjali. While some scholars think it was around 3100 BCE (Narayanan, p. 1), others indicate that Patañjali probably lived in the second century BCE (Feuerstein, 2001, p. 214). Yet others suggest that the Yoga Sutra was collected sometime between the first century BCE and the fourth century CE (White, 2014, p. x).

Patañjali, the compiler of the Yoga Sutra, is a complete mystery; through the years, debate continues over his identity. Some sources claim that the same Patañjali who compiled the Yoga Sutra also wrote a treatise on Sanskrit grammar as well as a text on Ayurveda, while other sources refute these claims. What we know – based on the Yoga Sutra – is that Patañjali compiled a complete, coherent set of ideas and practices that is not dogmatic, that has no allegiance to any school of philosophy, and is not tied to any particular religion. His work is beautiful for many reasons, not the least of which is that the Yoga Sutra is abstract enough to permit several interpretations, while the content is specific enough to be used as a handbook for practice.

The Yoga Sutra is arranged in four chapters or *pada*, consisting of 51 aphorisms, 55 aphorisms, 55 (or 56) aphorisms (depending on the source), and 34 aphorisms, totaling 195 (or 196) *sutras*. Chapter One, Integration (*Samadhi*), includes the meaning of yoga; a classification of human patterns; strategies for creating equanimity; paths and steps towards increasing clarity; the effects of distractions and ways to overcome them; and a list of the deeper aspects of meditation. The first half of Chapter Two, Practice (*Sadhana*), defines yogic action as a way to remove afflictions and to increase inner peace; explains the cycle of karma, the causes of suffering, and the removal of suffering; and proposes discernment as the way to avoid future suffering. The second half of Chapter Two introduces the eight-limb path of yoga as an effective way to decrease inefficiencies, increase wisdom, and establish discernment of one's true nature. The second chapter concludes with an explanation of the first five limbs. Chapter Three, Magnificence (*Vibhuti*), addresses the last three limbs in the yoga path for deep meditation, through which the practitioner gains insight into all aspects of internal and external phenomena. The third chapter also lists the many possible results of applying deep meditation to numerous focal objects and warns of the potential pitfalls in misusing advanced meditation techniques. The chapter closes enumerating the highest effects of meditation. Chapter Four of this ancient treatise, Emancipation (*Kaivalya*), illuminates the nature of existence, including the relationship between awareness and nature as well as the interactions between experiences, memories, and their manifestations as tendencies and specific circumstances. The interplay all of these elements becomes the context for developing a keen sense of discernment that leads into profound wisdom and eventual liberation.

The conciseness of the Yoga Sutra, each aphorism a type of cosmic shorthand, gave rise to systematic commentaries (*bhashya*) offering explanations and examples. Over the centuries, some of these *bhashya* have become virtually indispensable aids to understanding the original text, Many commentaries studied today hand-in-hand with the Yoga Sutra have themselves been around for at least a thousand years. As

David Gordon White eloquently demonstrates in his history of the Yoga Sutra, Patañjali's work has a fascinating history of interpretation, rich, varied and ever evolving.

Claude Maréchal, teacher and longtime student of T.K.V. Desikachar, offers a perspective on the Yoga Sutra based on knowledge handed down from legendary 20th century teacher, T. Krishnamacharya (Desikachar's father). In this view, each chapter of the Yoga Sutra is a complete course of study, designed for students at specific levels of aptitude and development. Maréchal suggests Chapter One, *Samadhi*, was for advanced students (*Kritanjali*) familiar enough with the techniques of yoga who used these methods to overcome many obstacles on the path to integration. Chapter Two, *Sadhana*, he posits, was for students who are dominated by suffering (*Baddhanjali*). This path is composed of the yoga of action and the first 5 limbs of yoga, also known as the external practices (*Yamas*, *Niyamas*, *Asana*, *Pranayama* and *Pratyahara*). Chapter Three, *Vibhuti*, he sees as intended for students who have mastered their minds (*Mastakanjali*). Their balanced and oriented minds can engage in the internal practices, *Dharana*, *Dhyana* and *Samadhi* to remain on the right path while uncovering the mysteries of life. Chapter Four, *Kaivalya*, Maréchal concludes guides accomplished and complete students (*Purnanjali*) who have attained complete detachment and are capable of understanding the intricacies of nature and the structure of life.

In ancient India, the source of yoga, and in contemporary India, the modern face of yoga, we recognize a wide diversity among practices considered to be expressions of yoga. As yoga has become known, explored, taught, and practiced around the world, interpretation and application of the Yoga Sutra itself is influenced by the mindset and needs of each individual practitioner. It may be argued that these local adaptations in contemporary practices are as natural and genuine as the ebb and flow of any river, or as intertwined as the warp and weft of a hand-spun fabric.

Patañjali's Yoga Sutra offers a concise, complete, yet complex map for explorers on the path to spiritual growth, transformation and true freedom. This chart is a navigational aid, a technical manual only activated through application. While interest in this text has waxed and waned over millennia, it has remained alive (beyond mere academic interest) because of its usefulness as a systematic approach for exploring the human condition, irrespective of the who, the when, or the where of its study. The wisdom offered within it must be tested by each student who tries to put it into practice with enthusiasm, intelligence and humility. Commitment provides the fuel to embark on this fascinating journey of exploration; consistency determines its rhythms. Each student innately possesses the resources needed to undertake this excursion toward enlightenment. Its measure of success is dependent upon how this cultivated wisdom ultimately is reflected, through daily actions and interactions in the world.

How to use this book

Famously terse and packed with meaning, the Yoga Sutra has the reputation of being challenging to read, understand, and apply. **Unravel the Thread** invites you to find your answers to the question *How can the Yoga Sutra be applied today?* As you unravel the meaning of the Yoga Sutra for you and for your own life, you discover intelligent, compassionate, and kind ways to untie the entanglements, knots and binds restricting the fullest expression of your true nature.

Unravel the Thread is organized into two sections, the first offering an overview of the complete Yoga Sutra; the second exploring the meaning and application of each one of the 196 sutras in the original text. Application activities, practice suggestions, and questions for reflection accompany each section of this book, providing practical exercises to bridge philosophy/theory with practice/process.

Section One: Overview
Together, we explore Awakening, Enlightenment, Liberation, Transcendence and Presence, and address the fundamental queries *What is Yoga?* and *Who am I?*

Section Two: Following the Thread
Chapters Six through Ten of **Unravel the Thread**: Integration (*Samadhi*), Practice (*Sadhana*), Magnificence (*Vibhuti*), and Emancipation (*Kaivalya*), consist of a summary synthesizing the major concepts in the chapter followed by an interpretation of each sutra with specific recommendations for practice.

The concluding Chapter Eleven offers specific guidelines for continuing the path of applying the Yoga Sutra, including suggestions for practicing the eight limbs of yoga: *Yamas* (Friendliness and Compassion), *Niyamas* (Purity and Sincerity), *Asana* (Intelligent posture and movement), *Pranayama* (Efficient Energy Modulation), *Pratyahara* (Inner focus and sensitivity), *Dharana* (Concentration), *Dhyana* (Meditation) and *Samadhi* (Integration). Here, we learn to weave the thread of yoga into life.

Unravel the Thread is a logical, heartfelt handbook for bringing the wisdom of the Yoga Sutra into your daily life, starting with the most accessible ways to practice. Through your commitment and your consistency, The Yoga Sutra will become a lifelong guide on the journey to living with wisdom, awareness, and compassion.

Let's begin.

SECTION ONE: OVERVIEW

अथ योग अनुशासनम्

atha yoga anuśāsanam

Now, yoga instruction

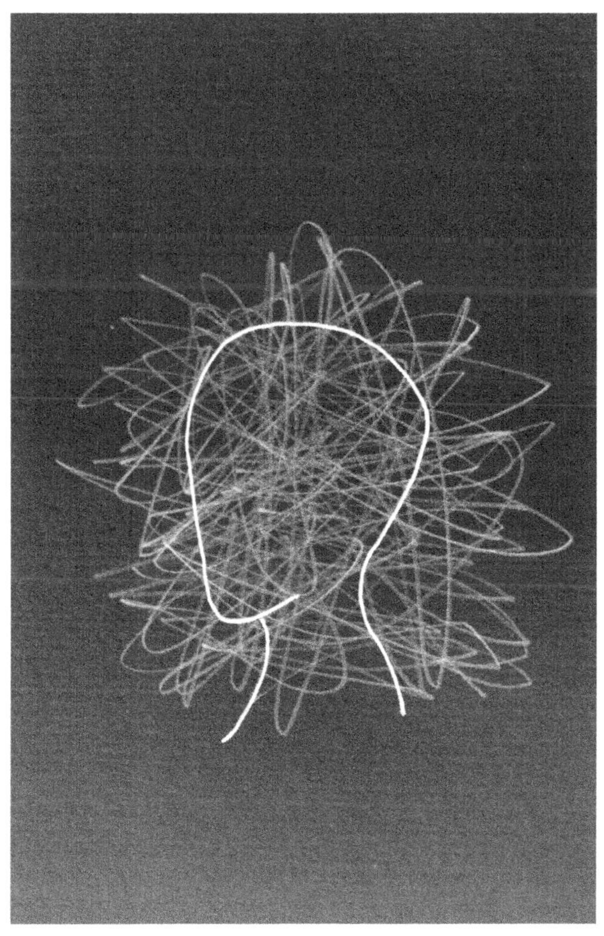

As we consistently try to meet ourselves where we are just as we are, we notice how often we get entangled by our habits, weighed down by our stories, and bound by our preferences and beliefs. We may also notice how many of our choices turn out not to be really ours. Although all this may sound discouraging, this shift in perspective carries with it the promise of transformation.

AWAKENING, ENLIGHTENMENT, LIBERATION AND TRANSCENDENCE

The words *awakening*, *enlightenment*, *liberation* and *transcendence* are used frequently in yoga circles. Far from casual jargon, these terms help us frame our discussions about yoga, and give us a common language for the important dialogues which arise from yoga study and practice.

Awakening is coming to realize that this moment is unique, because it has never happened before, and it will not be repeated ever again. Regardless of how much you want to be in a different moment, you can only be in this moment, right here and now. Indeed, this moment is the culmination of your whole life up until now. At the same time, this moment is the starting point for the rest of your life. *By being in this unique moment you are experiencing the effects of all your previous actions while also planting the seeds for your own future.* This moment is all that you have and the only moment in which you can act. Awakening is to recognize that you have never been in yesterday or in tomorrow, and that you are always, only in today. Awakening to that simple and irrefutable fact can be all the motivation you need to show up and do the best you can – instead of living in your head, in the *what if*, *what used to be*, and *what could have been*. This realization urges you to make your presence in the world matter today. The opposite of awakening is continuing to go through your life as though sleepwalking. Awakening is the recognition that the present moment is the most important moment of your life. Are you open to experiencing directly what awakening feels like?

When you keep repeating the same beliefs and opinions over and over and over, you eventually convince yourself that those thoughts, feelings, and views are facts, that your viewpoint is actually, inarguably *the* truth. Acting from that perspective may lead you to seek only others with similar opinions, or impel you to be hostile to those who do not share your beliefs. History is laden with examples of dogmatic ideologies serving as tools of oppression and violence. In yoga, **liberation** is your conscious decision to relinquish your beliefs and opinions so that you can experience your life directly, perceiving what is happening with as much clarity as possible, without the interference of your preconceived ideas. Liberation also refers to freeing yourself from your attachments and your constant inner commentary. Yogic practice provides ways to uncover these unhelpful, often obstructive patterns. A deep understanding of yoga leads you to recognize patterns in your ways of thinking, and allows you to see tendencies in your emotions, with the ultimate goal of removing these inefficiencies and restrictions. As you free yourself from ways of being that weigh you down, you'll notice changes to your inner life and to the ways you participate in everything you do.

Enlightenment is a lightening of your attitude, allowing you to touch everything gently, with kindness and compassion. You lighten your load in life by modulating your ways of being to minimize restrictions, leading to wholehearted and mindful living. A simple embodiment of the notion of enlightenment is to experiment with making your daily physical movements as graceful as possible, and then to notice how that simple physical change leads to lightness within. Another suggestion: Consider if you might be taking yourself too seriously. Often, just bringing a smile to your face and your heart can have a similar lightening effect. From this perspective, enlightenment would mean to make your smile your default mode of being. Enlightenment can also be understood as flooding the present moment with the light of your undiluted awareness. Rather than trying to predict how enlightenment will feel for you, feel it directly in the wondrous interactions between your body, your mind and your emotions, as well as in your daily interactions with the people and world around you.

Another word you hear often used in relation to yoga and its goals is **transcendence**. In addition to the common definition of transcendence as "going beyond material experience," there is also a very practical aspect of transcendence – surpassing your current limitations. Learning, for example, is a process of transcending your present levels of understanding so that your perception expands beyond its current limits. *In order to grow past your current level of knowing, it is essential to be able to sit with the discomfort of not knowing.* Without acknowledging what you do not know, it's unlikely that you might even consider venturing outside the boundaries of what you do know. Be curious to discover what is beyond your current levels of presence, awareness and understanding. And you must learn to discern between bearable discomfort and pain. Pain produces a protective response, that feeling when your body, breath, and mind brace for impact. This pain response is useful and relevant, alerting you to avoid potential injury. Bearable discomfort, though, is different than pain; it makes you uneasy, yet it doesn't tighten your muscles or restrict your breathing. Bearable discomfort often emerges when you go against the grain of habit or step out of what is familiar. You may even label what is unusual as pain, when what you are experiencing is actually the discomfort of not knowing. As you advance in your study and practice of yoga, you'll develop a heightened sensitivity to distinguishing clearly between bearable discomfort and pain. This is the key to transcending beyond your current ways of being, not just in yoga, but in every aspect of life.

Yoga is not inherently good or bad, harmful or beneficial. Yoga practice contains techniques to amplify your ability to show up to your life with integrity, grace and enthusiasm. That's why an open mind and open heart are useful – they enable you to show up unencumbered by preconceptions. Yoga may serve as a vehicle for your release from the physical, mental and emotional ways of being that restrict your life experience. Yoga can become a journey of optimizing your participation in life with grace and kindness. Yoga does not relinquish your responsibility for your decisions and actions.

It may be tempting to see yoga as a way to remove yourself from life and living in the world; however, yoga is an invitation to establish clear, coherent and harmonious relationships between your body, breath, mind and emotions. Yoga is witnessing the natural symbiosis of all your systems working in unison. Moreover, there is no time when you are absolutely alone and in isolation from everything else. The belief that you are only what is confined by the boundaries of your skin denies the fact that there is a deep interconnection between yourself and everything else. As Lawrence Krauss (Atom: An Odyssey from the Big Bang to Life on Earth...and Beyond) suggests, *every time you breathe you are connected to almost all of life on Earth today, in the past and perhaps even in the future.* Because of the interconnectedness of everything, your life is a constant dance between you and your circumstances. How you choose to participate in this dance resonates directly or indirectly with everything that exists. Yoga provides a system to guide your choices for treading through life with awareness and kindness.

Agency: you choose

As you immerse more deeply in the Yoga Sutra, you'll recognize that Patañjali offers you a framework but does not make decisions for you. This respect for your own judgment pervades the Yoga Sutra, and may be one of its most helpful and empowering aspects. It may also be one of the most challenging, because it requires you to be an active agent in your life, to be responsible, to choose your intentions, decisions, and actions consciously and deliberately. In this way the Yoga Sutra may be seen as a handbook offering you options for self-regulation. It will be the quality of your life which confirms or denies the accuracy of your yogic understanding. The agency, or action, of your existence is for you and you only to choose.

It is important to emphasize that nowhere in the Yoga Sutra are you asked to give up your capacity to decide for yourself. On the contrary, you are encouraged to continually cultivate your capacity to discern, so that your own internal clarity and peace can inform your actions and interactions in all environments and circumstances. You are in charge of your life and decisions, and regardless of the choices you make, you will have to live with their consequences, including your successes and your mistakes. Yoga provides context, guiding you to establish truth through exploration. By living your life, you've been conducting an experiment throughout your life; this yogic framework offers you a viable path to continue your experiment with intelligence and compassion. It bears repeating that your study and practice **do not deprive you of your ability to choose**; you remain committed to making your own decisions as best as you can. Since nobody else can fully know your experience, why would you let anyone else choose what's best for you? Making your own choices and facing their consequences is, arguably, your main responsibility in life.

These concepts of agency (making choices), awakening (living in immediacy), enlightenment (being in lightness), liberation (letting go) and transcendence (surpassing limitations) comprise a process rather than a destination. This process begins as you choose to participate in your life consciously and proceeds as you begin to notice that your thoughts, words, and actions generate feedback. The feedback you receive may trigger a reaction – bearable discomfort indicating that your previous perspectives, attitudes, and habits no longer fit who you are in the present moment. Choosing to ignore the feedback is an *easy* way to deal with it, but overlooks the fact that your feedback is exquisitely calibrated to your current situation. Ignoring the feedback (continuing living your life as you have been) results in more powerful feedback being generated. The harder you try to stay with your old habitual ways of being, the more discomfort you will experience. The message gets louder with each repetitive refusal to change, to ensure that it gets through. This is how identity is reshaped. Every traditional culture has rites of passage marking these life transitions as a transformation, often a symbolic death of the old ways of being. Although it is sometimes a forceful process, it also happens in a gradual and less dramatic way every single day when you learn something new. Remember, this is a lifelong process of growing in awareness. Trust that the process happens at the pace that you can handle.

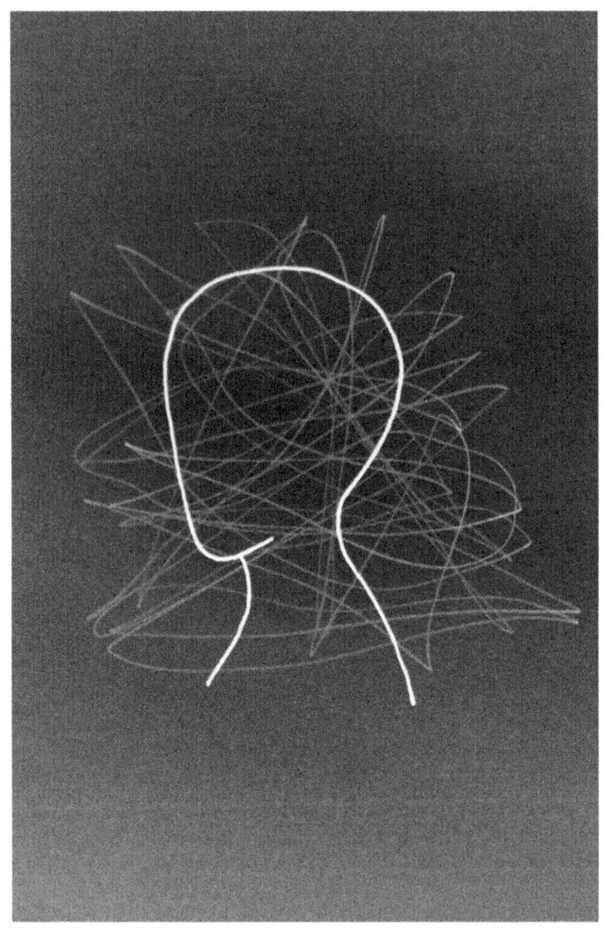

There is nothing as vital, essential, and empowering as presence. Presence of mind and heart communicate aliveness to intentions, actions and interactions, thus enriching life with enduring meaning, inspiration and responsibility.

PRESENCE

One word summary: Atha (अथ)

Several texts in the yoga tradition begin with the Sanskrit word *atha* (अथ). The "th" is pronounced like the "th" in ho*th*ouse or ligh*th*ouse. *Atha* can be defined both as "now" and as an exclamation used to draw attention. From the simplest point of view, all yoga techniques offer ways of bringing your complete and undivided attention to the moment you are in. The words "awareness" and "mindfulness" point to this quality of attending the present. *Atha* is both a reminder to embark on the journey as well as a pointer to its destination: Presence. Deshpande, a contemporary commentator on the Yoga Sutra, suggests *atha* be interpreted as "and now," which acts both as a reminder to be in this moment and a suggestion that life consists of the imperceptible passing of *this* now into the *next* now. *Atha* as "and now" also reminds us that even in our most earnest efforts to be present, we'll find ourselves facing distractions from this specific, unique moment. Your practice, then, is about continually, fully coming back to the now moment that is the present.

BEING PRESENT IS THE ESSENCE AND GOAL OF THE PRACTICE

Yoga is about being present. In other words, yoga is about showing up for your life with the intention of doing the best that you can. Since presence can only be experienced directly, talking or reading about presence (studying) is not presence itself; but study helps clarify the map pointing to your destination.

$$Yoga = Presence = Awareness = \ Being\, with\, what\, is$$

FIGURE 1. YOGA IS PRESENCE

Presence, yoga, is being with what is. When you attend to what is happening you notice that the present moment, "what is," is Presence – yoga – is being with what is. When you attend to what is happening, you notice that the present moment, "what is," is dynamic. It's a paradox, because you are always only in this moment, right here and right now, but this present moment keeps morphing into a brand new and unrepeatable moment. The present is a fleeting instant in eternal transformation. It is both a single point in time and all the different times that you have ever been in, as well as all the potential moments that you will ever be in. Take a moment to close your eyes and take this in.

Life is a precious gift delivered as the present, an always-new moment. We are free to do with that gift whatever we want, and anything we want. For instance, we can choose to ignore this moment because we think that a previous moment was/is the most important moment in life. So, we may choose to invest attention, energy, and money trying to go back to that previous moment. We could also choose to ignore this moment by projecting an idea, thought, emotion,

Presence, Being Present, Being with What Is, Mindfulness, Consciousness, Attention, Awareness
Think about all of these words as focusing only on the task at hand; concentrating on a single activity; paying close attention to your actions; acting consciously and deliberately; to do what you are doing; being here now; conscious awareness; remaining focused on what is actually happening right where you are.

or experience into the future. Regardless of which avenue of avoidance we choose– and many of us are trying to do both at the same time – we are still choosing to ignore, rather than be in, *this* moment.

Isn't it remarkable that you can choose whatever approach you prefer for participating in your life? You are choosing what you do with this precious gift of life all the time. For yogis, the destination is being in the eternal present moment. If you find yourself constantly thinking about other times and places as more desirable or more important than the moment you are in, or always planning the future or projecting outcomes of yet-to-be moments, remind yourself three things about the present: first, this moment is the culmination of every single moment in your life so far; second, the moment you are in is the only moment in which you can act; and third, this moment is the starting point for the rest of your life. The actions you take right here and now will influence the rest of your life. Reflect on these three characteristics of this very moment. Do you recognize the invitation to show up fully, to be wholly present, to *live* every moment as it occurs?

If you are already present all the time, or most of the time, you may already be in the state of yoga and have figured out a few effective ways to stay present. Many of us, however, frequently notice that we keep getting distracted from the present moment. I get distracted much of the time. Indeed, that is the main reason I practice yoga regularly.

Life is an experiment

I profess that I am both an optimist and an idealist. So, up until not very long ago, I used to assume that everyone who appeared successful in my eyes had figured out answers to at least some of the mysteries of life. By observing and listening more attentively to people and by removing my assumptions, it became apparent that each person is conducting an experiment with life. For instance, even when you have a recipe for a dish that you like and that you have made many times, every time you make it, in spite of following the recipe to a T, life in its ongoing newness and uniqueness brings variations, large or small, that influence how the recipe turns out. Of course, that is the essence of life: ongoing newness ever transforming.

All of us are currently conducting an experiment with our lives. As Samuel Butler said, "Life is like playing a violin in public and learning the instrument as one goes on." Some people are successful dealing with the uncertainty of not really knowing how the experiment will turn out, while others become good at pretending they have it all figured out. In truth, since nobody has ever been in this moment before, *every single person in the world is constantly improvising*. Two helpful concepts in navigating your individual life experiment are *framework* and *attitude*: a framework is a system that provides a sound structure for your experiment, and attitude is the way in which you choose to go about it.

Yogic Framework

The yogic framework simply asks you to act consciously and deliberately. Not unlike with the scientific method, there are helpful guidelines for applying it:

- Keep your mind open. Choose not to assume or predict.
- Notice your biases and keep them in check.
- Use your direct experience to establish what is.
- Be aware that internal activities such as narrating, describing and complaining are not *what is*; they are only your *reactions* to what is.

Attitude

The attitude you choose influences what you do and what you experience. You may choose the attitude of a seeker. In that case, you are searching, or looking, for something. The challenge is that to look for something, you need to know what you are going to find. For instance, when I misplace my keys, if I do not know what they look like I won't be able to find them. When you let go of preconceived ideas, predictions and assumptions, you are better able to notice what is actually happening, instead of dedicating energy to try to find out why things are different from your expectations. When free from preconceptions, you can actually experience directly what is taking place. If you already think you know, you are more likely to focus your perception on being right and on seeing what you think you "should" see. So, for this journey it is helpful to adopt instead the attitude of an explorer, scientist, or artist, as captured in Pablo Picasso's words, "I do not seek. I find." Another key attitude is curiosity. Curiosity is a genuine desire to understand, which infuses your actions with the energy of discovery. Curiosity tends to be more fruitful in supporting your full participation in your own life. Since life is changing all the time, nobody knows what will happen. Nobody has been in this moment before, so we are all improvising! What happens when you shift your energy from predicting to being curious? And, since your life is your own project, it is essential that your attitude embraces making your own choices instead of letting others decide things for you. Of course, having a useful framework and attitude is helpful only if they make sense to you… and if you actually use them.

Throughout this book, the application exercises are invitations for you to explore your internal environment. None of these exercises tell you what you should feel or find. Rather than trying to elicit a specific answer or experience, these exercises create opportunities for you to experience presence directly in your life. Because you are unique, and your life is unique, the experience of being you is specific. Thus, you may find some of these exercises and techniques helpful, while others may not do anything for you. In each instance, you are the one who decides if you want to use a particular tool on your unique journey.

PUTTING IT INTO PRACTICE: AM I PRESENT?

Take about 15 minutes to complete this exercise.

PAUSING & FEELING

Find a position where you can be comfortably alert for three to five minutes. Consider setting a timer. Close your eyes and notice what happens. When time is up, open your eyes.

CLARIFYING

Take a few moments to write down answers to the following questions. Use the questions to understand and digest the experience. There is no pressure on you to write "correct" answers; simply reply.

- What did you feel?

- How would you describe the experience you just had?

- Did any sensations capture your attention?

- Did your attention stay in the moment or did it go to other times and places, such as your to-do list, or some project you are working on?

- What was your general attitude?

- Overall, how did you feel?

You may have found this exercise relaxing, or frustrating, or annoying, or enjoyable, or some combination of these and other feelings. You may have even noticed something you had not noticed before, like an ache or a pain, or some underlying preoccupation. Many of us feel busy inside. Perhaps you heard an internal voice constantly talking, describing, liking or disliking, narrating, endlessly giving opinions, and asking "Is time to stop?" Often, this exercise helps us see that our experience of the present moment seems fragmented, and that our mind keeps running between the past, the future and the present. If that was the case for you, welcome to being human in the 21st century. Despite all these internal activities, I assure you: **There is nothing fundamentally wrong with you.**

Guidelines for the Journey

The heart of your practice is to choose to be here. You attend to whatever you are feeling right here and now. You choose to feel what is happening, rather than to engage in internal dialogue. There's no need to compare this moment with other times and places, because this experience is unique. This experience as valid, if only because you are having it *right now* – whatever is happening is what your life is at this very moment. Mindfulness (paying attention) teaches us that what we are feeling is mutable from one distinct moment to the next. Your journey may include exploration of how your attitude, posture, breathing, thinking, and feelings influence your perception of what is happening. (More on that later.) The suggestions I offer here invite you to study and practice yoga as the approach to conducting your life experiment, using yogic tools for living a conscious and deliberate life that is and feels meaningful, joyful, and vibrant.

DESIRE: SHOW UP, ONLY YOU CAN DO IT

Seeing the word *desire* may prompt conflict with some traditional ideas in yoga and Buddhism, which say that all suffering results from desire. In the long history of philosophy in South Asia, there have been innumerable debates over the question of desire, including the question *Is it possible to have no desire whatsoever?* One of the ancient critiques of Buddhism argued that wanting to be enlightened is itself a desire. For the average person living in the world, not having any desire at all could result in never getting out of bed in the morning, or never doing anything at all. Even if it were possible, this "desireless" life is quite impractical for most of us. Without desire, there is no motivation to do anything.

Every day, consciously and unconsciously, we make choices, big and small, about what to wear, what to eat, what to do, etc., etc. Throughout your exploration of the Yoga Sutra, you'll have to make some choices, and those choices will likely be influenced by what you want to accomplish, what you desire. In this context, desire is a meaningful and heartfelt aspiration, carrying with it the spark of energy to move you toward what you find meaningful and inspirational. Awakening to the undeniable fact that this moment is your life, that your life does not happen at any other time or place but right here and now can be a powerful reminder that ignites your commitment to show up to your life. Nobody else can do it for you! Anything you have achieved in your life happened because it was important enough for you to commit your time and energy to accomplishing it. Yoga is a commitment to show up to your life, ready and willing to give it your best try. Can you think of a better way to participate in the source of all creativity, life itself? Besides, being present in your life is both your inalienable right and your inevitable responsibility.

PUTTING IT INTO PRACTICE: WHAT DO YOU WANT?

Take about 10 minutes to complete this exercise.

In a comfortable position, close your eyes. Take a few moments to soften any tension from your eyes, mouth and jaw, neck and throat, shoulders and arms, abdominal and lower back area, and hips and legs. Invite yourself to investigate your desires by asking yourself:

- What do I want?

- What motivates me to get out of bed every morning?

- What is meaningful to me?

- How am I contributing my uniqueness to the world?

Your answers to these questions may change over time, or you may discover answers here which remain constant on your lifelong journey. Observe if anything you've written helps you feel more alive, awake and energized. Consider choosing those energizing answers to use as affirmations reminding yourself what you care deeply about. These affirmations may be statement like, "I participate fully in my life," or "I am present and full of compassion," or "I offer support and inspiration to myself and others," or "I am contributing to make the world a better place by…." The most powerful affirmations will be ones that are most meaningful to you, because they reflect your personal goals and values.

Attitude: Open Mind and Open Heart

"We see the world, not as it is, but as we are." anonymous

In the context of meeting each moment just as it is, our attitude plays a decisive role. For example, a few years ago, my wife and I were meeting a friend in a city we'd never visited before. We agreed with our friend to stay at a bed and breakfast close to the city center. The two of us arrived first, checked in, and marveled at how charming and lovely we found our accommodations. Upon returning from a quick stroll around the city center, we found our friend had arrived at our B&B. While the two of us very much liked our place, our friend kept pointing out things that were, in her opinion, inadequate or lacking. It struck me how the same place, during the same day, could be seen in such different ways by different people. This encounter demonstrated clearly how our individual attitudes influence how we feel as well as what and how we see.

Recognize that this is a unique moment, a moment in which you have never ever been before and a moment in which you'll never be again. This mentality is what is sometimes known as "beginner's mind." It's just like visiting a new place – our senses sharpen, we pay close attention to what is happening, and we see the moment in its uniqueness. That is our invitation to genuinely appreciate it. Think about the first time you traveled to a new city and how everything captured your attention, from the quality of the light, to the local architecture and color, to unfamiliar foods and aromas. **Newness invites awareness.**

On the other hand, if you travel to the same location again and again, or if you move to that place, some of the features that were new become familiar over time and, therefore easy to ignore, partly because you think you already know the place. Similarly, even though you have only one chance to be in each day, you may assume, because you have seen so many other Tuesdays that you already know what will happen or how you will feel on this Tuesday. Predicting what will happen (projecting the known onto the unknown) is a way we remove anxiety triggered by uncertainty. Trying to predict is also a way of living in the past, because predictions are usually based on previous experiences and on what you *think* you know. Since life is always changing in unpredictable ways, it is impossible for most of us to accurately predict what will happen in just 48 or 72 hours. Having an open mind enables you to come to each moment appreciating that you have never been in this moment before, so that you can approach this moment with curiosity and awareness.

The complement to an open mind is an open heart. Have you noticed how arguments with our loved ones and friends often result from somebody holding on tightly to his or her way of thinking and feeling? It is difficult to be receptive while feeling defensive. Inviting the mind to open is also an invitation for the heart to open, releasing the tendency to decide beforehand how you "should" feel. Believing that the world is a hostile place closes your heart, and filters everything you see through fear and anxiety. Seeing the world as a place of cooperation and connection creates possibilities for communication and community.

Take a moment to reflect on how you see the world. Is it a hostile place or a friendly place? Does life require you to be aggressive and competitive, or does it ask you to be helpful and cooperative? What direct evidence has informed your current views? How do your ideas influence your attitude, perceptions emotions and interactions?

To uncover some of the unconscious ways of thinking and feeling that influence your attitude, consider these questions, too. Are there obstacles preventing you from showing up to each moment with an open mind and an open heart? What assumptions color your mind, and what predispositions color your emotions? What would it take for you to invite yourself to participate in your life with gentle curiosity, gratitude, and enjoyment? What happens if you see that this day will never come back? What happens if you act as if you had infinite time for what you are doing?

Offering yourself the gift of Time

Giving yourself time is an essential skill for engaging in meaningful projects and for establishing meaningful relationships with yourself, with others, and with the world around you. In contemporary life, we tend to treat time as a commodity, a luxury that not everybody has. It seems unusual, certainly for urban dwellers, to find people who have plenty of time. On the contrary, a great majority of people feel pressed for time. Despite having more and more technological tools to help us "manage our time" and increase our productivity, time remains scarce. Believing that "time is money" urges us to stop wasting time, to save time and to gain time, as if time itself was a coin or coupon or a physical currency. The existence of "daylight saving time," when clocks are advanced or reversed at certain times in the year reminds us that time is just a convention, a tool we created for our convenience.

Author Joe Marshalla points out that time is just a way to measure the passing of now. Regardless of what day of the week or what time of day it is, **you are always only in the right here and right now**. Right here and right now is the most important moment in life, because you can only act in the present moment; actions that happened before or may happen in the future are mere mental memories and notions, lacking effect on the world. Accepting that this moment is unique and precious can be enough to offer ourselves the gift of time; however, feeling busy often gives us a sense of self-importance, a sense of being needed in other times and places. So, you must inquire: What does it take to give yourself permission to be fully present? Will life elsewhere continue its endless movement even when you are not there? Can the world survive without you? Have you considered that there are tens of thousands of different circumstances that had to happen in order for the moment you are in to be exactly as it is? Pondering these complex questions can create a unique opportunity for you to participate consciously and deliberately in this moment, inviting you to take part in life in the only way that you can – by being you.

Learning to see that your own life deserves your undivided attention is vital. Otherwise, it's highly unlikely you can be present. You are important. You have something unique to contribute to the world, something that no one else can give. Offering yourself the gift of time enables you to dedicate your attention and energy to what really matters.

RELAX

Knowing that you can be effective *only in the place where you are* enables you to let go of other times and places. How often do you take time just to be? When we try to be still and quiet, we may notice a constant stream of thoughts and opinions running through our minds. Many (if not all) of those thoughts are related to the past or the future in the form of regrets, worries, plans, dreams, and fears. One way of redirecting your attention and energy is to ask yourself if there is anything wrong that is within your power to change right where you are. If there is something that needs fixing and you can fix it right there and then, do it. Otherwise, if whatever needs to be fixed is out of reach at this point, then just drop it. Let it go. Releasing what is out of our control efficiently frees up the energy being used as tension, stress and worry.

Being relaxed is not the same as feeling sleepy or exhausted. Actually, redirecting energy away from mental, emotional, and muscular tension and towards being in the present moment has the dual effects of helping you feel relaxed and energized at the same time. The energy that was previously allocated to tension suddenly becomes available for presence. Try this now for a few minutes. Redirect your energy away from planning, remembering, or worrying by asking this:

Is there anything that is wrong, right here and now, that is within my power to change? Then, fix whatever needs fixing, if anything. If there's nothing to fix, then smile and enjoy being in a time and place where nothing is wrong. Notice how you feel afterward.

Distractions

It's a sign of your humanity, not an indication of inadequacy, that you will become distracted. Distractions will happen, sooner or later, either a few times or countless times. Distractions may be either external or internal. They come in many forms, like memories and emotions. Some distractions may be enticing, while others may not be welcome at all. Regardless of what the distraction is, to the best of your ability, just drop it. It may help to remember that this is the only moment you have and thus, no other moment can be more important than this. Let go of the distraction and **return to this irreplaceable moment without any struggle, strain, or self-judgment**. This attitude may be the single most important skill to cultivate. Notice that you got distracted, and just return to now, without agitation, without complaining, without self-criticism. I would even suggest that this is what the practice aspect of yoga is about: letting go of what is not here and calmly choosing to be in the only place where we can act and make a difference. Struggle, strain, and self-judgment are completely the opposite of being with what is. In yoga, we practice presence.

I've discovered the process of presence is easy and simple. We wake up to the fact that the moment we are in requires and deserves our undivided attention. We choose to be here, doing what we are doing.

I'll repeat this: It is simple, and it is easy. To bring your awareness into this moment, just chose to pay attention to one of your senses, take a conscious breath or move in a deliberate and slow manner. It is simple. What seems difficult is noticing how often distractions happen. If we have expectations like "I should be able to be free from distractions for at least X minutes," frustration will emerge as soon as we notice that we got distracted. All human beings tend to develop patterns of thinking, feeling, and moving. Some of those patterns are more useful than others. Noticing that you are getting distracted, that your attention is not focused on what you intended, is not a failure. On the contrary, noticing distractions is proof that your practice is working because you are becoming aware of your inclinations – your ways of being. Remember, what is important is to keep returning to your focal point, this moment. And, returning without struggle, strain, or self-judgment and with a gentle smile helps lessen your level of frustration. Over time, your ability to return to presence will become its own helpful pattern.

PUTTING IT INTO PRACTICE: ATHA

Recall that *atha* is a call to attention. In Sanskrit, one of the meanings of the word "*mantra*" is "instrument of thought." A *mantra* is a reminder, a word used to engage your mind and to collect your attention. You can use any word as your *mantra*. *Atha* can be the simple reminder to return from distracted mind to presence. The practice is simple: Every time you notice that you are distracted, either by thinking of other times or places or by listening to one of your internal "stations" fighting for your attention, say *atha* aloud or mentally. Once you return to being with what is, let go of the *mantra*. You can choose to combine the previous exercise, "Am I present?" with this one and notice if it is helpful in returning to presence. Please keep in mind that no one else is keeping count of how many times you get distracted, nor should you. The only thing that matters is to keep coming back to presence. Sometimes, you may think you should keep using the *mantra* all the time. But just like you exit the train or get off the bus once you reach your destination, you can let go of the *mantra* once it has served its purpose of bringing you into presence again. Of course, if you get distracted again, you may use the *mantra* again, as many times as you get distracted.

SMILE

When I was growing up, my father often reminded me to smile. His reminders took a while to take hold, but now I am grateful for his advice. During my time living in Thailand, I was inspired by the beautiful, heartwarming, and genuine smiles of Thai people. It made a lot of sense to me that Thailand is often called "the land of smiles." Often, during my day, I still remind myself to bring a smile to my face, my eyes, and my heart. It's still amazing to me to feel how simple and powerful a smile can be. When you are walking around, what happens when you look at someone and smile gently? How do you feel? To what extent do your attitude and experience change when you smile?

PUTTING IT INTO PRACTICE: HOW DOES A SMILE FEEL?

Take about 5 minutes to explore this exercise

Find a place where you can relax in a comfortable position. You may keep your eyes open or closed as you choose, but remember, your optic nerve is one of the major sources of stimuli to your brain, so choose wisely. Try to feel as best as you can what it feels like to be you right now. Then bring a gentle smile to your face and pay close attention to any changes in your internal environment. First, notice the physical changes that happen when you smile. Then notice if there are any associated changes in your mental and emotional states. If the changes are beneficial in any way, would you consider making a smile part of your regular mode of being? It is simple, it is inexpensive, and it is often useful, not only internally but also in your interactions with others. Relax. Notice the climate in your internal environment. Smile. What happens? How do you feel?

Would it make sense for you to make a habit of bringing a smile to your face?

PUTTING IT INTO PRACTICE: I AM HERE NOW

Take 5 minutes or more to complete this exercise.

Another *mantra* we can use is saying to ourselves "I am here now."

Find a comfortable position where you can be relaxed and attentive. Close your eyes. Invite your body to relax and your mind to attend to the ongoing sensations taking place in this moment. Observe your body breathing at its own natural rhythm. As you feel your breath, you can say to yourself, "I," when you notice your body inhaling. On the exhalation say, "AM." As the following inhalation begins, mentally say, "HERE." And when you exhale the next time say to yourself, "NOW."

Stay with the *mantra* for the duration of the exercise. Most likely there will be distractions. As you become aware that you are distracted, simply return to saying the *mantra* with the rhythm of your natural breath. Then release the *mantra* and take a few moments to notice the effects.

This simple technique gives you the opportunity to tune into presence. This happens as you feel your natural breathing process and through giving your mind a very simple task that follows your natural breathing. The meaning of the words reinforces your intention to bring yourself to this moment.

Results

Like with any other activity, it is essential to be able to tell if your practice is working. When you define yoga as presence, your yoga practice consists of choosing to show up to your own life, every day for every moment of it. It is a self-reinforcing cycle that starts with your decision to participate consciously and deliberately in your own life. Increasing the quality of your participation in your daily activities has a direct influence in the quality of your life. You know that your yoga practice is working because your life experience improves: You feel healthier, happier, and more energetic.

If, on the other hand, any aspect of your yoga practice is generating more agitation, negative self-talk, pain, and complaining, then the techniques you are using, or the approach you are following, may not be the most appropriate for you at this time. In that case, you can return to the notion that yoga is both a practice and a state. To start the cycle, choose to be present. Second, notice the distractions that take you away from this moment. Next, choose to drop the distractions. With a friendly attitude, keep returning to the only moment when you can act, the moment you are in. Knowing that whatever decisions you make in this moment have ramifications that will influence the next moment (and the rest of your life) may be enough motivation to make intelligent decisions right where you are. Ultimately, it is your responsibility to participate in your own life, because it is your life, and nobody else can decide for you what is best or what to do. Make conscious and deliberate decisions, if only because you are the one who will have to live with the consequences. A question that can direct your exploration is this: Do I notice a growing tendency to participate actively in my life instead of endlessly entertaining myself with my opinions and internal dialogue?

$$Yoga \rightarrow Quality\ of\ Life +$$

FIGURE 2. YOGA RESULTS IN INCREASED QUALITY OF LIFE

SUCCESS

Success can be defined as accomplishing goals. As a living being, staying alive is your main goal. The fact that you are alive, breathing and reading this, means that you have navigated successfully all the previous moments in your life. Indeed, every single moment in your life, every single decision and action, including triumphs, mistakes, and everything in between, have brought you to this moment. This moment is the culmination of your whole life. It needs repeating and remembering that this moment is the single most important moment of your entire life.

THIS MOMENT IS IT

There is no other moment. This is the only time you can act and participate in your life. How you attend to this moment is a choice (conscious or unconscious) that you make. Your actions will influence every single moment after this. Of course, since it is your life, you are free to choose whatever you want to do. Being fully present in this moment is essential.

The other definition of success is to keep trying. As a normal human being you will be distracted many times. Just keep returning to this moment with gentle friendliness and cultivate everything that is conducive to living a vibrant, joyful, and meaningful existence. As you continue exploring options for living consciously, remember that you *are* a success and remember that presence can be invited, but it cannot be forced.

As you continue on this path, consider keeping a journal of your explorations as a space for reflection. This may offer you some insights into how your journey is unfolding.

PRESENCE GUIDELINES

- Set your meaningful intention
- Show up with open mind and open heart
- Give yourself time

Presence

- Relax and cultivate being with what is
- Distractions will happen
- Keep returning to this moment
- Release any strain, any struggle, and any self-judgment
- Smile
- Feel the effects

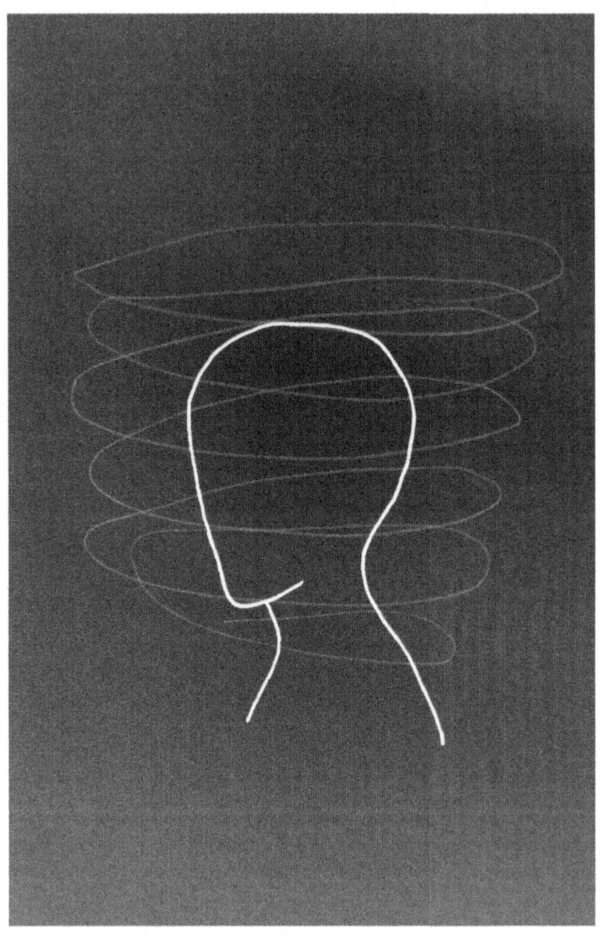

Know yourself thoroughly so that you can make conscious decisions instead of being at the mercy of your opinions, habits, and tendencies.

WHAT IS YOGA?

YOGA: regulating our ways of being

Yoga is awareness. Oftentimes, though, we discover when trying to be fully present in daily life we repeatedly get distracted. When you find distractions pulling your attention away from presence, try the four-word summary offered by Patañjali in Chapter One, aphorism two of the Yoga Sutra:

योगश्चित्तवृत्तिनिरोधः [1.2] yogaścittavṛttiṛttinirodhaḥ

When separated into individual words and transliterated into the Roman alphabet from Devanagari script (the characters used to write the Sanskrit language), the sutra above becomes *yoga citta vrtti nirodha.* Different translations of the Yoga Sutra offer these interpretations:

- Yoga is the uniting of consciousness in the heart (Nischala Joy Devi)
- Yoga is the control of thought-waves in the mind (Swami Prabhavananda & Christopher Isherwood)
- Yoga is the restriction (*nirodha*) of the fluctuations (*vrtti*) of consciousness (*citta*) (Georg Feuerstein)
- Yoga is the ability to direct the mind exclusively toward an object and sustain that direction without distractions (T.K.V. Desikachar)
- Yoga is the cessation of the turnings of thought (Barbara Stoler Miller)

- The restraint of the modifications of the mind-stuff is Yoga (Swami Satchidananda)
- Yoga is the stilling of the changing states of the mind (Edwin Bryant)
- Yoga is to still the patterning of consciousness (Chip Hartranft)
- Yoga is the suppression of the modifications of the mind (Swami Hariharananda Aranya)

In Sanskrit, each of the words *yoga citta vrtti nirodha* has multiple meanings. For example:

- ***Yoga***: yoking, joining, attaching, harnessing, using, remedy, cure, manner, method, way, device, supernatural means, charm, incantation
- ***Citta***: (pronounced *cheet-ta*) intention, aim, attending, observing, thinking, reflecting, wish, heart, mind, memory, intelligence, reason
- ***Vrtti***: (pronounced *vrt-ti*) way of behaving, course of action, tendency, nature, comment, explanation, maintenance, activity, mode of being, character, disposition
- ***Nirodha***: (pronounced *nee-rod-ha*) Preventing, checking, destroying, restraining, suppressing

Not only does *each word* have various meanings, *combinations of these four words* can be interpreted in a variety of ways. If we craft one all-encompassing interpretation based on the above, we may say,

Yoga is a method of aligning intentions, goals, and actions at the level of heart, mind, memory, and intelligence, through monitoring and regulating our tendencies, character, and ways of behaving.

Although that definition, arguably, can be put into practice, a simpler interpretation may be better, since complexity invites ambiguity (which itself invites distraction). Let's examine a more condensed interpretation,

Yoga is attending to and integrating
our heart, mind, memory, and intelligence.

Or, even more succinctly,

Yoga is regulating our ways of being

In your practice of some of the previous three exercises ("Am I Present?," "Atha," and "I Am Here Now"), you may have noticed distractions taking your attention away from the moment. For instance, the posture you originally thought was pretty comfortable may have become less so after several minutes. Or you may have found that there are some internal "radio stations" playing in your head: the "planning station," trying to remind you of the things that you need to accomplish today; or maybe the "worrying station," coming up with reasons to be concerned about this or that; or even the "complaints station," which seems to find fault in everything. Perhaps your internal radio is tuned to the "drama *du jour* station," where a new reason for being upset is served up fresh daily. If you're like me, there may be a cacophony of stations competing for your attention most of the time. In your regular practice you may notice some of these distractions keep coming back, as well as perhaps discomfort in your shoulders or neck, or feeling tired, sad or worried.

These internal activities are encompassed in the Sanskrit words *citta vrtti*. To expand on the small sample of translations of sutra 1.2 above, *citta vrtti* may be interpreted as consciousness, thought-waves in the mind, fluctuations of consciousness, mind distractions, turnings of thought, changing states of the mind, patterning of consciousness, and modifications of the mind. Translating *citta vrtti* as "ways of being," therefore, synthesizes all of the ways in which we take part in our life. This helps us move beyond the dichotomy of mind/body, favoring instead a holistic understanding of ourselves as complete, whole beings. Our ways of being include our intentions and thoughts, our attitudes, and actions, and even how we breathe and move.

Ways of being (*citta vrtti*)

Inclinations, tendencies, and habits that manifest in body, mind and emotions. These tendencies influence the ways in which we perceive and respond to internal and external events, many of which are unconscious. Effective yoga techniques have two purposes: First, they make you aware of these inclinations and preferences; second, yoga techniques help you regulate these habits to enhance your internal and external harmony. Even though some of these tendencies might be beneficial at times, eventually, all of them will be eliminated.

Most people trying to be present notice all of these internal activities taking place in interrelated ways at all levels – physical, mental, and emotional. Yoga, according to our simplified definition as regulation of our ways of being, is our learning to modulate these activities, so that we can be with what is. In other words, yoga is a system for creating internal and external harmony. To foster harmony, yoga leads us to inquire into our own natures. Since we do not exist in a vacuum, this inquiry will, by necessity, also lead us into exploration of the nature of reality and of life itself, as will be discussed in other chapters.

The yogic process starts by paying attention. When you pay attention, you notice your internal climate. You also notice some attitudes, opinions, and tendencies that influence how you perceive your experiences. Those opinions and attitudes are sometimes useful. Other times they are obstacles. Awareness is instrumental in discerning if a tendency is useful at this moment or not. Your awareness can also reveal how your choices are influenced by your own stories, beliefs, and preferences. Then, you increase the chances of making intelligent decisions right where you are. Awareness makes it easier to intelligently choose your actions.

Yoga is regulating your ways of being, to enhance the quality of your participation in your own life. Still, there will be plenty of times when distractions will prevent you from choosing consciously. This is where it helps to hone the most important skill in yoga: your ability to return to presence without strain, struggle, or self-judgment, and with a gentle smile. Getting good at this skill can make the difference in how effective – and how enjoyable – your practice is. Eventually, you grow in your ability to choreograph the dance between your two modes, being and doing, so that they coexist in integrated harmony.

Experiment, Exploration & Regulation

In the previous chapter, we reflected on the fact that all people are conducting an experiment with their own lives. For some of us, this is an unconscious experiment, while for others, it may be a more deliberate inquiry. Patañjali's Yoga Sutra offers a comprehensive handbook for conducting your life experiment. Yoga is a complete system to explore your body, your breath, your mind, your emotions, and your relationships. Since you're not a machine made up of separate parts, but an organism developed from a fertilized cell, these different aspects of you are interconnected and can influence one another. At the same time, you are connected to everything that exists. There is never a time when you are not interacting, consciously or unconsciously, with the world around you.

The yoga perspective asks you to notice what you are doing, to clarify what contributes to presence and what doesn't. Learning this distinction is a fundamental skill for making life-affirming decisions, so you may downplay ways of being that are not currently useful or that no longer serve a purpose.

A practical example: Most of us pay some attention to the weather, if only by looking out a window, so we can make intelligent choices, like taking along an umbrella if it looks likely to rain. That simple weather event – rain – can generate two distinct reactions from the same person. For example, if I've been working in my garden planting seeds, I may be quite happy when the first raindrops fall. But if I have plans to meet friends for a picnic, I may feel frustrated or upset at having to change or cancel my plans due to precipitation. Same person, same meteorological event, two quite different reactions.

When the weather outside aligns with our preferences, we feel happy, or at least in a good mood. (Of course! It is easy to feel happy when everything is going according to our liking.) When the weather turns, must our mood turn as well? Is the person who finds today's weather lovely the same person that complains tomorrow because it is too hot, too humid, too cold, too windy, or too wet? How do you react to the weather outside? One tendency may be a desire to control the weather. Another would be to try to predict everything that could happen with the changing weather. While the first approach may cause frustration because we can't control what is happening outside ourselves, the second option tends to generate anxiety from constantly trying to account for all possible outcomes. Self-regulation requires us to distinguish between what is within and what is beyond our control, because worrying about what is beyond our control is, simply, a waste of our life's energy.

The tools of yoga can assist us in turning our attention to what is within our control. Practicing the wise guidelines for behavior known as the *yamas* and *niyamas*, we may find that it is challenging to act with kindness and contentment all the time. Practicing postures and movements (*asana* and *vinyasa*) can show us that we have limited control over our body. Practicing the breath regulation techniques (*pranayama*) can show the limits of our ability to control our breathing processes. Attempting to practice inner sensitivity (*pratyahara*) may demonstrate our shortcomings in mastering our senses. Practicing concentration (*dharana*) and meditation (*dhyana*) will likely show us that it's quite difficult to keep our attention in one place for just three or four minutes. All these tools of yoga are directed to remove inefficiencies. In fact, every yoga technique uncovers inefficiencies and obstacles and facilitates their removal. And in the process of identifying and eliminating those obstacles, we will likely also learn humility.

As we learn to shift our attention from trying to control the world outside to directing our energy where it can be effective, our internal environment, we begin to notice just how much external events beyond our control influence how we feel and think. Letting our attitude and outlook be at the mercy of external phenomena is a recipe for constantly being on an emotional rollercoaster. Seeing yoga as a system to regulate our ways of being means that yoga practice enhances our ability to respond congruently to life. In this way, yoga practice empowers you to become responsible for your own internal climate. To start moving in that direction, we must first become aware of our ways of being.

PUTTING IT INTO PRACTICE: MY WAYS OF BEING

PART 1

Pause for a few moments at different times throughout the day over the next three days.

Over the next three days, keep your journal handy and pay attention and notice your ways of being by observing how you:

- Walk, sit, stand, move, eat, talk
- Work, rest, relax
- Handle things and situations

As you make notes, try to be as objective as possible, by describing what you notice, as if you were observing a person you have never met before.

PART 2

Give yourself between 10 and 20 minutes for this section.

At the end of the three days, go over your notes, and try to remember as best as possible your activities during the last three days. Then write answers to the following questions:

- What did you notice?

- What did you pay attention to?

- How was your attitude over the last 3 days?

- How would you describe your attitude and actions to somebody else?

- What are some of the words that you used most often during the past 3 days?

- Do you talk to yourself (aloud or mentally) when you are alone?

- What did you learn about your ways of being?

- Were your usual ways of being influenced by the fact that you were observing yourself?

This exercise offers you a glimpse into your life and how you live it. If yoga is regulating our ways of being, then bringing awareness to our ways of being is the first step. When you bring awareness to your actions, you are orienting to the present moment. Throughout your journey you'll find that the tools of yoga serve both as ways to come into presence and as ways of assessing your actions. It is possible that by the third day, you may have already found some patterns in your ways of moving, thinking, breathing, feeling, and interacting with others. You may have also discovered some other patterns you were not consciously aware of.

Watching your actions may make you uncomfortable at times, especially if your actions contradict some of the ideas you have about yourself. Noticing something you don't like may cause agitation or frustration, which interfere with your ability to choose your actions consciously. Remember the suggestion to cultivate the attitude of returning to this irreplaceable moment without struggle, strain, or self-judgment. This skill will grow into the ability to better regulate your internal climate.

Noticing your ways of being informs you about yourself and is a resource for awareness. This is not an exercise to make you feel good or bad about yourself; those feelings are choices you make. Instead of feeling good or bad, it's better to determine which ways of being are helpful and which are unhelpful. Then you make intelligent choices, like applying a way of being when it's helpful or downplaying another way of being that's not helpful at this time. For instance, energetically projecting your voice is quite useful when you are addressing a group of people in a large space; projecting your voice with energy, however, is probably less desirable when you are talking to your beloved in the confines of your small living room.

Yoga is self-regulation: knowing ourselves well, and consciously choosing the most appropriate way of being for a specific time and place, so that we create harmony in life and in the world.

PUTTING IT INTO PRACTICE: COMPLAINING

Consider practicing for one day or longer

Set your intention to observe and note what you complain about.

At the end of the time you allocated for this practice, notice the patterns:

- Do you complain?

- What do you complain about?

- When do you complain?

- Did you notice a tendency to express your complaints in veiled ways?

- How do you feel when you complain?

- What is the purpose of your complaining?

- What part of you seems to be complaining?

- Do your complaints indicate assumptions about how things "should" be?

Reflect on the amount of time and energy you invest in complaining and on how complaining affects the quality of your life experience. If complaining is not useful for you, can you find ways of being that will redirect your energy in a more useful way? The next practice can be a viable alternative.

PUTTING IT INTO PRACTICE: GRATITUDE

Allocate 5 to 10 minutes for this practice. Strongly suggested as a long-term daily practice.

Sit in a comfortable position, with your spine erect but not rigid if possible. Close your eyes. Give yourself permission to offer yourself your undivided attention. Allow your breath to flow at its own pace. Take some time to feel, hear, and savor your own breath for several rounds of unhurried inhalations and exhalations. With each exhalation let go of whatever is not part of this moment. If you notice any tension in your shoulders or face, for example, just let go of it as you exhale. As you feel ready, ask yourself if there is anything in your life to be thankful for. Don't think too hard or concentrate too intensely. Instead, let the question resonate with your whole being. You may find some reasons for gratitude emerge into your consciousness without effort. If nothing seems to come to mind, notice if there is anything in your immediate life that you appreciate, such as the ability to breathe, sleep, smile, feel, taste, laugh, and love. Feel the sensations associated with gratitude and remain aware. Try to keep this attitude of thankfulness and notice how it makes you feel.

As you continue finding reasons for being grateful, remember to also give thanks for obstacles, challenges, and difficulties, because they provide you with opportunities to learn about yourself and others and to grow beyond present limitations in your knowledge and understanding. Each time you give thanks, draw a gentle smile on your face. Invite your gratitude to expand gradually beyond your physical body and out into the whole universe. Can you enjoy how it feels to be you right now? For the last few moments, immerse completely in the sensation of gratitude.

Notice how you feel. You may feel relaxed, renewed, and more in contact with yourself and with the world around you. On the other hand, you may notice that it is difficult to find reasons to give thanks. This may be an interesting avenue to explore, to find out what are the obstacles preventing you from giving thanks.

Try this practice for 2 weeks, just for a few minutes each day, and notice its effects throughout the day. You can also take short "gratitude breaks" during your day, by pausing for a few moments to express your gratitude as it feels best to you.

Consider: is there a difference between your regular attitude and your attitude during this meditation? If you find differences, pose this question to yourself:

What would happen if my usual attitude is an attitude of gratitude?

This question is an invitation to find the answer through your own direct experience.

The journey so far

Until this point, we have defined yoga as presence, as the simple act of being with what is. We have a few exercises that invite us to be present. Recognizing that it can be challenging to stay present, we now have a complementary definition of yoga as the system that brings us into presence through regulating our ways of being. Since we can only regulate what we know, it is fundamental to develop the habit of observing attentively and without judgment as we establish our practice. We also tried a couple of techniques for helping us clarify the way we participate in our own lives. Here are some questions to guide your exploration:

- What are your ways of being?
- What tendencies do you notice in your ways of moving and in your posture?
- What are your tendencies when you breathe?
- What are the stories that you are more willing to believe in?
- How do those stories influence your perception and your choices?
- Do you notice patterns in your emotions?
- To what extent can you regulate these patterns, tendencies, and inclinations?
- When you get distracted, can you try to return to whatever you are doing without strain, struggle, or self-judgment and with a gentle smile?

Now, it is time to expand our understanding and practice by delving deeper into yoga and its relationship to who we are.

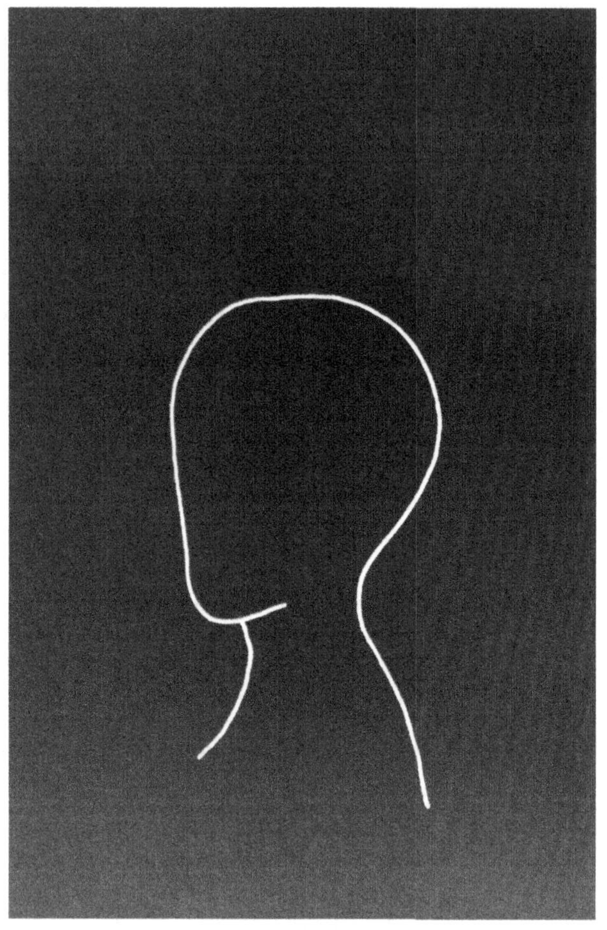

Who am I?" If you take a look in the mirror, it is very difficult to deny the changes constantly taking place in your body. Often, we get caught up in our reactions to those superficial changes. However, as you observe yourself without judgment, it becomes apparent that there is something within that has remain unchanged over the years. This begs the question, "Who am I?" Patient persistence in exploring this question gradually unveils the fundamental difference between who you are and who you think you are. Discerning the difference is the essence of yoga.

WHO AM I?

Connecting to our true nature

Yoga is a practice with a long history, perhaps because in its entirety, yoga relates to one of life's fundamental questions, a question every human being ponders sooner or later: *Who am I?* Practicing yoga is an empirical way to explore this essential question, through our ways of moving, breathing, thinking, feeling, and interacting.

In this chapter, we continue our gradual progression through the Yoga Sutra, considering the first four sutras in Chapter One of the Yoga Sutra as a complete summary of the essence of yoga.

Four sutra summary

> Now, yoga practice. [1.1]
>
> Yoga is regulating my ways of being. [1.2]
>
> As a result, I am embodied awareness, presence. [1.3]
>
> Otherwise, I think that I am my ways of being. [1.4]

These four sutras offer the foundation for all yoga practices.

The first aphorism asks you to show up to your life. As we explored in the previous chapter, yoga is about making the present moment the most important moment of your life. Doing so, you come to each moment alert and ready to participate with an open mind and an open heart. The second sutra defines yoga as a process of self-regulation. It hints at the human condition, especially at our shared tendency to get entangled in habit patterns. The third sutra presents the results of yoga, presence. To be fully present, you must become aware of your patterns, so you can monitor and modulate them. And the fourth aphorism points out what happens when your ways of being go *un*modulated. Without modulation, patterns may pull you away from participating actively and deliberately in your life. By being present you are able to respond to the flow of life with harmony and grace. Otherwise, you might end up believing the stories you are constantly making up about yourself and about the world, thinking that you *are* your ways of being.

Embody, embodiment

The direct experience of life as it manifests through your body. The wholeness of your being, which is not composed of different parts. The indescribable interconnectedness of all your different aspects in your physicality and all your internal life. The aliveness that you share with all of life and the whole Universe.

In these four simple aphorisms, Patañjali presents a framework for the whole life project (journey) of yoga. On one hand, there is life, the always ongoing phenomena that keep changing from one now moment to the next now moment. On the other hand, there is consciousness, what makes us aware. Neither life nor consciousness can be captured, isolated, or synthesized in any way. Life manifests as *all the changing experiences that are happening*, regardless of our noticing them— or not. Awareness is the manifestation of consciousness as *the light that makes it possible for us to notice that we are conscious,* and that enables us to feel bodily sensations, emotions, and thoughts.

Imagine an old movie theater. We'll use it as a metaphor to clarify these two ideas. The movie projector and the film running through it are the necessary elements for a movie to be projected onto the screen. The movie projector and film represent life. The movie projector includes a lamp whose light is concentrated by a lens and passes through each frame of the film. The light is then magnified by a second lens to project that image on the screen. **Consciousness** is like the electricity that powers the projector. Without electricity (consciousness), the film will not run through the projector and no movie will be seen. Awareness is the expression of consciousness – light flowing through the light bulb. If applied to this metaphor, the fourth sutra says that the lamp may end up believing, erroneously, that it is the electricity. However, without electricity, the lamp will still be in the projector, but the film will not be projected onto the screen. Life includes the changing phenomena, the screen, the projector and the movie that is projected on the screen. Life also encompasses everything else that makes up the movie theater. As you watch the movie, it is your own awareness that enables you to experience the images, soundtrack and dialog, as well as the sensory stimuli in your body when you see the movie, hear the sounds and noises in the theatre, feel the texture of the clothes you are wearing and the firmness of the seat you are sitting on. Life also includes your emotions and thoughts as you watch the movie. Yoga helps you modulate your internal activities and reactivity so that even as you watch the story unfold on the screen you remember that *you are not the temporary emotions and thoughts going through you,* because when they dissolve you still are here, and you still are you.

Our organism and the whole Universe around it are the site where the ongoing dance between life and awareness takes place. In these four aphorisms, the Yoga Sutra states that *our true nature is consciousness.* Consciousness enables us to recognize that we are alive. Our tendencies, however, may lead us to think that we *are* the fluctuating sensations, thoughts, and opinions that we experience; instead, our awareness facilitates our perception of these temporary phenomena.

The first four sutras offer us a simple and potent suggestion for practice and life: Find out who you are. Since some aspects of you, like your body, your ideas, opinions, and emotions keep changing, inquiring into these changing dimensions of who you are makes yoga a lifelong journey of self-discovery.

PUTTING IT INTO PRACTICE: WHO DO YOU THINK YOU ARE?

Allocate about 10-15 minutes to complete this exercise.

Take a moment to write down words that you use to describe yourself. Free write, so that there is no editing or censoring. Simply write down whatever comes to mind.

Now, review each word you wrote and ask yourself:

- How long has this word been an accurate descriptor of who I am?

- Have I always used this word to describe myself?

- When did I start using this word to describe me?

- How long will this word accurately describe me?

- Can you think of similar labels you used in the past, but that you no longer use?

- How many of these words are essential, the complete essence of who you are?

- Are there any labels that have **always** been accurate to describe you?

Who am I?

As you go through this inquiry, contemplate the different ideas you identify with, and notice how ideas may have changed over time. Some of the descriptors may be recent additions to your self-description, while others may no longer accurately describe how you see yourself. Reflect further on these ideas by asking:

- To what extent do these labels define, or influence, what I think I can and cannot do?

- Are these labels at my service, or am I at the service of these labels?

- Do these labels enhance the quality of my life, of my energy and awareness?

Pondering these questions helps illuminate the main concept presented in aphorism 1.4, which is the human tendency to identify with our ways of being, such as our education, age, upbringing and origin, as well as our pain, worries, anxieties, accomplishments, beliefs, and circumstances. Many of us identify with our belongings, our bank accounts, our titles, or professions. As we reflect, we may hear a couple of questions in our heads: Are you trying to tell me that all those things I have worked so hard for (like my degrees, position, status and belongings) are not who I am? And, if I am not all those things, then who am I?

Often, at the end of a program of studies, or after doing something that we'd been planning for a long time, or after finally getting something we've wanted for a long time, the whole experience feels somehow anticlimactic. The reality of the experience seems anticlimactic because we were building it up so much in our head that those expectations were not reached. In fact, even when our expectations are reached, we may feel that the experience could have been even more special, exciting, rewarding. Moreover, because the ideas in our head are only ideas, we keep changing them all the time. Our experiences and our ideas about our experiences belong in two different planes of existence, one never crossing into the other. Remember, *experiences cannot be encompassed fully by anything other than the experience itself.* Words are ways of trying to express our thoughts about the experience. Yet, no matter how accurate or precise our thoughts and words might be, both words and thoughts are merely artifacts pointing to something that happened in the past, whether immediate or distant. Experiences belong to the realm of presence, whereas words and thoughts are ways to try to comprehend what has been experienced.

We live in a world where we are constantly bombarded with messages selling something, whether products, experiences, or ideas. Often, these messages tell us either directly or indirectly that there is something missing or wrong in ourselves or in our lives, and that we can be "more, better, improved, enhanced," if only we would buy whatever is being sold. When we hear this message repeatedly, we internalize it, and we come to believe that acquiring more things, experiences, or labels will make us more whole, more complete human beings. Sutra 1.3 offers an antidote to that toxic artificial message:

As a result of regulating my ways of being, I am embodied awareness, presence.

Being embodied awareness is one way of saying *I am fully present and at peace with what is, exactly as it is, and with myself just as I am.* This aphorism is also translated "As a result, the seer abides in its own true nature." Which brings us to our next inquiry, *what is your true nature?*

PUTTING IT INTO PRACTICE: WHAT IS MY TRUE NATURE?

Take 10-15 minutes to complete this exercise.

Find a quiet space and a very comfortable position. Sit, recline, or lie down. Close your eyes and give yourself permission to disconnect from the world completely by remembering that there is no other place where you can act, and then choosing to be right here. Next, ask yourself *What is my true nature?* Be curious and calm and listen for an answer. Invite yourself to relax as completely as you can. Notice the sounds and noises coming from outside, away in the distance. After a couple of minutes, notice sounds and noises that are closer to the building you are in. Notice without having to identify or describe, just hear the sound and its own internal structure. Attend to the sounds closer to you, in the room. Don't describe or narrate, just hear, becoming aware of the multilayered soundscape all around you. Invite yourself to explore your own internal environment. Start by listening intently to the sounds inside of you. Listen without judgment or narration. Be curious and notice what is happening inside of you without trying to edit or censor what you notice. What internal activities do you notice? These internal activities may be sensations in your body, thoughts, or emotions. If it seems like there are any words in your inner environment, can you choose to let them just flow without trying to control them? Focus your attention on the way your body is breathing, feeling each inhalation and exhalation from the moment you notice air starting to flow into your body, to the transition between your inhalation and your exhalation. Follow the sensations that let you know you are exhaling until you feel the last molecules of air flowing out of your nose. There is no need to control anything. Just stay focused on the natural rhythm of your breath. From time to time, you may find your mind going off on some tangent, into some internal dialogue or description. Perhaps your mind starts planning the rest of your day or week, or maybe it is remembering something that happened recently. Whatever it is, let go of it and choose to attend to your breath with the curiosity of someone who knows that each breath is unique and irreplaceable. Be as relaxed as possible, just as if you were about to fall asleep. If you doze off, or get distracted, gently – without any struggle or strain and without any self-judgment – return to savoring this moment, when there is nothing else to do and no other place to be. Once you feel ready to finish, gradually stretch, breathe more deeply, and open your eyes.

Even when you try to be very relaxed and make time to do nothing but relax, you'll notice how your ways of being, like your tendency to complain, plan, comment or narrate, will pull you out of just being with what is, and into the complex ideology you have been constructing in your head throughout your whole life. Most people teeter between being and doing. In doing mode, the mind gets busy by trying to make sense of whatever it is noticing. However, in being mode, the mind settles and observes without reactivity. The internal activities you noticed in the previous exercise, your ways of being, keep changing, coming and going throughout the day. In order to go to sleep, you release all those ways of being. But very soon after you wake up in the morning, they seem to start on their own again. In fact, quite often, it seems that those ways of being are in charge of running your life. You can further your inquiry by asking yourself:

- If there are ways of being that can be turned on and off, are they essential?

- Are these ways of being fundamental to being who I am?

- Since some of these ways of being have not always been part of my internal environment, does that mean that they are not necessary?

- What is left when those ways of being are turned off? Does that even happen, ever?

- Where are all those ways of being manifesting?

As with other exercises on this journey, the only way to find out if this line of inquiry is useful for you is to explore it.

At the end of the day, when you are ready to fall asleep, you may find some lingering thoughts, perhaps some plans about what you are going to do tomorrow, or maybe some thoughts related to how the day went, or maybe some regrets about the things that could have been done differently. Eventually, all of us, in order to go to sleep, have to let go of all of those internal activities. When that finally happens, body, mind, and emotions surrender and relax fully. That is the moment when we fall asleep. Sleeping soundly enables your body to shift its focus from the world outside to the internal experience. This enables you to invest resources in healing, restoring, and replenishing. The converse process happens every morning when, right before opening your eyes, you realize, "I'm not asleep anymore." Soon your internal space is filled with a rush of ideas, tasks, thoughts, plans, and things to do, and the daily race begins anew. I suggest that all those internal activities that occupy your inner space are temporary and not essential to your being. If they were essential, it would not be possible to let go of them.

Yoga is a state of being

Yoga is the state of being when you consciously and deliberately let go of all the nonessential internal activities and you get to just *be*, inhabiting the boundless calm and inner peace where all those temporary activities take place. Most people have, at one time or another, experienced that simple state of being and recognized it as something that has been with them all of their lives. It's often expressed as the feeling of coming home. I would even go as far as to claim that one of the main goals in life is to establish an intimate connection with that state. Because, even though we may have all experienced that state, and indeed, even though we get close to experiencing that state unconsciously every night during dreamless deep sleep, most of us find that our thoughts, ideas, emotions, feelings, regrets, worries, anxieties, and plans draw our attention so strongly that we tend to forget that underneath all of those internal dialogues and opinions there is deep peace and tranquility within us. That state of deep tranquility becomes so elusive that we come to see all the activities we engage in as our life and our essence. This is what Patañjali is saying in sutra 1.4:

Otherwise (when I am not embodied awareness), I think I am my ways of being.

Even when there is a deep identification with our temporary ways of being, sooner or later we keep feeling that something is missing. What is missing is the connection to the basis of our being. *If that connection to our true nature is not there, everything becomes unsatisfactory.*

Think of your true nature like the sky – spacious, open, and boundless. The sky is always there, even if sometimes there are so many clouds in the sky that you cannot see it at all. If clouds cover the sky day after day for several weeks, you may even start thinking that there is no sky. Yet the sky is still there. Awareness is like the sky: spacious, open, and boundless. Awareness also enables you to notice the energy that animates you and your ways of being. Your ways of being are like clouds in the sky and sometimes these clouds obscure your perception, leading you to identify with the clouds (your job, your titles, your stories, and your opinions.) Rest assured, clouds come and go, but the sky remains. Throughout the Yoga Sutra, Patañjali states that confusing your true nature (the sky) with the temporary phenomena you experience (clouds and meteorological events) is the root cause of suffering. Perhaps most, if not all, of **the causes of suffering arise from the gap between who you are and who you think you are**.

Who am I?

Who you are is the direct, undiluted experience that is happening right where you are; the experience brings with it sensations, emotions, and thoughts. Presence (the state of yoga) is experiencing yourself fully as you are. Your experience is not necessarily good or bad, it just is. The embodied awareness of sutra 1.3 is sometimes called the natural state. The opposite "unnatural" state is to think about what you are experiencing, stepping out of moment-to-moment embodied awareness and trying to make "sense" of what is. That is the space of who you think you are, and it includes who you think you should be and who you think other people expect you to be or think you are.

By asking "Who am I?" you may to notice a gap between who you are and who you think you are. The answers to these questions may help aid your exploration of that potential rift:

- Are your desires, choices, and actions resulting from who you are or from who you think you are?
- What are the noticeable differences between the two?
- Where do you allocate your energy?
- Is awareness the underlying space where all of your internal activities take place?

The first four sutras present the foundation of yoga. They are an invitation to show up to your life from a place of peace and balance, so you can flow wholeheartedly and intelligently with the ever-changing newness of life. This approach to yoga requires a change of mindset from seeing yourself as incomplete and defective to recognizing that you are complete and whole. In other words, you know with certainty that *there is nothing fundamentally wrong with you.*

Yoga practice can be the simple act of seeing beyond your ways of being and remembering who you are, by directing your unclouded awareness to witness the exquisite interconnections between all your systems and the intricate interrelatedness of your life, and all of life, everywhere.

Equipped with the foundation provided by the first four sutras and the insights from the exercises we have tried so far, let's continue exploring more deeply on this journey to the core of our being.

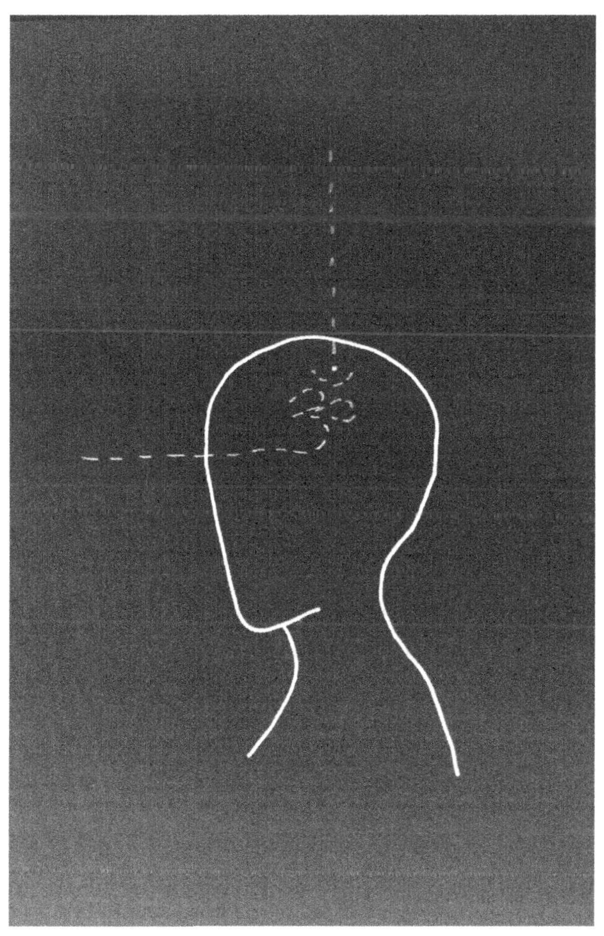

Sincere yoga practice asks us to stand naked in front of a full-length mirror. As we choose to look at ourselves honestly, a major obstacle emerges when we come face to face with our attitudes, beliefs, actions, and habits. It will no longer be possible to avoid, ignore, or cover-up the aspects of ourselves that we dislike, are not proud of, or are embarrassed by. Yoga practice requires strong commitment as well as kindness and compassion.

FOUNDATIONS OF YOGA

Yoga is a call to Action

Whatever you practice you get better at. Every time you practice, whether practicing consciously or unconsciously, you strengthen the patterns you are cultivating. Yoga is presence, and presence can be practiced, so the more you practice being present, the more present you will be.

As we attempt to participate fully in life, distractions attempt to draw our attention elsewhere. These distractions often arise from our opinions and beliefs, with opinions manifesting as objections to what is happening, and beliefs emerging as conditions we impose to accept ourselves as we are in order to accept life exactly as it is. Accepting *what is* not the same as resignation or a call to inaction. Instead, accepting *what is* the prerequisite for having the necessary clarity to act with wisdom.

Yogic actions call for participating in each unique moment with enthusiasm, intelligence, and wisdom. As a result, distractions and limitations diminish, and movement, breathing, thinking, and feeling are optimized. Wholehearted and conscious living awakens recognition of the magnificence of life within you, around you, and everywhere. Through practicing awareness, yoga makes evident the patterns you have cultivated, consciously and unconsciously, in your attitudes, thoughts, emotions, breathing and movements. Knowing your patterns and tendencies empowers you to choose the options most conducive to keeping your heart and mind open and expanding in awareness, love, and compassion. *Liberating yourself from the limitations imposed by your beliefs enables you to flow in harmony with the miracle of life.*

YOGA is AWARENESS

FIGURE 3. YOGA IS AWARENESS

As a reminder: the philosophy of yoga we're exploring is the art of living with wisdom, and living with wisdom is predicated on living with awareness. The Yoga Sutra invites us to show up to each and every single moment of life, knowing that each of us is the only one who can commit to living life with awareness. Awareness begins with exploration of what is closest to us, hence yoga is awareness of body, breath, mind, emotions, and their interdependencies. Because all humans have the tendency to develop habits, one of the most universal and important skills to cultivate is knowing our own tendencies. Being aware of our tendencies enables us to gauge if a particular tendency manifesting at this moment is helpful or unhelpful. For instance, being meticulous is quite helpful when preparing a tax return, but not so helpful when brainstorming or improvising a dance.

As awareness of our tendencies grows, it's inevitable our shortcomings will become more apparent to us. In fact, as this awareness expands, it becomes more and more difficult for us to continue to ignore attitudes and actions that are detrimental to our physical, mental, and emotional wellbeing. Far from being a system for torturing ourselves by exposing unyielding personal flaws, yoga provides a way of approaching ourselves – flaws and all – with kindness and understanding. Every single person on earth is a work in progress; all of us are trying to learn and trying to do the best that we can. Each and every one of our actions has effects, some positive and some negative. The effects of our actions provide accurate feedback to everything that we do, even when we act unconsciously. When we experience discomfort and agitation, we may choose to react by getting aggravated or by thinking that the world is unfair. Another option is to see our discomfort and agitation as teachers, offering perfectly calibrated, appropriate feedback to our actions. Indeed, *everything that is happening around us is constantly providing feedback to fine tune our attitudes, intentions, and actions.* Yoga invites us to act with enthusiasm, wisdom, and humility to resolve every situation we encounter – event those situations triggering discomfort and agitation – with awareness and grace.

Awareness of your tendencies naturally leads you to notice how one of your systems influences another. For example, worrying about something will probably have some effects on your physical posture as well as on your breathing and your emotions. Similarly, changing the pace of your inhalations and exhalations can help you feel energized, or agitated, or relaxed, in body and mind. Pay attention to how you feel at all levels when you are inspired and hopeful as opposed to when you are sad or filled with negativity. Yoga is a system for becoming a connoisseur of the exquisite interactions among all your systems, so that you may regulate them expertly, according to the changing circumstances of every single (unique) moment.

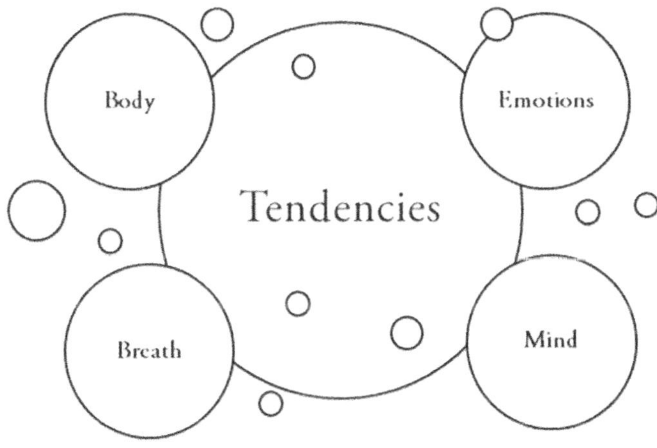

FIGURE 4. YOGA IS AWARENESS OF YOUR TENDENCIES

Becoming an expert on how your organism works will help you optimize your actions. Bear in mind, becoming an authority on how your systems interact and interrelate is not an exercise in narcissism. Yoga is not about developing an excessive interest in, or admiration of, yourself. On the contrary, yoga is about seeing yourself quite clearly, including being aware of what you don't know. Knowing yourself well helps you see the difference between who you *are* and *the stories you believe about who you are.* The less your investment in those stories, the more clearly you can see yourself. Separating your self-awareness from the stories and beliefs that inhibit your vision allows you to *be*, without having to be right or wrong, or better or worse than anyone else. The more you know yourself, the more you see the similarities between you and everything else around you. You recognize that you have never truly been isolated from anything around you! Yoga is a system for cleansing your perception and clarifying the ways you interpret what you experience. Yoga empowers you to explore yourself and your life without preconceived notions and without expectations. Since it is impossible to ever know what will happen next, you then invite the spark of curiosity to guide you in greeting each new moment with clarity, enthusiasm, and peace.

As you refrain from coloring your perceptions with stories and predictions, your own inner-connectedness begins to highlight the interconnectedness between all that is. You start to see yourself not as an isolated individual, but in terms of relationships. Once you consciously attend to your relationships, you become cognizant of your relationships to self, to others, and to the Universe around you. *Yoga is realizing the unity with all that is.* This growing awareness of being deeply embedded in the ever-changing web of life suggests a question to guide your life: How can I be useful?

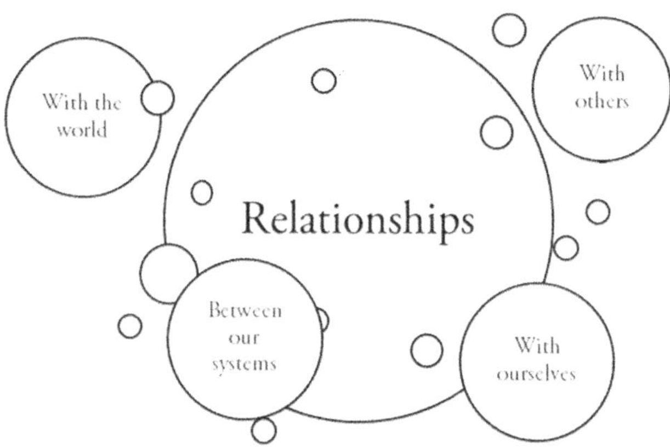

FIGURE 5. YOGA IS AWARENESS OF YOUR RELATIONSHIPS

Method for Presence: Self-Awareness, Self-inquiry, Self-care

It seems paradoxical to need a "method" for something as "simple" as being *present*. It should be easy. But most people who try to be attentive and aware for every moment of each day find it challenging to *remain* present, because of distraction-creating tendencies. When someone points out that you are hunching your shoulders, you have an immediate reaction to release tension and relax your shoulders. Simple and easy. But what if it's your *tendency* to hunch your shoulders? Then even when you notice the tension and relax it, your shoulders may get tense again in a few moments. It may be the same when we are trying to be present: if our tendency is to be distracted, we may become frustrated not so much by actual distractions, but by the fact that we are noticing we are getting distracted. In those moments, the skill of **returning to this irreplaceable moment without struggle, strain or self-judgment** is invaluable. One way to polish that skill is Pause-Notice-Respond.

When doing a thing – anything – you can choose to briefly **pause** and invite self awareness, creating space for awareness in between the constant stream of your internal thoughts, opinions, and stories. Then you **notice**. How does it feel to be you right where you are, doing what you are doing? Is what you are doing enhancing the quality of your participation in this unique and irreplaceable moment? Then, depending on what you notice, you can choose the most appropriate **response**, a conscious and deliberate choice to either continue doing what you were doing, or to adjust your attitude or actions as needed. These three steps align with three central aspects of the system of yoga, namely: Self-Awareness, Self-Inquiry and Self-Care. Self-Awareness is aligning with presence and feeling the fundamental truth that you are embodied awareness embedded in the endless interaction between life and consciousness. Self-Inquiry is the investigation of your nature and realizing the differences between who you are and who you think you are. Self-Care encompasses the actions that you take to enhance the quality of your participation in the flow of life. Yoga is a continuous cycle of self-regulation, leading you into greater presence and awareness and a feeling of deeper interconnectedness to yourself and to everything around you.

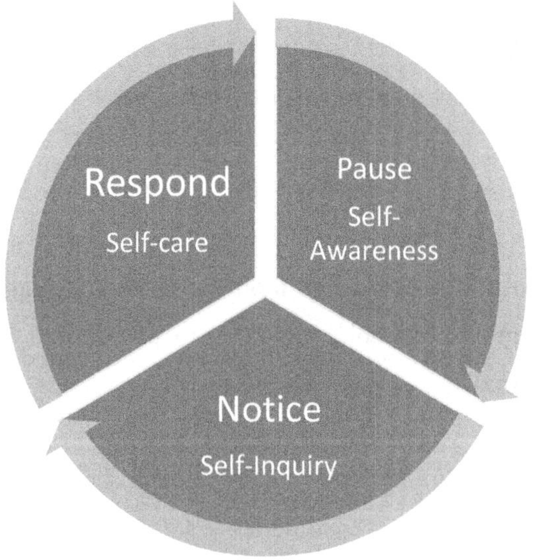

FIGURE 6. AWARENESS PROCESS

In the process of coming to presence, expect to find distractions pulling your attention away from life as it is manifesting right in front of you. These distractions often come out of the stories, beliefs, and opinions that you carry with you all the time. Distractions may also serve as a way for you to avoid a situation you are facing, making you feel like you are escaping something unpleasant or unexpected. Trying to escape the moment you are in, however, plunges you deeply into the complex entanglement of stories, opinions, and preferences in your own mind. All ideas about moments in life other than the one in which you are present (even projections into the future), are based on the past. Even when you are thinking about the future, your thoughts are based in your memory – an interpretation of past events. Distractions, therefore, lead you to choose, consciously or unconsciously, to ignore the unique moment that you are in. This lack of attention to the present moment generates feedback that frequently manifests as a subtle hint, suggesting a way to shift direction. Ignoring this feedback increases its intensity, indicating that you do not understand the important message you are receiving: *Participate consciously in this moment, because it is the most important moment of your life.* The feedback you receive is a compassionate message guiding you to flow harmoniously with the flow of life.

To make this process more specific, we'll expanded it into a step-by-step approach to embody presence:

- Pause
- Notice
- Feel
    - Validate
    - Clarify
    - Choose
- Respond

If there are no distractions, there is no need to do anything, just stay present with the almost imperceptible transition from one moment into the next. When distractions arise, clarify if action is needed. Let's go through a brief explanation of the steps and then put them into practice.

Pause

"He who can no longer pause to wonder and stand rapt in awe, is as good as dead; his eyes are closed." Albert Einstein

Many of us feel that it's difficult to take time for ourselves because we have too much to do that just can't wait. It's possible that feeling busy gives us the sense that we are important and needed, but the very fact that we are alive is confirmation enough that we are indeed important and needed. **Pausing is a way to create space for presence,** because it is our presence that's needed in our lives and in the world. Without presence it is highly unlikely that you can participate consciously in your life. Invite awareness into the moment you are in

Feel

"To come to your senses, you have to go out of your mind." Alan Watts

Once you pause, you connect to the direct experience of the present moment by feeling what is happening. When you pause and feel, you may notice your internal voice narrating or offering opinions about what you are doing, as well as about what you are feeling. Clearly you are already *experiencing* this moment, so there is no need for a narrator. And no need to create a story about your sensations. Shift from thinking about what you're feeling and **attend to the ongoing stream of changing sensations**. In other words, you are changing from thinking and doing to being and feeling. Literally *coming to your senses* is a direct way to return to presence.

VALIDATE

"Be yourself; everyone else is already taken." Oscar Wilde

When you validate, you remember that nobody else can have the experience you are having because each of us is a unique being. Similarly, you cannot have the same experience as anybody else, no matter how hard you try. Even if you are in the same space with another person, your physical vantage point is different and the filters through which you experience each moment, such as your personal history, are also unique to you. This step, after pausing and feeling, helps you recognize that **the experience you are having is valid simply because it is happening to you**. This is also a reminder that you are valid, that the fact that you are alive confirms undeniably that there is a reason for your existence, even when you are uncertain about what that reason may be. You validate by acknowledging that you are unique and that you have something unique to offer to the world.

Validating a moment doesn't mean you have to like the moment; by seeing this moment as a valid experience, you choose not to struggle with what is happening. (Thoughts of "This is not what I expected," or "This should not be happening," or "Why is this happening to me?" are indications that you are struggling with this moment.) To validate is to make a conscious choice to acknowledge that your experience is valid, even if what you are experiencing is anxiety, fear, or happiness.

Validating your experience is also a way to let go of self-judgment. Basically, you are coming to this moment, whatever the moment might be, **choosing to be with your life just as it is, and to be with yourself just as you are.** In this moment you witness whatever is happening with as much clarity as possible.

Clarify

"For me the greatest beauty always lies in the greatest clarity." Gotthold Ephraim Lessing

We invest a lot of time and energy creating a coherent story of our lives and of who we are. It makes sense that any inconsistencies between our story and our actual experience create a disruption, a wrinkle in the fabric of our story. Thus, many of us are continually editing our story in our minds for consistency. Writing and rewriting our life story is a way to bring a sense of coherence into our lives. However, when you attend more to the story in your mind than to the moment-to-moment development of life, you are not truly present. To clarify is to make sure that rather than living in the story in your mind, you are participating in your life to the best of your ability. In this step you confirm if there is a gap between what you are doing and what you think you are doing. A couple of useful questions for clarification are **Why am I doing what I am doing?** and **Am I doing what I think I am doing?**

Choose

"We are our choices." Jean-Paul Sartre

As you show up to your life, it's vital to exercise your free will. You are constantly making choices – even when you choose *not to choose*, you've made a choice! Ensure that you make choices that are meaningful to you, if only because you will have to deal with the consequences of your choices. You've invited awareness to the moment that you are in; it's time to decide whether action is required. For instance, if you notice that your intention and actions are aligned, you choose to continue on the same path. If, on the other hand, your intention and actions are not aligned, you can decide to align them, either by changing your actions or your intention. Moreover, even when your actions and intention are aligned, you can choose to change course if you find that the results are not what you intended originally. A simple question to help this part of the process is: **Is this action contributing to enhance the quality of my life?**

Additionally, it is important to notice the attitude you're choosing for your participation in this moment. Are you resisting? Are you enthusiastic? Are you overexcited? Do you think you know everything already? Or are you choosing an attitude of wonder and curiosity?

Respond

"Happiness is when what you think, what you say, and what you do are in harmony." Mahatma Gandhi

Responding is taking a conscious, deliberate action. Rather than your thoughts, it is your actions that make you who you are; your actions (and interactions) accurately reveal both who you are and what is important to you. **This is how you participate in life.** Acting deliberately and observing your actions can teach you a lot about yourself. How you respond to events in your life is all about responsibility. Response-ability means acting on your conscious choices. Paying attention to the motivation for your response and noticing the effects of your actions enable you to discern if what you are doing is useful or not. You assess if there is a difference between the way you felt before taking action and the way you feel after.

Life is a continuous feedback loop where your actions generate internal and external feedback. This feedback offered by your body, mind, and emotions, as well as by your environment, provides useful information for making intelligent and heartfelt decisions. Your actions enhance the quality of your life if they contribute to make you more aware. And at the same time, since you don't spend your vital energy being agitated and reactive, you end up being both relaxed and energized.

Awareness (Yoga) is a cyclical process to inquire into what is happening right where you are. If going through the complete awareness process shows you that nothing is wrong or that nothing needs to be changed, stay where you are, doing what you are doing. The diagram below summarizes the process.

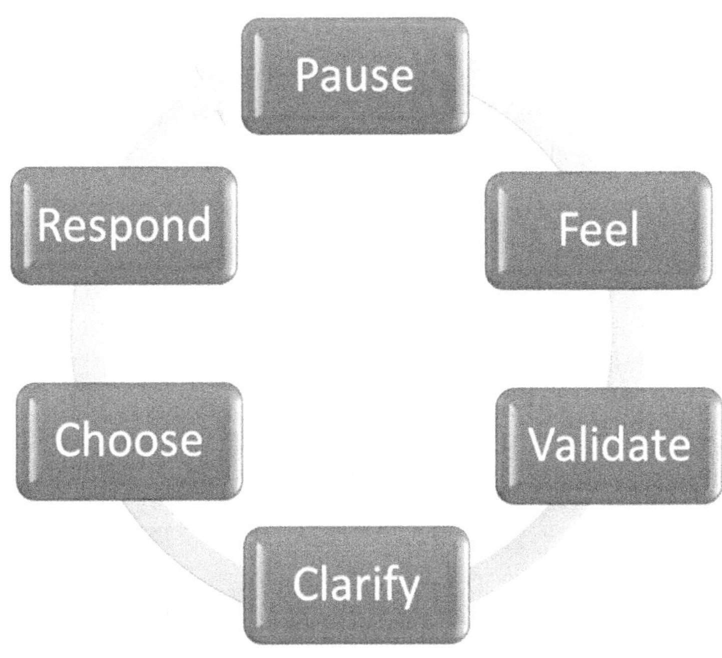

FIGURE 7. COMPLETE AWARENESS PROCESS EXPANDED

Activating the method

The most effecting way to learn this process is to use it. Then, you can test how effective it is for you. As with anything else, it takes practice to develop this way of being until it becomes an effortless way of participating in each moment. As you try to cultivate this useful way of being, your actions are fueled by your desire to show up to your life with an open mind, an open heart, and with an attitude of curiosity.

- Pause – Am I here?
- Feel – What sensations, thoughts and emotions are part of this experience?
- Validate – Whatever I am feeling is valid
- Clarify – Why am I doing what I am doing? Am I doing what I think I am doing?
- Choose – Is this helpful or not?
- Respond – Act consciously and ask, "How do I feel now?"

Now you can apply this method to all the practice exercises in this book. The following exercises are designed to demonstrate the different elements of the method. Implicit in each exercise is the noticing step. As usual, you are in charge of noticing the effects so that you can choose if the exercise may be useful for you. One directive in this process is to engage in a heartfelt inquiry leading you to presence – engaging in every moment with open mind and open heart.

PUTTING IT INTO PRACTICE: PAUSE

This exercise takes only 5 minutes. Consider practicing it 4 times a day.

Whenever you have a chance, take a moment to pause and take in the experience you are participating in. Feel whatever is happening, including what is happening outside of you and inside of you. Briefly notice your attitude and take a few minutes to reflect:

- What happens when you choose to pause?

- What do you observe?

- When you do this exercise with some consistency, do you find any patterns in your ways of being? (Remember that your ways of being arise in your posture, movements, breathing, thoughts, emotions, and attitude)

- Does the pause have any effect on you, or on the experience you are having?

Notice the effects of this brief pause, then resume your activities. Be aware that quite possibly, even though you may have the best intention to try this exercise four times a day, you may only remember once, or you may even forget it altogether for a few days. If that happens, recall that there is no need for struggle, strain, or self-judgment; just take a pause whenever you can. Use your own direct experience to decide if you want to add this exercise to your repertoire of techniques for presence.

PUTTING IT INTO PRACTICE: FEEL

Allocate about 5 minutes to complete this exercise.

Whenever it makes sense for you, choose to pause, and then focus your attention on the actual sensations taking place in your body. Your hands, fingers, feet and toes, eyebrows, eyes, jaw, and lips are productive places to focus your attention because of the number of sensory receptors in those areas. *As you pause and feel, it may be good to remember that you are not trying to describe or comment on the sensations.* All you are doing is feeling. Quite likely you may find that the sensations keep changing from one moment to the next, and this may invite you to stay focused.

Take a few moments to digest the experience:

- What did you observe?

- Does anything change in your internal environment when you pause and feel?

- Is this exercise helpful or not helpful?

- Would it make sense for you to try this with some consistency over the next week or two?

PUTTING IT INTO PRACTICE: VALIDATE

Take about 10-15 minutes to complete this exercise.

In a place without distractions, find a comfortable position where you can close your eyes and relax. Take your time to really feel at ease. Give yourself permission to direct all your attention to yourself. Bring into your mind the memory of a recent event that caused you **minor** frustration or discomfort, perhaps a moment that was embarrassing for you. Remember the event as clearly as possible and try to focus on what you are feeling rather than on trying to explain what happened. Perhaps try to locate the actual sensations in your body. Can you stay with what is happening right now and see whatever you are feeling as valid? Remember you do not need to like, approve of, or condone what happened. What does it take to see whatever is happening in your internal environment as a valid set of thoughts and emotions? Take a few moments to really contemplate this idea. Let it swirl around your internal environment and witness what develops. Can you withhold the tendency to comment and just feel? What happens when you stay with the sensations: Do they change? How?

Sometimes we react to unkind or uncomfortable memories by berating ourselves. That is not what validating is about. Some other times we may try to avoid or to fix what we are feeling. That is not validating, either. *Validating is choosing to be OK with what you are feeling.* It is a way to process your experiences and to make peace with yourself by making peace with your past. As you feel again the sensations of discomfort, you may notice that they lose some of their potency. If you remain focused on feeling, eventually those dis-comforting sensations dissolve. When you can think of that memory again and it does not generate reactivity, you have allowed it to consume its own emotional energy. Then, it is only a memory that you have integrated and have made peace with. Without being at peace with yourself right now, it is unlikely that you can move forward toward greater integration. Some people find it useful to channel their internal sense of discomfort as a source of energy that drives them in a more productive direction. What works best for you?

The next technique consists of four progressive parts that build upon one another. Using this specific technique provides an opportunity to clarify something that is fundamental both at the level of application of the technique and at a much deeper level related to our general outlook in life.

PUTTING IT INTO PRACTICE: CLARIFY - WHAT IS IMPORTANT TO ME?

Allocate 20 minutes to complete this exercise.

PART ONE: WHAT IS MY NATURE?

This is a free writing exercise. Just write whatever comes to mind without editing or judging. Write down answers to the questions below.

- Who am I?

- What are my values?

- What is important to me?

After you finish writing, read what you wrote. Being as impartial as possible, underline the words that resonate strongly with you. Take a few moments to focus on those underlined ideas and notice your inner responses to those ideas. Then, select the three ideas that best represent what is important to you.

PART TWO: MY ACTIONS

Once again, without filtering, write answers to the following questions.

- How do I spend my time?

- What do I do with my energy?

- How do I spend my money?

When you feel you have written enough, take a moment to pause, close your eyes and enjoy a few rounds of natural breathing. Then open your eyes and read your answers.

PART THREE: CHOICES

Now, as accurately as possible, make a list of your activities during the past 3 or 4 days.

PART FOUR: CLARIFYING

Your answers to the previous sets of questions offer you an opportunity to reflect on what you think is important, what you think you do, and what you actually do: your choices and actions. Notice how your actions over the last few days reflect your inclinations, preferences and priorities – some conscious, unconscious. As you compare these answers, notice if your thoughts and actions are in alignment. *Did your activities of the past few days reflect accurately what you think is important?*

If your intentions and actions match very well, enjoy the feeling of finding congruency between who you think you are and who you actually are. However, if you have doubts about your ideas and actions being in alignment, then you can try the following exercise. And even when you already think there is alignment, the Minding the Gap technique can be quite illuminating.

PUTTING IT INTO PRACTICE: MINDING THE GAP

Use this technique for the next two weeks.

WEEK ONE

At the end of each day, take at most 5 minutes to write down in your journal how you invested your time, energy and money that day.

DAY 1

DAY 2

DAY 3

DAY 4

DAY 5

DAY 6

DAY 7

At the end of the week review your entries for the past week. Are there any patterns in your actions?

WEEK TWO

Just as you did during the previous week, at the end of each day, take no more than 5 minutes to record what you did during the day. Then, take 2 or 3 minutes to jot down what you need and want to do the following day. At the end of each day compare your intentions for the day with the activities that you engaged in.

DAY 1

PLANNED ACTIVITIES ACTUAL ACTIVITIES

DAY 2

PLANNED ACTIVITIES ACTUAL ACTIVITIES

DAY 3

PLANNED ACTIVITIES	ACTUAL ACTIVITIES

DAY 4

PLANNED ACTIVITIES	ACTUAL ACTIVITIES

DAY 5

PLANNED ACTIVITIES	ACTUAL ACTIVITIES

DAY 6

PLANNED ACTIVITIES ACTUAL ACTIVITIES

DAY 7

PLANNED ACTIVITIES ACTUAL ACTIVITIES

AT THE END OF THE SECOND WEEK

Take time to review your journal. To what extent are your thoughts and actions aligned? How often does it happen that you think or say one thing but do something different? For instance, did you write down that you wanted to go for a walk the next day, but other things got in the way and you never got around to going for a walk?

Upon completing this exploration, many of us find that there are inconsistencies between what we think and what we do. Are those inconsistencies inescapable? For instance, when I find one of those gaps, I can deal with it by saying "That's too bad, but that's just the way I am. I have always been that way. Besides, it's too late to change that now..." However, anytime I hear myself thinking that, I can also pause to consider if I may have other options, so that I can choose to empower myself to act in ways that are truly meaningful to me. In addition, some of us may be surprised by inaccuracies in our perception. For instance, we may think or say to ourselves, or to other people, that we are working on some project, yet when we look at our actions, we may find that we have not been investing any actual time or energy on that project. Or we may think that we are not accomplishing enough, but then discover that we are actually much more productive than we give ourselves credit for. Clarifying is one way to be certain that there is consistency between what we think and what we do (our choices and actions).

PUTTING IT INTO PRACTICE: CHOOSE & RESPOND

Allocate 5-10 minutes daily for this exercise.

From the previous exercises (or from what you already have observed about yourself) choose a way of being that is not very beneficial. For instance, driving on a regular basis, I have noticed my tendency to make a quick (and probably inaccurate) judgment about the drivers in other cars based on a bumper sticker, a personalized license plate or the way they are driving. Having noticed that pattern, realizing that it doesn't enhance the quality of my life and that it instead pulls my attention away from my intention (which is driving with awareness) I set an intention to pause my judgments as I am driving. Then I notice if that brief pause has any beneficial effects. For me, refraining from judging immediately helps to declutter my mind and encourages me to focus on driving more mindfully. For this exercise, choose a pattern that keeps you from investing your time, energy, and money on something that is meaningful for you. Then write down your intention below.

For the next ____ days, I …

To activate your intention, every day choose to remember and to honor your intention. Pay attention during the day to the different distractors pulling you away from your objective. Whenever you find yourself getting distracted, acknowledge what you are doing by mentally saying what you are doing, and then gently redirect your attention towards your meaningful objective. Notice what happens. Beware that some deeply entrenched patterns may recur more frequently than you might like. If that is the case, remember the 4 Ss, *strain not, struggle not, self-judge not* and *smile a lot*. Just as it took some time for that unhelpful pattern to become established, it may also take some time to implement a more useful pattern. What is important is to make your choice and to try to stick with it despite the many distractions that may emerge in the process. After a few days, assess your progress and decide if it is helpful to continue this practice.

Summary

At this point, you have approached the Yoga Sutra gradually. You have become familiar with the general theme running through the whole Yoga Sutra: knowing yourself well, starting with knowing your tendencies. Because this is a handbook for practice, you have also found several ways of applying these ideas into practice in your own life. Moreover, in this chapter you have engaged in a meaningful exploration of yoga practice in a way that is smart and potentially beneficial to all aspects of your life. As a result, your practice can be enjoyable, which contributes to making your practice sustainable. Remember the abbreviated version of the method for presence:

- Pause – Am I here?
- Feel – What sensations, thoughts and emotions are part of this experience?
- Validate – Whatever I am feeling is valid.
- Clarify – Why am I doing what I am doing? Am I doing what I think I am doing?
- Choose – Is this helpful or not?
- Respond – Act consciously and ask, "How do I feel now?"

You are now equipped to continue your journey of self-exploration by diving into the details of each chapter in the Yoga Sutra. Each aphorism will offer you suggestions and questions to put into practice.

SECTION TWO: FOLLOWING THE THREAD

तपः स्वाध्यायेश्वरप्रणिधानानि क्रियायोगः

tapaḥ svādhyāyeśvarapraṇidhānāni kriyāyogaḥ

Yogic action (kriya yoga) combines enthusiasm (*tapas*), intelligence (*svadhyaya*) and humility (*ishvara pranidhana*)

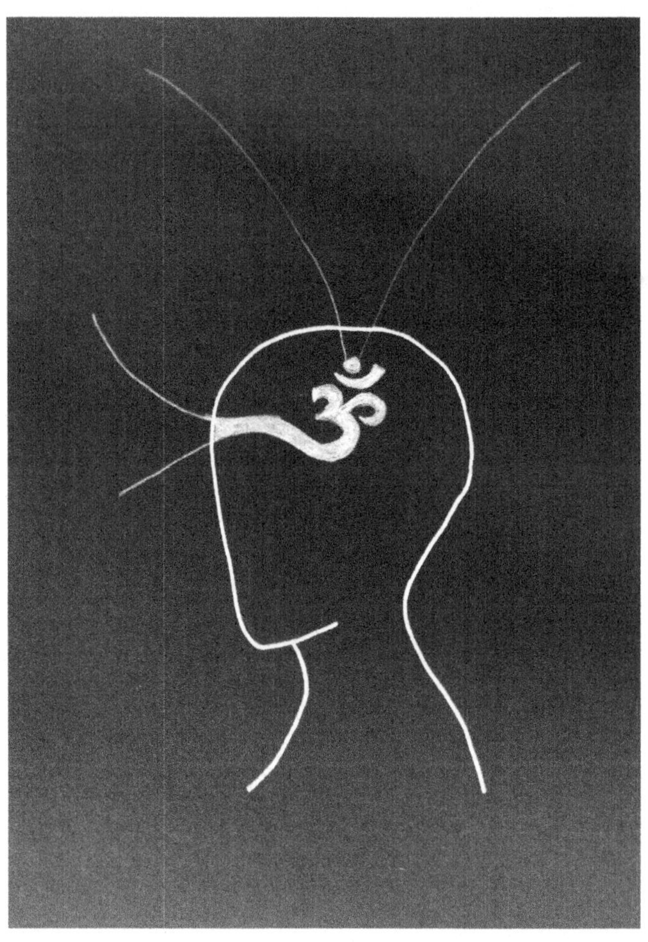

Presence is the essence of the practice and its objective. Presence is dynamic.

YOGA SUTRA SUMMARY

Before we dive into the meaning and viable applications for each sutra, let's summarize a representative selection of aphorisms to paint an overview of the complete Yoga Sutra. The numbers in brackets point to specific sutras; the first number is the chapter and the second number is the specific sutra.

General Overview

Chapter One: Integration (*samadhi*)

- What is yoga? [1.1-1.4]
- Ways of being [1.5-1.11]
- A method for self-regulation [1.12-1.22]
- An alternative approach, humility [1.23-1.29]
- Distractions, their symptoms, and removal [1.30-1.39]
- The progression of insight into liberation [1.40 - 1.51]

Chapter Two: Practice (*sadhana*)

- Yogic action [2.1-2.2]
- Afflictions [2.3-2.11]
- Effects [2.12-2.14]
- Suffering [2.15-2.17]
- Awareness and experiences [2.18-2.22]
- Discernment [2.23-2.27]
- The limbs of yoga [2.28-2.55]

Chapter Three: Magnificence (*vibhuti*)

- Concentration, meditation & integration [3.1-3.8]
- Transformation [3.9-3.15]
- Meditative integration & its effects [3.16-3.37]
- Warning [3.38]
- Subtle energy [3.39-3.44]
- Highest attainments [3.45-3.50]
- Freedom [3.51-3.52]
- Purpose [3.53-3.56]

Chapter Four: Emancipation (*kaivalya*)

- Awareness & nature [4.1-4.5]
- Impressions, tendencies & consequences [4.6-4.11]
- Realm of experience [4.12-4.17]
- Consciousness and awareness [4.18-4.24]
- Emancipation [4.25-4.34]

Summary

Yoga is regulating my ways of being [1.2] so that I am embodied presence [1.3] instead of identifying with my changing ways of being. [1.4] With deliberate intention, [1.13] gradually, over a long period of time, I practice continuously with sincerity and without interruptions [1.14]; while at the same time I cultivate clarity that releases assumptions, opinions and expectations from my mind and heart. [1.15]

Planting the seeds of humility, I let go of the illusion of control. [1.23] To counteract the ongoing tendency to get distracted, I choose a meaningful single point of focus. [1.32] I notice my biases and remove judgment by opening my heart and mind through friendliness, compassion, inspiration, and equanimity. [1.33] I grow the roots of presence by bringing joy [1.36] and love to my heart. [1.39]

Yoga is showing up to my life with enthusiasm, intelligence, and humility. [2.1] My yoga practice removes obstructions in body, mind and heart, while enhancing my inner harmony and integration. Not knowing my own nature causes confusion (*avidya*) which leads me to believe stories I and others make up about me and about the world (*asmita*). These opinions generate likes (*raga*), dislikes (*dvesha*), and a sense of self-importance (*abhinivesha*) that leave impressions in me and result in a never-ending cycle of suffering. [2.3-2.15]

My yoga practice is a complete and systematic journey for the gradual removal of limitations, inefficiencies, and suffering. As a result, I establish clear discernment between my ways of being and my true nature, thus removing misidentification and suffering. [2.15-2.27] Observing the *yamas*, I release strain and cultivate appreciation for the interdependence among all of life through love (*ahimsa*), truth (*satya*), generosity (*asteya*), reverence (*brahmacharya*), and abundance (*aparigraha*). [2.30, 2.31, 2.36-2.39] Observing the *niyamas*, I release struggles and cultivate inner harmony through clarity (*shaucha*), contentment (*santosha*), enthusiasm (*tapas*), self-awareness (*svadhyaya*), and humility (*ishvara pranidhana*). [2.32, 2.40-2.45] When unhelpful thoughts, memories and emotions arise, I respond by directing my awareness to uplifting thoughts, memories, and emotions (*pratipaksha bhavana*). [2.33, 2.34] My *asana* practice optimizes posture and movement through balancing stability with ease, removing struggle, strain, and self-judgment and through an attitude of having infinite time. [2.46- 2.49] My *pranayama* practice purifies my nervous system through breath regulation that enhances my awareness and invites my attention inwardly. [2.49, 2.50, 2.51, 2.52] My *pratyahara* practice enhances my internal sensitivity facilitating meditation. [2.54, 2.55]

Concentration and meditation prepare me to transition from sustained single-pointedness to effortless mindfulness that gradually develops into direct insight into the mysteries of life and true wisdom. [Chapter Three] Meditation eliminates distractions and disturbances [1.32], neutralizes obstacles [2.11], transforms my body, mind and senses [3.9], prevents the generation and storage of emotional impressions [Chapter Four], cultivates discernment and clarifies the distinction between individual awareness and pure being. Yoga leads me to experience the world as it truly is, without misidentification or misperception. Eventually the mind can become a purely reflective surface that offers awareness a mirror to itself. With this extraordinary clarity, and without any further distractions, all afflictions and impressions cease. [Chapters Three and Four]

Now, we will continue our journey in living the wisdom of the Yoga Sutra by exploring interpretations of each individual sutra as well as suggestions for putting them into practice.

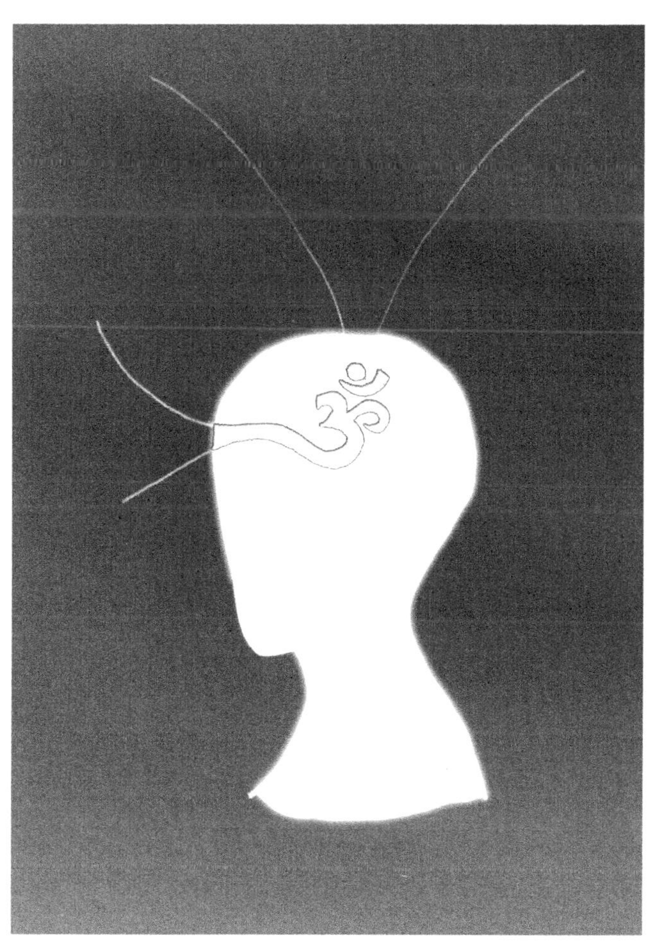

Integration means to become a receptacle for wholeness and fullness. Noticing our inclinations and how they influence our attitudes, intentions and actions enables us to regulate our ways of being to release distractions, inefficiencies and agitation. This gradual process will test our resolve as well as our capacity to keep returning to presence time after time.

INTEGRATION (*SAMADHI*)

The title of Chapter One of the Yoga Sutra is *samadhi. Samadhi* can be translated as perfect *meditation, abiding in inner stillness and inner silence or integrated harmony. Samadhi* is also translated as "being," and that definition is the theme of Chapter One. This first chapter consists of six interconnected topics:

- What is yoga? [1.1-1.4]
- Ways of being [1.5-1.11]
- A method for self-regulation [1.12-1.22]
- An alternative approach, humility [1.23-1.29]
- Distractions, their symptoms and removal [1.30-1.39]
- The progression of insight into liberation [1.40 - 1.51]

Remember that application is the path of direct experience to embody the wisdom of yoga into your life. As you read the Yoga Sutra by chapter and aphorism, explore the questions and suggestions for reflection and practice in each section.

WHAT IS YOGA?

1.1 Now, yoga practice.

As with any journey, the journey of exploring who you are can start only after you decide that you are ready for – and committed to – this endeavor. You must set your intention to be present in your own life, and you make yourself available to the ever-changing flow of life by withholding your tendency to object or put conditions on this moment. Ask yourself: Have I prepared for this journey? Can I make yoga (being with what is) my intention and purpose? Can I make a commitment to deepen my connection with myself? These questions can become gentle reminders to keep returning to your intention every time a distraction pulls you away from presence.

The lifelong journey of self-discovery is profoundly affected by your attitude and state of mind. In fact, your attitude may contribute to pull your attention away from showing up fully to the moment you are in. It happens often that a strong commitment may be fueled by ambition. However, ambition can derail you by making you rigid or by pushing you beyond the limits of what you can do consciously and sustainably. Moreover, ambition tends to generate expectations that preclude you from seeing the whole spectrum of options available to you. When you really want to understand something, kind and playful curiosity helps you explore with awareness. This attitude invites an open mind to consider everything without preconceived ideas. How can you cultivate your playful curiosity?

It's also quite common that we are particularly harsh critics of ourselves, even having an exacting tone we use only with ourselves – probably because nobody else would stick around if we behaved the same way towards others that we do to ourselves. Gratitude can be a doorway to shifting perspective and opening your heart. Can you be grateful for the opportunity to embark on this journey? In addition, forgiveness and compassion are instrumental in softening your attitude, especially when you recognize *you are sincerely trying to do your best.* Can you plant the seeds for unconditional love by practicing gratitude, forgiveness, and compassion?

The practice in yoga is practicing **presence**. Remember, you have a variety of options to keep coming back to presence. For instance, you can always use *ATHA* as a mantra to keep you coming back to presence, recalling that *ATHA* can be translated as "And now." You can ask *Am I focused on doing what I am doing?* and *How am I doing what I am doing?*

1.2 Yoga: regulating ways of being.

Yoga asks *Is it possible to regulate our own internal climate, by choosing how we respond to what is happening outside?* To answer, we start by becoming aware of our ways of being. Then, we let go of what is beyond our control. The next step is to notice what is within our control. With playful curiosity, we learn to modulate our attitude, bodies, breath, senses, and minds. The more attuned we are to our inner climate, the easier it will be to determine how our thoughts, emotions, movements, attitude, posture, movements, and breath are influenced by what is happening outside. Simultaneously, we increase the probabilities that we can learn how all these aspects of ourselves influence our intentions, choices, and actions.

Yoga is being with what is: instead of fighting this moment, you choose to accept this moment as it is, and yourself as you are. As you attempt to be in this moment, you notice if your ways of being, manifested in your posture, movements, thoughts, emotions, and attitude, contribute to wholehearted and unconditional participation in the moment you are in. If so, you continue flowing harmoniously with life and its ever-changing circumstances. Otherwise, if your ways of being are obstacles to presence, you are in charge of regulating your ways of being so that you can be fully present. Yoga is self-regulation.

On the journey of yoga there are two options: the first is to be in the state of yoga; the second, to move towards that state. You can do the latter by asking yourself, "Am I fully present?" and "How is this posture/movement/thought/emotion/attitude conducive to presence?" It's essential to be aware of your own ways of being in order to be able to regulate them. Thus, yoga requires you to be aware of your tendencies by noticing your inclinations and predispositions and then asking yourself, "Is this tendency useful right now?" and "Is this tendency helping me move towards my objective?"

1.3 As a result, embodied presence.

Often translated "As a result, the seer abides in its own nature," this sutra tells us what happens when we successfully regulate our ways of being or internal activities. Where the previous sutra (1.2) defined the active aspect of yoga, this sutra complements it by providing a definition of yoga as a state, best summarized as **being**. In other words, sutra 1.2 presents the "doing" side of yoga and 1.3 presents the "being" side. We may see yoga as a dynamic process of balancing our *doing* with our *being.*

In the state of yoga, when body, mind, and emotions are integrated and focused, you experience your true nature, the aspect of you that has not changed at all throughout your whole life.

Presence is a deep connection to this fundamental aspect of your being. At the end of every day, you return to the core of your being when you relax deeply and fall asleep. In your dreams, you are still processing some of your daily experiences. In dreamless deep sleep you release all the ideas you have about who you are (or should be) and the notion of being separate from everything outside of you gets blurred. Yoga, regulating your ways of being, makes your ways of being more evident and helps you connect to the presence that underlies all your actions, thoughts, movements, and emotions. Yoga strengthens your ability to *consciously* access your deepest awareness. This may prompt you to recognize that you are not, and have never been, alone in a seemingly hostile world. Instead, you are deeply interconnected to all that is. You can contemplate with profound curiosity and patient persistence "Who am I?" and "What is my true nature?" and "Am I the changing phenomena I perceive?" and "Is there something in me that does not change?" Remember that pondering these questions is more productive than rushing to come up with conclusions, opinions, beliefs, and stories to entertain yourself.

To abide in your own true nature seems like such a simple idea. Simple things tend to be powerful ways to examine ourselves, because their simplicity prevents us from getting entangled in the process itself. The following exercise can be an effective inquiry into your true nature:

Find a position that is comfortable, so that you can be very relaxed yet attentive. (Lying down may be so relaxing that you fall asleep, which would be fine, but would not help you explore what your true nature is.) Close your eyes softly. Notice the sounds and noises and other sensations like the temperature, level of humidity and the scents around you. For the following questions, try to answer based on your direct experience as it is happening *right here and now*. Your mind will try to offer answers based on what you know or think you know. Invite your mind to help you focus on feeling the questions and their possible answers. Be open to the possibility that there are no clear-cut answers to these questions. Be as still as possible.

First question:
How tall do you feel? Savor the question and try to feel your height. Notice how tall you feel you are without referring to a number that you think you know. Just try to feel your height.

Next question:
What is the color of your eyes? Can you feel the color of your eyes? Is there a way to feel the color of your eyes without referring to anything else other than the actual internal experience you are having right now?

Now, can you feel your age?
Rely only on your current sensory experience. Without going into stories or ideas, can you feel your age? What does your age feel like?

You probably know your name better than anybody else, but can you feel your name? Notice any tendency to want to have an answer in words or stories and choose to just stay with the sensations of your name.

Although height, eye color, age and name serve as identifiers to associate with who we think we are, what happens when you choose to stay with these wordless sensations and the combination of everything that you are feeling without having to add an opinion or a story? How does that feel?

Can this exercise be a portal to experience your true nature? No words can ever fully describe your true nature. But you can experience your true nature directly. Is it possible that your true nature feels spacious, formless, ageless, and nameless? Might it be possible that your true nature feels timeless, without beginning and without an end? Is it possible that this sutra is encouraging you to know your true nature through your direct experience?

Another avenue of exploration:
First thing in the morning, as soon as you discover that you are awake but before you get up, notice the first thoughts and emotions that arise. Is it possible to delay the onset of internal and external activity, just for a few minutes so that you can deliberately experience the state of transition between sleep and being awake? Can you stay in the deep peace that you retire into as you sleep? Can you keep a subtle connection to that deep peace throughout your day? What do you discover as a result? Can this exercise influence your mood and set the tone for your day and your interactions?

1.4 Instead of identifying with ways of being.

This sutra suggests that there is a fundamental difference between who you are and who you think you are. Your true nature is presence, but when body, mind, and emotions are not integrated, the tendency is to get distracted by your ways of being. Your ways of being include the habits you have developed in your attitudes, posture, movements, breathing patterns, and in your sense awareness. You probably have developed ways of being in your interactions with others. These ways of being manifest often as internal chatter in your opinions, emotions, and memories as well as in the way those opinions influence your perceptions and your actions. This sutra states that you may end up believing that you are your external and internal activities. For instance, as you listen to yourself talk and think, pay attention to your "I am…" statements, such as "I am happy," "I am worried," "I am a student," "I am employed by…." When you examine these labels, can you find out to what extent they create a sense of identity, a sense of who you are? Additionally, are you aware of how much energy, time, and effort you have invested in making that label part of who you are? How much work does it take for you to sustain that portion of your identity? You have acquired most, if not all, of these labels at some point in your life. If the label has not been a part of you all the time, what were you before you had that label? In other words, those labels are temporary because at some point in your life (in the past or future) each one of those labels will not describe you accurately. In fact, every night, in order to fall asleep, you let go of all labels and ways of being. Not being able to let go of some label or internal activity will probably keep you from falling asleep.

This pair of sutras, 1.3 and 1.4, offer two options. Sutra 1.3 says that your true nature is embodied presence. When you are called to act in the world, you participate in each moment with an open mind and an open heart. Sutra 1.4 says that the alternative is to misidentify with the habits and tendencies that you have developed. Consider how your internal dialogue and your interactions contribute to crowd your inner world with more labels. Each label places demands on your time and energy. Furthermore, the labels you and others have chosen to describe you serve as filters that deeply influence how you perceive yourself and your environment. For instance, if you have often heard that you are not creative or intelligent, these ideas will affect what you think you can and can't do. Some of the most inaccurate and toxic misconceptions you may hold include *I am not enough*; *there is something fundamentally wrong with me; I am incomplete*; *I am not good enough*.

Becoming aware of these statements invites you to contemplate how your own ways of being contribute to the quality of your participation in each moment. Are there some ways of being that are not essential to your life? You may answer this question through some of the previous exercises like, Who do you think you are? (page 80), What is my true nature? (page 85) and What is important to me? (page 113).

As you consider your ways of being and labels, remember that a label that is useful in one situation may be unhelpful or irrelevant in a different context. Besides, the label is most likely not *essential* to your being. Understanding this enables you to use these labels without believing that they make you who you are. Every day you can explore this aphorism by paying attention at the end of each day to the process of consciously and deliberately releasing all of your labels and ways of being. Notice how you feel as you let go. Beware of emotional attachments to some of those ideas. Practicing this regularly can give you insights into your ways of being and into how you feel when you release them as well as into how they influence the quality of your sleep. You can make note of the labels that you feel attached to and find hard to let go as they may suggest fruitful paths of inquiry. You can combine this practice with the practice suggested for the previous sutra.

Remember that, in addition to ways of being in attitude, emotions, and thoughts, our bodies are molded by our postural habits and by our movement habits. If you wore the same pair of pants for a full week, when you took them off you could easily see the shape that your body is most frequently in. *You are actually shaping your own body with your activity patterns.* So, if you sit for many hours a day in front of a computer, your body may be taking a certain shape. That shape will likely condition how you move as well as where your tension accumulates. It will also influence the movements that you can and can't do. If you identify with your body, are you identifying with the conscious or unconscious shape that it has right now? Notice also that the definition of ways of being would suggest that your emotional patterns, like feeling inadequate or overconfident, will influence your thoughts, mood, breathing, choices, and actions. Similarly, your thoughts, such as thinking that the world is a place of hostility or cooperation will influence your attitude and emotions as well as how you interact with other people.

Recall, sutras 1.3 and 1.4 suggest two basic modes of operation – being and doing. Being is an inward orientation, doing is an outward orientation. Yoga regulates your ways of being at all levels to strike a dynamic balance between being and doing that is conducive to living in integrated harmony, inside and outside.

Ways of Being

1.5 Ways of being manifest in five different ways, sometimes helpful, sometimes unhelpful.

Prior to Sutra 1.5, our attention is summoned (1.1), yoga is defined (1.2), we learn what happens when we are in a state of yoga (1.3) and that when we are not in a state of presence we get confused by our ways of being (1.4). Sutra 1.5 then enumerates the ways of being and indicates their effects.

Patañjali's definition of yoga is commonly translated as controlling or suppressing the activities of the mind. If we think about ways of being as thoughts, we may assume a separation between body and mind. Instead, let's consider that the original Sanskrit words, *citta vrtti,* can be translated as a combination of the meanings of *citta* (intentions, thoughts, reason, and memory) with the definitions of *vrtti* (behavior, action, tendencies, and disposition), an articulation of mind and body. Is it possible that your own cells, tissues, organs, and systems have their own intelligence, dispositions and tendencies?

Sutra 1.5 suggests that your ways of being can be painful or not painful. Rather than thinking about your ways of being as static tendencies that are active all the time, it is more accurate to understand your ways of being as dynamic. For instance, some of your tendencies may be primed by your context and circumstances. When you are socializing with a group of risk-taking friends, you may be more willing to take some risks yourself. Conversely, you may respond by reinforcing your risk-averse inclinations. Some of your ways of being may apply in one aspect of your life but not in another. For example, you could be fine with taking risks in your professional life, but you may be conservative in how you manage your finances. This variability of your ways of being may be a reason to choose to focus on the effects of your ways of being to assess their potential utility. Perhaps on some occasions it is wise to remain silent, so that you do not create confusion or offer unsolicited opinions that may bring up hostility or pain. Other times, it is important and necessary to express your perspective so that you act according to your conscience.

This sutra is an invitation to know your own tendencies. The more entangled you are on your preferences and habits, the more difficult it will be to have a critical distance to choose consciously the most appropriate and life-affirming action for each situation. Attending to your inner state and noticing your reactions and responses to external events and internal activities can reveal if some of your tendencies increase your levels of internal disharmony, causing pain, lethargy, or agitation. Conversely, you may find that some of your tendencies enhance your level of harmony, clarity and effectiveness. As you explore your own tendencies and their effects, pay attention to levels of pain. Keep in mind that, as mentioned before, there is a clear difference between pain and bearable discomfort. Pain serves as a warning sign alerting you to avoid the risk of injury. Bearable discomfort often indicates that you are reaching the boundaries of what is familiar to you.

These questions will guide your inquiry on the meaning and relevance of this sutra for your life:
Am I aware of my tendencies?
How do these tendencies manifest physically, mentally, and emotionally?
Do my tendencies influence my interactions?

Do my tendencies influence other tendencies?
At this moment, is this tendency my best friend or worst enemy?
What are the effects of my preferences on the quality of my life?
How do my habits influence my participation in my life?
Are there some tendencies that are sometimes useful and other times painful?
Can I regulate my own inclinations?

1.6 They are knowledge, misperception, imagination, deep dreamless sleep, and memory.

This aphorism lists the five manifestations of our ways of being, the patterns that develop consciously and unconsciously in posture, movement, breathing, thinking, feeling, and interacting. Systematically observing these patterns can help us uncover when some of them are helpful and when unhelpful. For instance, there are moments when it is quite useful to be detailed-oriented, such as when you are following a specific set of instructions to assemble a piece of furniture or when proofreading an important message. At other times, like when you are thinking creatively or when you are trying to focus on the goal of a project, getting lost in the details may cause you to lose perspective.

These five categories – knowledge, misperception, imagination, deep dreamless sleep, and memory – are ways to classify our internal activities. The simplest approach to this sutra is to reflect on each one of these words, its meaning and its influence on your thoughts, emotions, intentions, and actions.

Knowledge.

Living in a time with overwhelming amounts of information available about all kinds of topics, it's useful to contemplate the difference between knowledge and information. How do you know which one is which? How do you know what you know?

Misperception.

Misperception is the opposite of knowledge. What happens when you fail to understand something correctly? To explore this notion, we ask ourselves: How do I know if what I think I know is true?

Imagination.

The third way of being is imagination including anything you think that does not exist in reality. Start with the simple question: What do I think? Is what I think conducive to being present in my life?

Dreams.

What are my dreams? Are my dreams offering me insights and guidance or are they cryptic and confusing? Do my dreams generate calmness or agitation?

Memory.

The last category is memory. What do I store in my memory? Is my memory accurate? What are the effects of my memories on my thoughts, emotions, desires, and choices?

Keep in mind that these five categories have been presented in the context of presence. Specifically, each of these ways of being influences your ability to be present as well as the quality of your presence. The basic idea is to pay attention to your ways of being. Then, it is easier to notice the relationships between your posture, movements, breathing, thoughts, and emotions – like when your posture influences your emotions, when your thoughts affect your breathing, or your emotions influence your posture. You can put this idea into practice by asking yourself: Is this posture useful? Is this way of moving helpful? Does this way of breathing contribute to the quality of my participation in this moment? Do these thoughts help me be present? Is this emotional attitude appropriate for this activity or for this interaction?

Those questions intend to create a gap in the habitual mental, physical, emotional, and respiratory activities to invite presence. The overarching goal is to enhance the quality of your experience. To assess the quality of your experience, it's helpful to clarify your intention by asking Why am I doing this? And then corroborating that what you are doing is what you intend to do. By shining the light of awareness on what you are doing, you can make conscious decisions. In addition, these questions foster recognition that the input you perceive delivers useful feedback to help fine tune your participation in whatever you are doing. In the following aphorisms, Patañjali provides definitions of each one of these five ways of being.

1.7 Knowledge (*pramana*) results from direct experience (*pratyaksha*), inference (*anumana*), and transmitted wisdom (*agama*).

It is often said that the lists in the Yoga Sutra start with the most important element. The first of the ways of being is knowledge. Knowledge is derived from direct experience, inference, and wisdom from an authoritative source. When you do something consciously on a regular basis, you acquire an understanding that is different from what you know because of reading about it or from listening to somebody else who has done the same thing. For instance, when you are learning to bake bread at home, you may find instructions telling you to knead the dough to the right consistency. Even though reading about the process or watching a video about it can give you some useful information, when you have never kneaded dough before, that directive may seem too vague. Listening to the advice of a master baker can offer you useful tips on how to knead. However, all that information will truly become knowledge as you actually try to knead your dough. As you knead consciously and consistently you will notice the different qualities of the dough and how those qualities relate to the final product. Then your direct experience will help you assess and corroborate the information you inferred or received from other sources. Over time, you may be able to tell the right consistency of the dough from several factors, including its appearance, its temperature, how it feels to the touch, how it responds when you press on it, and so on. Even if you read a dozen books about the right consistency of bread dough, all that information does not compare to your first-hand experience. Your direct experience is embodied knowledge. Being a whole-body event, the knowledge resulting from your direct experience is almost impossible to describe accurately in words.

Next, inference or logical deduction (*anumana*), is the second component of correct perception. You use your inferences every single day. For example, if look out from your window and you see dark heavy clouds approaching you might infer that it will rain later. Sometimes your inferences are correct and other times they aren't.

The third source of correct knowledge, *agama*, is what you know from the wisdom transmitted by a trustworthy source. It is critical to ensure that both conditions are fulfilled, first that it is true wisdom, and second, that the source is trustworthy. These three sources of knowledge are best triangulated to corroborate what you know. You ensure that what you know is verified by your inferences and by the testimony of someone you can trust. In general, correct knowledge is confirmed by common sense. You may find, however, that common sense is not as common as you might think, and that some of us may be inclined to rely on our beliefs rather than trying to gather information through our direct experience. In fact, the current tendency to search on the internet for all kinds of information may not always include a critical analysis of the quick answers found online.

To embody this sutra, consider what you know and how you know it by asking yourself: How do I know what I think I know? Is my knowledge correct and accurate? Are the sources of my knowledge trustworthy? How do I corroborate what I am told? Are my beliefs and opinions true knowledge? You may also investigate if your beliefs and opinions are truly yours. Another avenue of exploration is to ensure that your direct experience, your inferences, and trustworthy testimony agree. When you pay attention to your words, actions, and interactions can you discern the kind of knowledge that they are based on? One more interesting avenue for reflection is to contemplate the question: What is common sense? Remember that these questions, rather than directing you to find a specific answer, are an invitation to discover your own assumptions, beliefs and habits and their role in your ability to be present.

Interestingly, one of the meanings of the word *pramana* in Sanskrit is oneness or unity. Contemplate the possibility that true knowledge creates a feeling of unity, harmony, and wholeness.

1.8 Error (*viparyaya*) results from inaccurate perception.

The next way of being is to be mistaken, or to be in error. As explained in aphorism 1.4, not knowing your true nature causes you to perceive yourself as the temporary phenomena coming and going through your internal systems. As a result, you might get entangled in an endless cycle, either chasing after some experiences that you like, or by pushing away what you dislike. Another typical manifestation of misperception is lack of awareness of the gap between what you are doing and what you think you are doing, such as when you claim that you are doing something out of love, but you do it because of self-interest. Or, when you think you are trying to help somebody, but your unrequested help is an imposition on somebody else so that you can feel better about yourself. The 'What is important to me?' exercise (page 113) provides one way of noticing if you are acting in error. You may also engage with the questions explored in the previous sutra (1.7). In addition, you can bring conscious awareness to your actions by asking "Am I doing what I think I am doing?" and then following through to find out.

In addition to uncovering our misunderstandings and misconceptions, it may be useful to explore also what we don't know. It sounds like a tongue twister or a riddle, but what we don't know includes both what we know we don't know as well as what we don't know that we don't know. When you visit a new city, quite likely you don't know many of the places and ways to get around from one location to another. This is part of the known unknowns. You know that you don't know how to get around the city. This information will prompt you to find a guide, a map, an app, or a book to guide you. There are also unknown unknowns. Many of us may know that photosynthesis is a process plants use to synthesize energy. However, if we needed to explain the process in detail, many of us would discover that we don't know that we did not know the specific details involving the chemical interaction involving photons from the sun, carbon dioxide and water. To what extent are you aware of both your known unknowns and your unknown unknowns?

Misperception also happens when you carry unresolved issues in your heart, such as regrets and guilt, because those emotions bias your perception and cloud your ability to be present. Finding ways to make lasting peace with yourself and your past, like practicing forgiveness and compassion, can empower you to move forward and act from a place of greater clarity and emotional maturity. Recognizing that even your mistakes have contributed to shape your current life, and learning from your previous erroneous actions offers you valuable feedback to enhance the quality of your current actions. Moreover, in order to prevent misunderstandings with yourself and with others, pay attention to your thoughts, words, and actions to ascertain if what you think is correct and true. Then, you are more likely to know why you are doing what you are doing as well as ensuring that you are doing what you intend to be doing.

1.9 Imagination (*vikalpa*) is the activity of the mind not based on direct experience.

After explaining knowledge and misunderstanding in the previous two sutras, this sutra continues the systematic inquiry into the ways in which human awareness works by defining imagination (*vikalpa*). Imagination is anything that is created in the mind that is not based on direct experience. Imagination belongs to the realm of ideas. Your imagination plays a role in recreating the stories you tell yourself and others. Other people's stories, as well as the stories you have heard many times through your upbringing, education, and social institutions all feed into your imagination. It often happens that you have heard your parents tell a story about you when you were 2 or 3 years old, perhaps about a memorable family trip or a funny event or a clever comment you made. Many people may not be able to remember such a remote story, but when you have heard it so many times (and may have even seen pictures of the event), you may construct an image in your mind and count it as one of your memories, when it is in fact one of the things that you imagine. Imagination is one of the ways in which people constantly arrange and edit their life story, what they've done, where they've been, including the contextual whys and hows of the story. This is an ongoing process that gives you a sense of coherence and that you are a logical and sensible person making decisions based on good information and sound reasoning. However, this constant editing of your own life story may cause you to end up believing your own stories, even stories that are not the result of your lived experiences. It may also be the source of misunderstandings with other people when there is conflict between each person's version of an event.

Notice how the things you imagine exist only in your head. As such, they can often seem "ideal." When we try to bring those ideas into being, we will probably find friction between the world of thoughts and ideas and reality as it is actually happening. It is usually in this gap between what we think and how it actually happens where we find sources of agitation. This is an example of what Patanjali was saying in sutra 1.5, that our ways of being can be helpful or not helpful. For instance, you start thinking about a place that you would like to visit. You even read about the place, its history, and why it's important to visit. When you get to the place, what you encounter may not match accurately your ideas about it. Sometimes what you find is much more exciting or beautiful than what you had imagined. Other times, what you find does not measure up to your expectations. Notice how each option will probably trigger thoughts, emotions and attitudes that might distract you from being fully present right where you are.

In yoga, because we are interested in being with what is, and not what could have been or should have been, it is important to distinguish between our direct experience and mind activity that is not based on our own experiences. You can make a point to observe closely the contents of your mind to differentiate what you know from what you imagine. You can also listen closely to the stories that you tell yourself and examine them for accuracy and relevance. Some of the questions that can guide you in this process include:

What stories do I tell myself?

What are the stories that I want to hear?

Do I believe the stories I tell myself (and others)?

Are my beliefs based on direct experience, or on my imagination?

You may also explore the contents of your imagination to find out if what you imagine is conducive to greater integration or to fragmentation. Are you using your imagination to visualize a meaningful goal for your life? Or, on the contrary, are you using your imagination to remove yourself from attending to your life consciously? Is your imagination distracting you by adding unnecessary things you "need to worry about," or by imagining what other people might be thinking? **Does your imagination contribute to the quality of your participation in your life?**

1.10 Dreamless deep sleep (*nidra*) is when the mind is empty of content.

The Sanskrit word *nidra* is translated both as sleep and as dreamless deep sleep. Sleeping is when you give all your systems a chance to relax, restore and rejuvenate. A lot of what happens during sleep is still a mystery, and thus a fertile ground for systematic contemplation. From the yogic perspective, the process of sleep is one of processing, digesting, and releasing thoughts, ideas, plans and beliefs. In fact, if you can't let go of some idea or worry, you will probably have a hard time falling asleep. As you fall asleep, your awareness turns inward, and reception of external sensory stimuli is turned off. During dreaming you witness what has left an impression in you during your daily activities and interactions. In this timeless space, impressions collected at different times combine in several ways. This combination of disparate memories is an attempt to digest, consolidate, and perhaps resolve some of the unresolved challenges you have faced. Clearly, the dream state is one form of internal activity (*vrtti*).

However, in dreamless deep sleep, even the subconscious activities seem to be turned off. During dreamless deep sleep, identification with temporary phenomena dissolves, and sensory perception is also turned off. Brain activity decreases to a minimum and even the strong associations with name, age, and other personal labels fade. The idea of being separate also dissolves. In dreamless deep sleep, the boundaries imposed by body, thoughts, and emotions disappear and you merge into spaciousness and oneness[i]. This is quite similar to stages of meditation, with the significant difference that during dreamless deep sleep we are not fully conscious.

Sleep is generally a time for recovery, repair, and renewal at physical, mental and emotional levels. Is the silence and stillness of deep sleep a way to connect to the pure consciousness underlying everything that exists? Is that how insight and inspiration blossom, offering simple and elegant solutions for the problems or challenges you might be facing? If this is so, you can ponder how your current ways of being facilitate deep sleep by noticing any patterns that foster or hinder your ability to rest and relax deeply.

Do you know how much sleep you really need? To what extent are your daily activities conducive to deep sleep? Are your sleep patterns conducive to regulating your internal clock? A simple experiment is making peace with your day. At the end of the day, when you are already in bed and ready to go to sleep, relax fully and take time to review your day with the perspective of this moment. Choose to make peace with your day, including what went well, what did not go so well, what turned out badly, and everything else. Then instead of starting to plan the next day, relax in the knowledge that you tried your best, so that you can make peace with yourself. This practice can combine nicely with the practices suggested for aphorisms 1.3, remaining with the peaceful calmness from sleep when you first wake up, and 1.4, becoming aware of the first thoughts that arise in the morning, to create a ritual that may help you sleep better and wake up rested and calm.

1.11 Memory (*smriti*) is retaining experiences.

The last way of being is remembering. Of the many impressions you sense in a single day, the impressions that have a strong emotion attached to them are the ones that will be stored. It is possible that you may know somebody who seems to be living in the past, longing for days long gone and how life used to be. The attitude of an "old" person can be defined as being attached to the past. It is not a matter of chronological age but of attitude. This attachment can result from wanting to retain what is no longer here, or from trying to push away the memory of something that happened before. In either case, this attachment may be so consuming that there may be very little energy left to invest in this moment. Consider also that fixating on your ideas about the future is one way of attaching or reacting to the past, because your predictions are probably based on something that happened before.

In contrast, the attitude of a "young" person could be defined as somebody who recognizes the newness of this moment and responds intelligently and with grace to it. Of course, it is not necessary to think that memories are bad and that you should eliminate them. Memories are part of your personal history. They contribute perspective. Rather than thinking that you should eliminate all your memories, consider your relationships to your memories. Do you hold your memories – or do they have a hold on you? Is it possible to have a healthy relationship with your memories? What would that mean for you?

One way of exploring this idea is to discover the emotional charge of a memory. Since emotion is the active element in creating an impression in your memory, you can gain insight by clarifying the emotional imprint left by an event. For instance, find a memory that defines you. Then, focus on the details of the memory like the situation and participants in the original event. Next, shift your attention from the superficial aspects of the memory to its emotional signature. What are the emotions this memory triggers in you? Do the emotions triggered by the memory brighten you internally, or do they dampen your physical, mental, and emotional energy? When you feel these emotions, do you react by pushing the memory away or by holding on to it strongly? Can you choose to just feel the sensations and emotions flow through you until they dissipate instead of trapping the emotions inside of you? When you practice this technique, can you notice similarities in the emotional imprint of your deeply held memories? Are those similarities indicative of memories with an unresolved emotional charge? When you reflect on those memories, do they offer you insight into some of your present attitudes, tendencies, and choices? Can you make peace with your memories and your past by releasing the emotional charge of each memory (regardless of it being positive or negative)? Can it help to recognize that previous events have contributed to shape your current perspectives and circumstances? Can you acknowledge that at every single point in your past you probably did what you thought was the best choice, even though you may not do the same thing again?

Method for Self-Regulation

1.12 Integration (*samadhi*) results from practice (*abhyasa*) AND freedom from attachments (*vairagya*).

This sutra offers a two-pronged approach for regulating your ways of being. It serves as a reminder that yoga is a dynamic dance articulating opposites into a fine balance between *being* and *doing*. This is a pervasive theme in the Yoga Sutra, appearing again in the suggestions for overcoming obstacles later in this chapter, in the definition of posture in Chapter Two, and in the definition of concentration (*dharana*) and meditation (*dhyana*) in Chapter Three. Sutra 1.3 indicates that quieting down your ways of being enables you to embody your true nature. That true nature is characterized by a dynamic equilibrium between your different aspects. This is present throughout the natural world. For instance, a tree cannot survive if there is no balance between its sky-bound branches and its roots digging in the ground. There is a similar harmony between the complementary aspects of breathing, where the inbound inhalation would be incomplete and ineffective without its corresponding exhalation. In the breathing process, each inspiration is a doing that brings air in, while each expiration is a letting go that releases what the body no longer needs. Our organism operates through many complementary processes like these: for instance, when some muscles shorten, other nearby muscles respond instinctively by lengthening. Our nervous system is constantly balancing out the outward orientation of the sympathetic nervous system with the inward orientation of the parasympathetic nervous system. In this sutra, Patañjali recommends articulating the complementary processes of practice (*abhyasa*) and release (*vairagya*) to move towards a deep integration of all internal systems for living in harmony with everything that is. This strategy combines doing, practice (*abhyasa*), with being, letting go of attachments (*vairagya*).

In the definition of yoga in aphorism 1.2, the idea of self-regulation was introduced, the combined strategy in this sutra offers a means for self-regulation. The first step is to notice your tendencies, the ways of being (*citta vrttis*) mentioned in 1.2 and explained in sutras 1.5 to 1.11. Keep in mind that **anything you practice, even what you practice unconsciously, will become stronger.** The practice (*abhyasa*) is to keep coming back to presence by attending consciously to the moment you are in. The ways of being will often generate distractions, pulling you away from presence. When that happens, you let go of attachments to the distracting ways of being. You also let go of attachments to the expected outcomes of your actions and, of course, you let go of self-judgment. This is *vairagya*. This strategy is encapsulated in an idea mentioned before, the practice is to keep coming back to presence without strain, without struggle, without self-judgment, and with a friendly attitude that brings a gentle smile to your face. The combination of practice and detachment can be summarized as acting with gentle persistence.

This strategy is a practical and effective approach to self-regulation. It is one way of choosing a balance between doing and being. Awareness of your own tendencies (ways of being, or *vrttis*) makes the process easier and more effective. In fact, this is a gradual process of cultivating sensitivity to internal and external feedback to determine how much to do and how much to let go of. The feedback also indicates if what you are doing is working or not. *Beware of the expectation that what worked before should work again in exactly the same way.* This is seldom the case. Perhaps the only formula that will work every time is "Be present." In practical terms, practice (*abhyasa*) is to align with your capacity for awareness, to respond to the specific situation that you are in, in the best way you can and then to be content with the results (*vairagya*), even when they are different from what you planned or expected.

Some questions for contemplation and for applying these ideas:
What are you currently practicing?
Of what you are practicing, how much is conscious and how much unconscious?
What are your tendencies in what you practice, too much, just right, too little? What are you attached to?
Do you take yourself too seriously?
How do you balance out what you do with just being?
To what extent do you try to manipulate the outside world to match your agenda?
How do you know that you have found a point of equilibrium between being and doing?

1.13 Practice (*abhyasa*) is established through deliberate intention.

In order to get started on any project, it is essential to have clarity on the goal of the project. Finding a goal that is meaningful and beneficial motivates you to get started. It also reminds you to let go of distractions and to stay on track. For some people the goal of yoga is fitness, flexibility, or relaxation. Others see yoga as a way to create inner harmony, or as a path to live authentically. Another option is to see yoga as a way to create balance in your life so that you can show up to your life with enthusiasm, kindness, and compassion. *What is your goal for your yoga practice? How is that goal similar to or different from the goals you have for your life?*

In the process of setting a meaningful intention, it's useful to distinguish if there is a difference between what you think (or say) is important to you and what you actually do. Revisiting the "What is important to me?" exercise (page 113) can help clarify your intention so that you can write it into a simple sentence such as:

I dedicate my life wholeheartedly to ......

or

I contribute ...... to the world.

Setting your intention in clear terms provides an easy way to assess if you are actually moving in that direction. As you read your intention aloud to yourself, notice how this intention feels. What type of response does your intention produce in you physically, mentally and emotionally? It is perfectly natural to feel some uncertainty or trepidation but beware of the tendency of the inner critic to crush what at this point may be only an idea. One of my favorite quotes is from Henry Ford: "Whether you think you can or you can't, you are correct." Thus, at least give your intention a chance. Planting your intention firmly by repeating it to yourself daily starts creating space in your awareness for that intention. Then you will be better able to notice ideas and information related to bringing your intention into reality. Also, know that moving towards your intention will probably require you to confront some obstacles and to move beyond complacency. This is how your determination gets tested. So, as you clarify your intention, it is a good idea to ask yourself:

What are my commitments?

Are my commitments aligned with my heartfelt purpose?

What do I allocate energy and time to?
What do I put on my "easy-to-ignore" list?
What do I put on my list of priorities?
Can you balance commitment with not taking yourself too seriously?

1.14 And is firmly rooted over a long time of continuous, wholehearted, and sincere action.

Remember that anything you practice will become firmly established, even what you practice unconsciously. Also, remember that nothing meaningful happens overnight. Everything in nature develops organically at a pace that is sustainable and manageable. This aphorism reminds you that realizing your meaningful intention will not happen automatically, because an intention not acted upon is just an idea. If your intention is dear to you, it deserves your best effort. Once you plant your intention in your space of awareness, you nurture it through your actions. Acting from your heart and with love will in itself provide sustenance for the journey. Presence is always available and the practice of moving towards presence is continuous. You move towards presence because you know it is a wise way to live your life. Practice, *abhyasa*, can be considered something done with the attitude of a ritual, stepping outside your habitual mindset to participate in something that is meaningful to you. **Consistent practice has the capacity to transform you.**

If it seems that there is not enough time to do all that you want to do, consider examining your priorities. This is what the "Clarify: What is important to me?" (page 113) and the "Minding the Gap" (page 116) exercises are for. These exercises help you clarify what you are making important enough to dedicate time to. As one of the teachers who came from India to the West, Swami Rama, pointed out, once your intention is clear then you can reinforce your desire to move in that direction by reminding yourself: "I need to do this, I can do this, I want to do this, I will do this."

Other obstacles on your way may be some patterns in your posture and actions, at the physical, mental, or emotional level. This is where the Method for Presence (page 99) can be useful: Pause and feel what is happening, validate what you are sensing and then clarify in order to choose the most intelligent and wholehearted action. Then, notice the effects. When you remember that there is only one time – here and now – you can enter the practice from a mindset of having infinite time, so that instead of rushing from one task to the next, you attend to what is happening right where you are. Remember, this moment is the culmination of your life and the portal into the rest of your life. Navigating this moment successfully will bring you into the next moment without agitation.

This is a lifelong journey. Developing any habit starts one step at a time. You will find that the more you commit to your meaningful intention, the more it makes sense to keep practicing, one moment at a time, one breath at a time. At some point you look back and realize how far you have traveled and how you have been getting better at regulating your physical, mental, and emotional tendencies so that they are less of a hindrance and more of a support to your goal.

Some of the questions that can be valuable include:
Do my actions reflect my intention?

Am I acting with joyful curiosity or with ambition?

What are the qualities of my actions?

Are my actions validated by true knowledge?

Since it is probable you will get distracted, for an instant, a few minutes, hours, days, months, or years; remember to keep returning to your intention without strain, struggle or self-judgement and with a gentle smile.

1.15 Freedom from attachment (*vairagya*) develops with an attitude of evenness that releases all cravings for external stimuli and internal dialogue.

When you try to give your undivided attention to the moment you are in, either in being mode or doing mode, most likely you will find your awareness pulled away from presence. In contemporary life there are endless streams of sensory stimuli competing for your attention. In fact, when you take a pause to rest and do nothing, quite possibly you will notice how you have been training yourself to shift your attention from one thing to another, and then to yet another. Your senses are constantly gathering information that your internal system decodes and interprets to decide if a response is needed. This continuous flow of information influences your thoughts, emotions, and attitudes. Quite often, the main filters used to process the sensory information received are two simple questions: *Do I like this?* and *Do I dislike this?* – as well as variations like *Do I want this?*

Sensory stimuli also evoke memories that may also bring up nostalgia, regrets, and longing. Sensory stimuli can also generate anticipation, anxiety, and worry. This sutra is an invitation to let go of the tendency to chase after sensory stimuli as well as to release the tendency to let sensory input generate internal dialogue and reactivity. This is not about ignoring what is happening. It is choosing to feel what is happening directly and consciously, noticing without getting entangled in your internal web of opinions and stories. This aphorism reinforces the idea of just being with what is, as it is (being mode), to counterbalance the doing encouraged in the previous two sutras about practice (*abhyasa*).

To put this sutra into practice, you can employ the method for presence. You choose to pause, feel, validate, and clarify if what you are attending to is aligned with your intention. If it isn't, then you can choose an option that enhances the quality of your participation in your life, right at that moment. In addition, you can make note of what distracted you. Over time you may start noticing patterns in your distractions. Examining distractions and attachments can be guided by questions such as:

What are the sources of distraction for me at home, at work, in my yoga practice and in my interactions with others?

What do I crave?

What are the expectations, beliefs and habits I am attached to?

Do I have a healthy relationship with whatever comes into my life?

Am I trying to control the world outside?

Do I have to have an opinion about everything?

Am I entertaining myself by making up stories about everything I am

experiencing?
Can it be enough to just feel what is happening with clarity?

You may also consider if, at a more fundamental level, the distractions you experience result from your sense of I, me, my, and mine.

As you ponder these questions and observe your actions, you gradually become more aware of how you allocate your attention, which is the key to redirecting your efforts to what is truly important. You also become better able to notice if you are reacting unnecessarily to whatever enters your space of awareness. Along the way, you may feel frustrated by how distracted you are on a regular basis. This is hardly unusual. In fact, every time you notice that you got distracted, that is a sign that the practice is working because probably you did not even notice getting distracted before. So, next time you get distracted, to promote detachment, you can ask yourself: Am I taking myself too seriously? And with a gentle smile you can redirect your attention and energy to presence without strain, struggle, or self-judgment. Another productive avenue for exploration is releasing expectations for the fruits of your actions: Doing for the sake of doing and welcoming whatever results. Is this possible for you?

1.16 Awareness established in Truth does not become distracted, even by the subtlest fluctuations in nature

A clear and firm intention is sustainable if it is directed towards something that lasts. The previous sutra helps you recognize the temporary and changing nature of wants and dislikes, so that it is possible to stop chasing after sensations, thoughts, and emotions. Almost inevitably questions arise: What is not temporary? Is there anything that lasts? As you attend to life processes, you are bound to notice that nothing seems permanent. Perhaps, the only thing permanent is the constant mutability of life in its ongoing variations. In fact, what aspect of you notices these endless changes? Is it simply a way of looking? As you stand in front of a mirror and look at yourself and then look at a picture of you from five or ten years before, you can see the changes in your external appearance. Yet, despite the changes in your body, in your ways of thinking, and in your emotions, it seems like every time you look in the mirror there is some part that does not change, that seems to remain the same. Is that part more lasting than all the temporary aspects of yourself? Is that aspect of you what is often called the Seer or the Witness? Is that aspect of you related to the state explored in aphorisms 1.3 and 1.4, the state of just being with what is, also known as the natural state? Another way of exploring this is to ponder what is left when temporary activities quiet down. Does contemplating impermanence influence your moods, thoughts and actions? As your explorations bring some experiential insight into these questions, you may expand your research to live with these questions. What is the background of all of life? If everything is impermanent, is there anything that is permanent and unchanging? If so, is that what Truth is?

INTEGRATION

1.17 A gradual progression towards deep inner integration (*samprajñata samadhi*) develops through subtle refinement of attention from reasoning (*vitarka*), to contemplation (*vichara*), to joy (*ananda*) and then to the sense of being (*asmita*)

This sutra presents the process of moving towards deep integration, *samadhi*. This high level of integration is presented by Patañjali in two sutras, 1.17 and 1.18. Towards the end of Chapter One, Patañjali elaborates on the subtle details related to these two types of integration. The first type, explained in this aphorism is *samprajñata samadhi*, integration with higher wisdom. As with all things in nature, and in life, nothing develops overnight. Everything is a process, moving from one step to the next in an organic manner. For example, if you want to grow your own mango tree in your backyard, it makes sense to find out the most suitable variety of mango for your climate. Then you will need to make sure that there is enough space in the backyard to accommodate a mango tree of that variety. Then it would be useful to go to your local nursery to get advice about the best soil preparation and times for planting. Next, you can get a seed or a sapling that you would need to plant and water as necessary. However, having planted your seed does not mean that you can go in the garden the next day to pick a ripe mango. It will take time for the tree to develop and mature so that it can produce flowers and then, when some of those flowers are pollinated, they may transform into potential mangoes. Each step needs to happen in the right season and eventually, if you are lucky, after some time passes you may get some delicious mangoes right in your backyard.

Similarly, there is an organic process towards deeper levels of integration. As you saw in the previous aphorisms, the process begins by removing distractions through establishing a clear intention and by committing your actions to your intention (*abhyasa*). You complement your practice by releasing attachments (*vairagya*) so that all your systems work in harmony facilitating a steady focus. Free from distractions, you choose a focal point to contemplate (*vitarka*), then your attention moves towards the subtler essence of that object or idea (*vichara*). At this level of subtlety, the mind is delighted, illuminated by its own stillness and silence (*ananda*). Beyond that level, you feel your own sense of self, or your sense of "I," in relation to the focal point chosen. These stages are the finer aspect of an even mind (*samadhi*). Rather than a reasoning process, this is a progression into refining your pure direct experience. Since it is not a thinking process, it is beyond the mind and thus impossible to represent fully with words. And, if you have to decide if you are in one of those states, that is already an indication that you are not. It truly is an organic process; it cannot be forced.

It makes sense that the twofold strategy of commitment and detachment is presented immediately before this idea of complete integration (*samadhi*), because it is exactly that balanced practice without attachment to the results (*vairagya*) that is most useful in moving towards this deeper level of integration. Moreover, relinquishing all attachments is what makes it possible to keep moving towards deeper levels of direct experience, because it will be necessary to let go of everything you think about. Furthermore, the previous sutra indicated that directing your attention towards Truth, the everlasting ground of existence where all the changes in life take place, removes all distractions and distractedness.

Letting go of constant internal commentary enables you to remain focused and gain a deeper experience of whatever object or idea you concentrate on. Eventually, you experience directly and with increasing clarity your own individual sense of aliveness. Just like the sun is not changed by the clouds in the atmosphere, your fundamental essence (being or individual aliveness) is not changed by your activities (doings or becomings). This sutra points out a gradual refinement of your connection to the sense of aliveness within you. Remember, your sense of aliveness is *always* within you. However, your sense of individual aliveness sometimes gets obscured by the activities, labels, and opinions in your internal space of awareness. The experience of integration (*samadhi*) introduced in this aphorism is the gradual process of refining your perception to experience life as it is.

One possible way of exploring this sutra is by focusing on one of your senses from its outward expression into its internal individual experience. For instance, when you are about to take a sip of water, you can slow down the perceptive process by pausing and focusing fully, with your eyes closed, on the contact between the water and your lips. Possibly some ideas about water will enter your space of awareness. Let them flow. Then focus on the sensations as best as you can. Then feel the sensations of water on your inner mouth, teeth, gums, and tongue. Instead of loading the experience with words or concepts, stay with the sensations in your mouth until you swallow the water as slowly as possible. Then stay with the very faint sensations lingering in your mouth. Notice what is happening, including any subtle processes being triggered, like related thoughts, feelings, emotions, or memories. What is the subtlest aspect of the experience? Does the experience illuminate with awareness your sense of being? Is the subtlest aspect of water highlighting your own subtle sense of aliveness? This whole process is wordless and indescribable. You can try this approach systematically with each one of the senses, noticing where each takes you. Obviously, choosing an inspiring and meaningful focal point is more likely to be uplifting.

As you engage in this exercise, the internal distractions will offer hints uncovering beliefs and ways of being that are active and have not been released yet. Remember, that this process of internal integration (*samadhi*) happens after the inner talk has subsided. Thus, if you are still dealing with internal commentary, choose to drop the internal dialogue. Patient persistence is essential to drop internal activity, especially because your ways of being tend to be deeply entrenched. This is where the skill of returning again and again without strain, struggle, or self-judgement is helpful. On the other hand, the experience of being is at the core of who you are, you are always connected to it. In fact, you cannot unplug from it. The practice is letting go of the ways of being that tend to take over your space of awareness. One of those ways of being is the need to comment constantly on the experience of just being. What do you find when you try this exploration? How does it contribute to the quality of your presence?

1.18 Resulting from practice, a higher state of integration (*asamprajñata samadhi*), with no thoughts remaining, only subconscious impressions (*samskaras*).

This aphorism describes a complementary type of deep integration, *asamprajñata samadhi*, integration beyond higher wisdom. Some commentators indicate that this type of integration is a transitional state between each one of the four stages mentioned in the previous sutra, *vitarka*, *vichara*, *ananda*, and *asmita*; other commentators suggest that this is a higher level of integration altogether. In this type of integration (*asamprajñata samadhi*), the yogi is fully absorbed in the direct experience of pure awareness without the need of a focal object. Reaching this stage requires that all ways of being are deactivated, at least temporarily. Although the ways of being are effectively neutralized, there remain latent impressions of previous experiences. This yogic process progresses from outward orientation to the exploration of internal landscapes uncovering increasing levels of subtlety in your own being. You go from a tendency to entertain yourself with constant opinions and internal commentary to enjoying temporary gaps in your inner talk. Gradually the gaps become longer and eventually, this new pattern of inner silence starts to take hold and grow. As your ability to focus grows, distractions subside. First, your focus feels like it needs to grip firmly to avoid getting distracted, until only gentle holding is needed. As it was suggested in sutra 1.17, even that softness of focus can become subtler, so that there is no holding. Then, an experience of calmness and ease blossoms and continues into the pure experience of being an individual, I.

Continuing into further refinement, even the sense of "I" dissolves, revealing a deeper stillness and silence when only latent traces of past impressions (*samskaras*) remain. At this level of integration there isn't even a focal object or any knowledge or wisdom to attain, thus its name – integration beyond higher wisdom. On the way towards this objectless level of integration, as you remain focused you notice stray thoughts, memories, and ideas crossing your space of inner awareness. Since you have chosen to focus on a specific focal point, these potential distractors are likely emerging from your subconscious mind. In other words, you are witnessing the fuzzy boundary between conscious and subconscious mind.

Where are those thoughts coming from? In Sanskrit one of the meanings of the word *samskara* is mental impression. During a regular day you are exposed to many sensory inputs. For example, as you walk from your home to the post office, you see people and many things, like plants, trees, houses, buildings, and cars. Many of these things you may not remark on. When you return home, you may not be able to tell exactly how many people you saw, or how many blue cars were on the street as you were walking. If somebody asked you how many people were standing in line at the post office when you arrived there, you may not be able to give a specific answer, unless you made it a point to count when you got there. A *samskara* is an impression stored in your space of awareness. If, on your walk, you saw something that captured your attention, like a beautiful garden with your favorite flowers in bloom, or a traffic accident that almost happened, or a group of children playing boisterously, you would probably remember.

Usually, what seems worth remembering is something that generated an emotional response. Emotion is the glue that makes a specific experience stick some place in your inner environment. Everything you pay attention to and every experience can potentially leave an impression. Well-rehearsed patterns of thought and action tend to become unconscious, so that you operate without even having to think about what you are doing. Think about how little attention you probably pay to the specifics of brushing your teeth, so that it's your "muscle memory" controlling those actions. In the same way, you store thoughts, expectations, and memories. Some of these impressions may be completely out of your conscious awareness. Yet, every action you engage in and every experience may leave some impressions in you, some stronger than others. These impressions can influence your choices, like when you try to recreate a set of actions and circumstances to cause, or to avoid, a specific outcome, like wearing your lucky t-shirt, or avoiding going by a place that reminds you of something painful. With every action generating an impression, each person carries many past impressions buried deep within, with more impressions accumulating every day. This aphorism says that even when you experience great calmness and stillness within, there will be some lingering impressions.

Consider if there are memories that still seem to have a grip on you:

Are you really at peace with your past, or are you holding a grudge, resentment, or regret?

Can you make peace with past events?

Can you make peace with previous versions of yourself?

Are some of your ways of acting a reaction, conscious or unconscious, to past experiences?

Are some of these past impressions obstacles to your current projects?

Do some of these impressions influence how you see yourself and how you perceive the world?

As you also contemplate the type of concentration described in this aphorism, it may be useful to think of it as a shift on the center of experience from I, to simply *being with what is.*

1.19 Higher integration results from objective existence for disembodied beings (*videhas*) and for those merged in nature (*prakritilayas*).

This sutra can be one of the most obscure aphorisms in this chapter because it mentions two types of beings: the disembodied and the ones merged into the essence of nature. Before exploring those types of beings, it's helpful to think about one possible interpretation of one of the cosmological views of the world in the yoga tradition. The world can be understood as a synergistic interaction between consciousness and life. The notion of consciousness is still a matter of debate today. From a simple, common sense perspective, consciousness can be thought of as the knowing or witnessing that gives us a sense of being alive. It is consciousness that enables us to sense and perceive. Life, on the other hand, can be understood as all the experiences and phenomena that can be sensed and perceived. Life is a process of endless change (doing) that happens in the all-pervading consciousness (being), which is the substratum for all that exists. If you think of life as doing and consciousness as being, what is the relationship between the two? This is a question worth contemplating.

The previous sutra says that after reaching a high level of inner silence (*samadhi*), there are still some subtle impressions left in the yogini's mind. Sutra 1.19 talks about two states of existence at a high level of subtlety before reaching the higher level of objectless integration (*asamprajñata samadhi*). The interpretation that follows is not the result of my direct experience (*pratyaksha*), but a combination of the two other sources of correct knowledge, traditional wisdom (*agama*) and inference (*anumana*), combined with pure speculation.

The first state mentioned is disembodied beings (*videhas*). These are the gods whose bodies have dissolved, and all that is left of them is the accumulation of their subconscious impressions existing at a very high level of subtlety, yet still as part of nature. The other state, the *prakritilayas,* are beings who have identified fully with one of the primordial elements of nature, and when their bodies have come to an end, have merged into the subtle aspects of nature. Although both the disembodied and the merged in nature have reached high levels of purification, being part of nature implies that these disembodied beings will continue to exist at these subtle levels while nature continues its never-ending cycles of change and transformation.

This sutra states that, eventually both the disembodied (*videhas*) and the merged in nature (*prakritilayas*) will have to take existence as an embodied being in order to reach complete liberation. If you are reading this, it is more than likely that you are still embodied. This means that you can still try to put this sutra into practice.

A practical way of interpreting this sutra is to see disembodiment as a way to release all identification with your body and with your ways of being. Practices such as yoga nidra and meditation on very subtle focal objects may facilitate gradual release of awareness of the different layers of your body from the most external, until you experience directly the subtlest aspect of yourself, your own awareness. In the state of yoga nidra and in meditation, you can effectively release body identification. One notion that is important here is that being attached to your preferences will keep you from moving to higher levels of integration.

It may also be possible to explore the experience of disembodiment by using a floatation tank. Also known as a sensory deprivation tank, it is a tank where you can float effortlessly due to Epsom salts dissolved in body- temperature water. Isolated from visual and auditory stimuli and free from gravitational forces, your awareness can release your body, entering a meditative state. Another way of practicing is to allow your sense of self to dissolve by contemplating a natural phenomenon. Some useful phenomena include a sunset, the endless flow of ocean waves, clouds floating effortlessly in the sky or a meteor shower. For instance, concentrate fully on the cosmos in its vastness. Gradually expand your focal point to invite the whole Universe to expand completely in your inner environment. Let go of your awareness of your own physical boundaries and allow your sense of self and associated processes to disappear. Keep releasing until eventually there is not even the sense of "I." Remain open so that all that you experience is your pure awareness. You may also choose to focus your attention on one of the elements, earth, water, fire, air or space, perhaps following the progression from coarse to subtle presented in sutra 1.17, going from external to internal and gradually to the subtlest aspect of the experience.

Consider:

What happens when you try these techniques?
Can these practices offer you a different perspective and, perhaps, even a way to re-evaluate some of your attitudes and preferences?
Can some of the inner stillness you experience be carried into your activities in the world?
Even if the experience does not produce a deeper sense of inner peace or integration, can it assist you in highlighting some of your current ways of being that are preventing a deeper experience of your awareness?

1.20 Others, rooted on trust and confidence (*shraddha*), that ignites vitality (*virya*); and on remembrance (*smrti*), that steadies their focus; grow into evenness of mind (*samadhi*) that leads to insight and wisdom (*prajña*).

This aphorism presents the alternative pathway toward higher integration, the path for the rest of us. Again, this is a *gradual* path. It begins with trust and confidence (*shraddha*). Although the word *shraddha* is often translated as faith, the connotation of blind belief may be misleading, particularly if it is interpreted as renouncing one's common sense or capacity for rational thinking. Faith can also be misinterpreted as a call for letting others make one's decision and choices. However, this sutra calls practitioners to root their practice in trust and confidence that grow out of truth, correct knowledge arising from direct experience, logical inference, and trustworthy testimony (1.7). True knowledge is a source of energy that ignites vitality, passion and enthusiasm (*virya*). This energy provides sustenance to stay on the path of personal discovery. What you know through your direct experience is easy to remember. Thus, true knowledge acts as a reminder (*smrti*) to remain steady on the journey and not to lose sight of the goal, embodying full awareness.

Engaging on your path with trust, vitality, and memory of your intention creates the ripe conditions for your mind to be calm, steady, and growing in inner silence (*samadhi*). As a result, being less distracted by the coming and going of temporary phenomena, you are better able to notice insight and wisdom all around you (*prajña*). This insight or intuition manifests as the silent whisper of your heart, or inner *guru*, guiding your intentions and actions. Thus, you can tune into pure common sense offered by all of life and recognize that your teachers are all around you – and that what used to feel like coincidences are actually synchronicities showing you the deep interconnectedness between all that is.

Check-in:

How are you cultivating your trust and confidence?
Are you energized by your life and choices?
How are you keeping your intention clear in your mind and actions?
What helps you remember your deeply felt intention?
Are you noticing a gradual decrease of distractions drawing you away from your objectives?
Is there slightly more evenness of mind?
Are you willing to trust the subtle guidance you receive in your daily interactions?

COMMITMENT AND INTENSITY

1.21 It is near for those who apply themselves with intensity.

1.22 There are three degrees of intensity within each level: mild, moderate and excessive.

After sutra 1.20 indicates a path towards deep serenity, the following two sutras further explain that the level of commitment in following the path will influence the results. Earlier in this chapter, in aphorisms 1.2 and 1.12, self-regulation appeared as a major theme in the Yoga Sutra. Self-regulation appears again here: evenness of mind and wisdom are near for the practitioners who apply themselves with intensity. The intensity itself can be mild, moderate, or excessive. *Each person, at each moment, is in charge of finding the right level of intensity balancing firm and unwavering commitment with a heartfelt and compassionate attitude.* Too much commitment may make you rigid or dogmatic, whereas too much detachment may lead you to avoid applying yourself to the best of your ability. Here is where being aware of your tendencies is invaluable because it enables you to fine-tune your level of intensity, so that it is an appropriate and sustainable way to achieve the perfect balance between doing and being.

Your actions provide an excellent mirror to notice the quality of your attention and the level of intensity that you bring into your daily activities. Yoga practice is often conducted in a space where sources of distractions are reduced, so that you can observe how you engage with your practice. Noticing your attitude and your drive gives you insight into your ways of being. In fact, all yoga techniques, whether they are directed to your body, breathing, mind, or emotions, can be quite effective in revealing your tendencies and ways of being. For instance, people who tend to overreach in their professional and personal lives are likely to also overreach in their *asana*, *pranayama* and meditation practices. You can use your practice as a way to measure your level of commitment and the right amount of intensity, so that your practice is sustainable and enjoyable. If the practice is not enjoyable, it becomes an exercise in self-torture, and that is very difficult to sustain over a long period of time. In fact, being consistent is a challenge for most of us.

Consistent practice is a test to your commitment. Sutra 1.21 highlights that each practitioner is in charge of the level of commitment to the goal of yoga. You choose. This means that it is totally up to you to decide how you apply to your practice. This is excellent news. At the same time, if you are the one who makes the choices, that means that you cannot blame anybody else for your lack of commitment. Is it possible that your level of commitment is proportional to the sense of urgency to be present in your own life? This is where it is critical that you clarify what is important enough for you to invest your time and energy on (Putting it into practice: Clarify - What is important to me? on page 113). Additionally, when you practice with awareness, instead of mechanically, some of your patterns and pains will become more evident. For example, the more you tune into the rhythms of your body, the discomforts and soreness that you have learned to ignore may become more apparent. This is a testament that your practice is working because you are shining the light of awareness into areas you have not addressed. Of course, you can choose to ignore those signs, or to sedate your senses not to feel discomfort. Or you can, instead, address the cause of your soreness. Each choice requires a different degree of commitment.

There are some obstacles that emerge for many of us. For instance, as we set our intention, we may immediately hear the inner critic downplaying the importance of that intention. How can you learn to trust yourself and your choices so that you can avoid self-sabotage? To what extent is there a sense of urgency in you to practice because your practice enables you to participate fully in each irreplaceable moment of your life?

Also, yoga offers a broad spectrum of practices to address challenges at the physical, mental, emotional, and interpersonal levels. Is your practice balanced and balancing?
If your practice leaves you exhausted, how is your practice enriching

your life?

Can your yoga practice offer you a daily opportunity to experience what enough is for you each day?

What are you committed to?

What is your level of commitment to yourself?

To living in awareness?

To growing out of the patterns that are no longer useful?

To showing up to every moment of your life?

What are the signs of your commitment?

AN ALTERNATIVE APPROACH, HUMILITY

1.23 Or, by wholeheartedly relinquishing the illusion of control (*ishvara pranidhana*).

After listing the twofold method of practice (*abhyasa*) and indifference (*vairagya*) and after showing the skills required to go on that path (including trust, vitality, remembrance, evenness of mind, and wisdom in 1.20; and the varying levels of intensity of application in sutras 1.21 and 1.22), aphorism 1.23 presents an alternative approach. The original Sanskrit, *ishvara pranidhana*, is often translated as "surrender to God." Some meanings of *ishvara* include queen, prince, god, king, lord, ruler, god of love, Supreme Being, supreme soul, and master. It's important to know that in the Yoga Sutra, Patañjali does not specify or suggest any particular religious tradition. From the perspective of seeing yoga as being with what is, one way of interpreting this aphorism, without interference from our preconceived notions or history with words like God, is to translate *ishvara* as Supreme Being.

Supreme Being is understood as *being* in its highest form, pure being, and also as the totality of Being. This "Beingness" is the quality shared in equal measure by all that is, a quality that is unbounded, pervasive, unchanging, and omnipresent. Being is, at the same time, particular and universal, local and transcendent. In other words, Being is happening everywhere, both as each individual instance of anything that is manifest, as well as the totality of all of existence. Regardless of how hard you may try, being cannot be grasped, manufactured, or even described fully with words. In fact, all the arts, literature, and sciences have been trying for millennia to describe some aspect of life, or being, in different ways; yet not even the complete aggregation of the works from these fields can encompass the complete picture of existence.

Pranidhana, the second word in this sutra, includes in its meanings: attention, vehement desire, profound religious meditation, great effort, prayer, endeavor, abstract contemplation of, assiduousness, vow, access, and entrance. The final particle in the sutra, *dva*, means "or," indicating that *ishvara pranidhana* is an alternative to the previous approach to finding deep inner peace and stillness (1.20). This sutra invites you to recognize that you did not create yourself or the Universe and, despite whatever you may believe, *you are not in control of the world.* Indeed, paying close attention to your mind, emotions, and body will soon remind you that you hardly have control over your own mind, emotions and body.

One of the challenges most practitioners face is the pressing urgency of their internal activities and agendas. Living in your own drama creates a myopic perspective that tends to blow every thought and idea out of proportion. This sutra provides the perspective of distance from our own stories. One simple practice you can explore is to contemplate yourself and your immediate environment. Gradually you invite your attention to zoom out of your immediate internal environment by thinking about expanding concentric circles rippling out from wherever you are. You think about your house, then your block, your neighborhood, your city, county, state, country, continent, planet, solar system, the Milky Way galaxy, the Local Group of galaxies, the Virgo Supercluster, the Laniakea Supercluster and beyond, all the way to the fringes of the known Universe. As you embody the paradox of containing the infinite expanse of the Universe in your individual mind, it may be easier for you to recognize how little control you have and how small our species and planet are. Entertaining this longer and wider perspective facilitates a gentle humility that can put your individual worries and anxieties into their proper perspective. More importantly, it can keep in check the self-importance that fills your inner space and very often pulls your awareness away from this moment. Moreover, seeing yourself from this larger perspective can be instrumental in letting go of the tension generated when you try to carry the world on your shoulders.

Gaining a more accurate understanding of you and your sphere of influence can be an effective way of redirecting your energy to act effectively in the world according to your capacity, level of skill, ability, and scope. Of course, for people who find solace in their own meaningful understanding of God, it may be easier to surrender themselves and their lives with complete devotion to God. Others, who may see god as true love, can choose to open their hearts and minds to love everything, without conditions. When you offer your love, noticing your conditions and objections provides you with insight into yourself and your worldview. You can choose to consider this information as an appropriate doorway, offering you a clear path to unravelling some of those objections and conditions.

There are as many ways of understanding this aphorism as there are people in the world. One more idea that might assist you is seeing this sutra as attuning to pure awareness. You may start by dropping your most external characteristics: your weight, height, eye color. Then release your beliefs, preferences, and dislikes. Then let go of your name and who you think you are.

What happens if you attune to pure being and drop your conditions on this moment?

If you anchor your awareness on the all-encompassing pervasiveness of being, what happens?

If you expand your perspective to acknowledge the magnificent miracle of life, can this assist you in cherishing yourself and your life and to release self-importance?

Whatever your choice, this avenue of exploration extends an invitation to living in harmony with life, both within and without. In your own understanding, is there anything that you can rest your trust on completely? Is there anything that offers you an unconditional sense of support, encouragement, and hope?

1.24 Supreme Being (*ishvara*) is a special kind of being untouched by afflictions (*kleshas*), actions (*karma*), consequences (*vipaka*) or their impressions.

After offering an alternative path to integration (cultivating our humility by surrendering our illusion of control and acknowledging that there may be a Universal Truth), Patañjali presents in this, and the following sutras, the characteristics of Supreme Being (*ishvara*), a technique to connect to *ishvara*, and the effects of using that technique. Sutra 1.24 says that Supreme Being is different from other beings. Supreme Being is not affected by pain and hardship, by actions, their effects, or any of their remaining impressions. Exploring these ideas is a fertile ground to disentangle some of your beliefs and personal baggage associated with the ideas of life, purpose, and God. A useful starting point is contemplating which word or words would be best for you to relate to the idea of *ishvara*. In this interpretation *ishvara* is rendered as Supreme Being. Other potential words could be Truth, Love, God, Life, Pure Awareness, Pure Being, Source, or Spirit. Is there one word that feels more meaningful to you? Explore your responses and reactions to this question. Then take whichever word resonates with you and contemplate how that word/concept relates to the notions of affliction, action, consequences, and impressions.

What do you discover?

Can you think of something that is not influenced by obstacles, actions, or their effects?

Is there anything that can be free of regrets and expectations?

Additionally, you can try to engage in a simple experiment over the next five days. On the first day, set your intention to notice if you are experiencing any afflictions in the form of grief, trouble, hardship,

distress, pain, or anger. What do you notice?
Do you know anything that is not affected by any afflictions?

On the second day, focus on your actions and notice if you are affected in any way by your actions.
To what extent do your intentions and actions manifest in your body, mind, breath, and emotions?
How do you act?
Are your actions influenced by your circumstances and environment?
What are your mood and attitude as you act?
Are your actions skillful?

On the third day pay attention to effects and consequences.
Can you trace the causes of the experiences that you are having?
To what extent are your experiences influencing your internal activities and mood?
Is your mood influencing your experiences?
When you sensitize yourself to your reactions, are your reactions automatic or impulsive?
Are you responding in conscious, wholehearted, and deliberate ways?

On the fourth day you can focus your awareness on the impressions left by your irritations, actions, and reactions.
What do you notice?
Does it ever happen to you that you feel annoyed or frustrated by no apparent reason?
Can your mood be a remnant of something beyond your conscious awareness?

On the fifth day of your experiment you can reflect on your previous days. You can zoom out of your immediate level of experience to reflect on the potential connections between your afflictions, actions, reactions, and impressions. Quite likely you will notice that some of your experiences vary according to your circumstances.

Do you notice any trends?

Can this process help you uncover some of the irritants that tend to generate more pain, reactivity and regret or resentment?

Are some of these irritants the buttons that other people activate in you, quite often unintentionally?

Are there ways for you to deactivate these sources of grief and anguish?

How are the afflictions, actions, reactions, and impressions you notice related to your ways of being?

After your experiment, return to the idea of *ishvara.*

Are you unaffected by afflictions (*kleshas*), actions (*karma*), consequences (*vipaka*) or their impressions?

Can you be open to the possibility that there may be something, some aspect of existence, that remains free of influence from these factors?

1.25 In Supreme Being the seed of omniscience is unsurpassed.

Omniscience is a fascinating word. Two of its meanings include infinite awareness and Universal knowledge. This sutra invites the question, is all-encompassing, pervasive awareness possible? From the ground of your own being you can start exploring the meaning of this word by contemplating *How do I know what I know?* Of course, this implies that you are already clear on the distinction between what you know and what you *think* you know. Remember that mere access to information is different from knowledge. If you ever get subtle helpful hints that provide insight or clarity, where do these hints come from? How do you actually perceive them? How do you distinguish between an idea and true insight? Do they have different mental, physical and emotional signatures? How does your conscience express itself to draw your attention to something specific?

When you are deeply relaxed, when you feel love, joy or gratitude, what dimensions do these embodied experiences stem from? Might it be possible that there is an ever-present all-encompassing field where all aspects of life, in all times and places, exist as potential or as manifestation? Is there something underlying all your thoughts, emotions, feelings, and memories? Rather than using these questions as way to create internal arguments, use them as points of entry into contemplation, to live with each question and notice what unfolds. One approach is to find a comfortable and relaxed position and then to formulate the question with the true intention of wanting to know the answer directly, through your personal embodied experience. Stay with the question for a while, allowing the answers to brew in your calmness and silence. Then, when you are ready to finish this exercise, silently repeat the question to yourself as an invitation to be with the question as you participate in your life. Notice if there are subtle and not so subtle answers – emerging as synchronicities – as your day progresses.

As you create a ground of openness within you through these questions, remember that life is flowing through you right where you are, all the time. Just as you are not compartmentalized into discrete segments, you are also not isolated from life. In fact, just like every single living being, you are an individual manifestation of life, interrelated, interconnected to all that is, all that ever was, all that ever will be. Then, does it seem possible that infinite awareness and Universal knowledge are possible?

1.26 Not conditioned by time, Supreme Being is the unequaled teacher of all times.

This sutra continues clarifying the nature of Supreme Being. So far, we know that Supreme Being is truly impartial as it is not affected by afflictions, actions, reactions, or impressions (1.24). We also know that Supreme Being is infinitely aware and all knowing (1.25). This sutra adds that Supreme Being is timeless and that it is the unsurpassed teacher of all time. At any moment, when you are fully present, especially when you are completely absorbed in something that captures your undivided attention, it seems that time stops. For instance, when you are engaged in a conversation on a topic that you are truly curious about, you remain focused without distractions. As the conversation ends, it is often difficult to say how much time elapsed. It is as if your awareness enables you to step out of the constraints of time. This is often described as entering the timeless present moment. At that moment, are your afflictions, actions, responses, and impressions automatically on hold? Does this relate to what sutra 1.3 talks about, that when you quiet down your ways of being you embody your true nature? Does your yoga practice transport you into the eternal present moment? Have you found ways to enter the timelessness dimension of life? From a different angle, what makes you feel bound by time? If you feel that you do not have time to do all that you need and want to do, it will be helpful to examine your priorities to notice what you are making important enough to deserve your time and attention. As you reflect on your own relationship to time, consider if there may be anything that can be free of the conditioning of time.

The second section of this sutra states that Supreme Being is the unsurpassed teacher of all times. Great teachers inspire you to explore the boundaries of your current understanding. As you reach the zone of bearable discomfort indicating that your current ideas are no longer useful, the teacher supports and guides you. Great teachers do not get caught in their own personal drama because that prevents them from guiding their students impartially and with caring awareness. In the process of growing as a human being, each person will find obstacles and challenges. These challenges are feedback, suggesting alternative options to move beyond where you currently are. As you engage in the deep self-inquiry that is yoga, it is instrumental to understand your own learning process; a teacher can create the situation that facilitates your growth, but it is completely up to you to go through the process of expanding the current boundaries of your understanding. How motivated are you to continue learning? Even if your teacher is outstanding, it is still you who does the learning. If you refuse to learn, nobody can make you. Can you harness the skills suggested in sutra 1.20 (trust, vitality, remembrance, evenness of mind, and wisdom)? In addition, notice how the obstacles you face are the perfect result of what has happened before. These obstacles are lessons elegantly calibrated to where you are, what you need and what you can handle. Most often your likes and dislikes become an obstacle to differentiating between what you want/like and what you need. This is the cause for a lot of drama and resistance.

Are you tuned into your own learning process?

Do you know how you learn best?

If you keep running against the same obstacles again and again, are you making conscious choices or are your likes and dislikes choosing for you?

Can the obstacles you face help you become aware of what you know and of what you know you don't know?

Since life continually adjusts the feedback to be most appropriate for you, is it possible that life is indeed the greatest teacher?

Are you making yourself available to life by accepting the lessons that it offers you?

1.27 OM is the sound that designates Supreme Being.

1.28 Chanting OM and contemplating its meaning.

After introducing the path of humility in sutra 1.23 through surrendering the illusion of control and honoring Supreme Being, the subsequent aphorisms explained the characteristics of Supreme Being. These two sutras, 1.27 and 1.28, offer a way to relate to and access Supreme Being. If Supreme Being cannot be defined in a few words, it makes sense to use a special symbol to point to all-encompassing and pervasive Being. OM is one way of transliterating the Devanagari symbol ॐ. (Devanagari is the alphabet used to represent the Sanskrit language). ॐ is also transliterated as AUM. The word used in the sutra for this mystic syllable is *pranava*, which relates the sound OM to the life force, *prana*. This symbol can be interpreted as a map to the whole journey to integration.

The *Upanishads* are a collection of philosophical texts that appeared over the span of many centuries. One of the shortest *Upanishads*, the *Mandukya Upanishad*, very concisely defines AUM as everything that is, including all aspects of time, past, present, and future. It also indicates that each one of the letters represents one of the four states of consciousness: awake, dreaming, dreamless deep sleep and a fourth state. (Although the transliteration includes only three letters, and the original symbol results from combining the equivalents of A, U and M, it is understood that there is a resonating echo implicit in the sound.) This fourth state is not even named, it is simply called "the fourth" to hint at the impossibility of fully encapsulating the all-encompassing transcendence of pure integrated consciousness.

Sutra 1.28 introduces a specific practice to embodying the path of *ishvara pranidhana*, the wholehearted cultivation of humility, by repeating the syllable OM. The practice consists of two aspects, *japa* and contemplation. *Japa*, is the practice of whispering or silently repeating a mantra like OM. As this aphorism explains, the basic idea is to use a sound, syllable, or phrase that is meaningful to you. This sutra also reminds you that it is not a mechanical repetition. The repetition is a reminder of your interest, motivation, and awareness, in the same way that the first word of the Yoga Sutra, *atha*, acted as an invitation to presence. Like other mantras, chanting OM is an instrument of thought, so the repetition is accompanied by a reflection and deep contemplation on the meaning of the word being chanted.

There are many ways of chanting ॐ. Consider these two simple approaches. The first one is to chant OM starting with a soft sound, gradually making the sound louder and, after a while making the sound soft again until it becomes a gentle whisper. Then continue chanting silently and explore with curiosity if it is possible to make the internal silent chant subtler each time until it barely seems that you are chanting. Traditionally people use a *mala*, a garland of threaded beads, to keep count of their chants. Since 108 is an auspicious number in the yoga tradition, you may try chanting for 108 rounds. If you want to refine your chant, you can try to cushion the sound in between breath. That is, you first let a little bit of breath flow out without sound, then the sound OM, and toward the end, you let the sound fade out and finish with a little bit of soundless exhalation. Feel the sensations before, during and after each chant. As you chant, open yourself up to the mind-transcending meaning of Supreme Being. And as with any aspect of yoga, there is no strain, no struggle, and no self-judgment. You may also consider finishing each chant focused on feeling the lasting "m" vibration inviting you to savor the experience, as if tasting something truly delicious, producing a gentle inner smile.

The second approach is to chant the sound as A-U-M. Notice how the A sound happens toward the back of your mouth, the U sound toward the middle of the mouth and the M sound is generated with your lips closed. In other words, the AUM sound encompasses the whole range of your mouth. You may also add an extra layer to your chant by imagining the A sound originates at the center of the pelvic floor, and that the vibration flows up along the center of your body. Then you imagine the vibration flowing toward your heart center, while transitioning smoothly from the A sound into the U sound. Continue imagining the vibration flowing up along the central axis of your body. As the vibration travels toward the center of your brain, the sound transitions to M. Of course, you can also explore changing the volume, from low to high, to low again, and finally to silent. It is important to also contemplate the meaning of Supreme Being and your direct experience of it.

What happens when you practice *japa* on ॐ as you reflect on its meaning?
Do you feel any difference between chanting OM and chanting AUM?
What happens when you chant with full attention, open mind, and open heart and with the intention to listen to whatever happens without expectations?
How do you feel?

1.29 Awareness turns inward, and all disturbances are removed.

As a reminder of the practical nature of this endeavor, in this sutra Patañjali indicates the effects of the practice introduced in the previous sutras. This is the completion of the section on the alternative path that started in sutra 1.23, relinquishing the illusion of control. Now you know this path of humility and how to practice it, and this sutra helps you verify that the practice is working. Cultivating humility is a process leading you from outer focus toward inward attention. It often happens that an attitude of seeing the world as a place of competition and hostility leads a person to react with increased internal agitation. Recognizing one's limitations can be conducive to seeing the need to connect to others and to create harmony with the world around us. Chanting OM is an invitation to turn inward and to using your own voice as a source of vibration for dissolving the misperceptions that cloud your understanding. As a result, you recognize your underlying nature, the radiance of your heart filled with kindness, compassion, and unconditional love; and the brightness of your mind able to perceive clearly whatever is happening. Then, all disturbances are removed because you recognize and honor that every moment is the prefect result of whatever caused it. Consequently, your natural calm and clarity enable you to perceive acutely and with increasing subtlety the situations that you face, as well as the most appropriate responses that will contribute to the harmonious flow of life. Please remember, this sutra is not asking you to withdraw from intelligent action or to become complacent. Notice how this aphorism echoes the message in sutras 1.3 and 1.4, *As a result, embodied presence* and *Instead of identifying with ways of being*, respectively.

It is useful to remember that yoga practice is a gradual journey so the progress may, at some points, seem slow.

If you recognize that you are not separate from life, and that, in fact, you are life embodied and that you are deeply embedded in the all-encompassing wholeness of the Universe, does your perspective change?

Do the temporary comings and goings of your ways of being decrease?

Are the distractions decreased?

Does anything change in your internal environment?

Can it be true that chanting OM helps to open your receptivity to insight and intuition?

Does it seem that you can listen better to the silent whisper of your heart?

Does it feel like you can trust a little bit more those unspoken gentle nudges suggesting movement or action in a direction that feels right, even when your rational mind hesitates?

Does chanting influence your worries and ruminations?

Also, as it was indicated in sutras 1.21 and 1.22, notice to what extent the results of your practice are influenced by your commitment and intensity.

Distractions, Their Symptoms and Removal

1.30 The distractions (*vikshepa*) and obstacles (*antaraya*) on the path to deeper inner stillness and inner silence are disease (*vyadhi*), dullness (*styana*), doubt (*samshaya*), carelessness (*pramada*), laziness (*alasya*), indulgence (*avirati*), confused perception (*bhranti darshana*), inability to be grounded (*alabdha bhumikatva*), inconsistency (*anavasthitatvani*).

The previous sutra presented the results of the *japa* practice using OM: awareness grows, and the obstacles are removed. This sutra now offers a comprehensive list of the obstacles mentioned. The sutras that follow will explain the symptoms of these disturbances and distractions as well as a strategy and a variety of methods to deactivate those disturbances. It is a fact that most, if not all, practitioners will find multiple distractions and obstacles pulling them away from a natural state of calm, integration, and inner harmony. Those distractions take many shapes and forms and may affect you at different levels. Almost certainly, all of us have experienced some or all these distractions and know that when we are not feeling well and have some illness (*vyadhi*), it is difficult to pay attention to anything else other than the pain or discomfort we are experiencing. In cases where there is chronic pain, this also generates feelings of helplessness and hopelessness. Similarly, stiffness, apathy, and rigidity (*styana*) disconnect us from feeling alive and vibrant. Hesitation, doubt, and uncertainty (*samshaya*) often undermine our intention and our commitment to our life. Negligence and carelessness (*pramada*) betray our disconnection from presence. Being unmotivated, idle and without energy (*alasya*) precludes us from participating in each moment with focus and intention. Overindulgence and chasing after our senses without moderation (*avirati*) will also keep distracting us from our intention. Confusion, wavering, and vacillating perspective (*bhranti darshana*) lead us astray from our goals. Feeling unsettled and without support (*alabdha bhumikatva*) makes it impossible to find traction on our path. When we feel like we are not connected to something that lasts (*anavasthitatvani*) it is challenging to find a meaningful objective to move towards, causing us to feel like we are just floundering in an ocean of irrelevant busyness. As a result, intermittent and inconsistent effort keeps us fluttering, inhibiting our progress. These distractions tend to band together. When one is active, it usually attracts other disturbances.

As you consider the following questions, remember that these are instruments for inquiry, not for finding fault and self-judgment.

What are the distractions that keep you from committing wholeheartedly to your life?

Can you see any patterns that result in you feeling unwell?

Where do you feel rigid or stuck in mind, body, breath, emotions, and life?

What causes you to doubt your goals and yourself?

What leads you to be careless?

What are the effects of your carelessness?

What circumstances or situations are conducive to your not giving your energy to what is important to you?

When and how do you tend to overindulge?

How do you know that your perspective is clear and accurate?
Are you doing what you think you are doing? How are you ensuring that you are moving toward greater balance and integration?
Are you physically, mentally, and emotionally stable?

One way of putting this sutra into practice is to make each question the guiding principle for your day or your week. In other words, you use each question as a filter to interpret what happens during your week or day.
What do you discover when you do this?
Does looking at your life through these filters suggest adjustments to your intention and actions?

1.31 The symptoms of the distractions include: distress (*duhkha*), despair, suffering, trembling, and abruptness in breathing.

This sutra explains that the symptoms of an obstacle or distraction manifest at the mental, emotional, and physical levels. They include pain, distress, feeling disheartened and hopeless, unsteadiness, shakiness, and uneven breathing. Feeling these symptoms is an indication that there is something that requires your attention. Rather than seeing the symptoms as shortcomings, it is more useful to recognize these symptoms as teachers offering you a pathway to address something that is creating disharmony. These distractions and obstacles test your resolve, and their symptoms offer you clear feedback that you can use to inform your actions. Remember, you are always in charge of your life experiment. From one moment to the next, you are constantly choosing what to do with the feedback you are receiving. Some of those choices are conscious, while others are unconscious. Whatever your choice, every action is part of a continuous cycle. If something is coming your way, even when you choose to ignore it or avoid it, it will find you and, quite possibly, the symptoms and feedback will become even louder to prompt you to act intelligently.

Remember, yoga is a practice of removing whatever obstacles keep you from being with what is unconditionally. Patient persistence in your practice helps you uncover inefficiencies restricting your optimal function at the physical, mental, and emotional levels. In addition to reviewing each one of the nine obstacles, as you did in the previous aphorism, you may find ways to decrease or remove these obstacles and distractions by engaging with the following questions:

Is there physical, mental or emotional dis-ease?

Is your pain increasing or decreasing?

Does one distraction generate further disturbances and discomfort?

How is your outlook: hopeful or hopeless?

Are you complaining more?

Are your movements graceful and smooth, or shaky and abrupt?

Is your breath steady and continuous, or labored?

Are you content?

As you explore your internal environment, remember that whatever is happening is valid, because you are feeling it. You can pause to bring your awareness to what is happening, then feel clearly what is happening without trying to make it into a drama or story so that you can respond consciously (Method for Presence: Self-Awareness, Self-inquiry, Self-care in page99).

This is one way of making intelligent decisions so that you can change direction when it is needed. Then you can feel the effects of your actions to verify if the change had the results you desired. Even when your actions decrease your current level of anxiety, pain, or agitation, you'll probably notice, sooner or later, that you keep reverting to the way of being you have grown accustomed to. **Recall that this is a sign that your practice is working, because you are becoming better at noticing how you feel and because you can perceive with greater clarity the connections between stimuli, actions, and reactions.** This is where no strain, no struggle, and no self-judgment can help you move forward without agitation. In the next aphorisms, you will find specific ways to address the obstacles and distractions listed in the previous sutra and the symptoms outlined in this sutra.

1.32 Practicing single pointed focus eliminates the distractions and disturbances.

This sutra offers a simple yet powerful idea for counteracting the distractions and disturbances listed in sutra 1.30, as well their symptoms (1.31): one-pointedness. But what is one-pointedness? Has it ever happened that you have gotten so engrossed in a book or a movie that you completely forgot about the world outside, when you didn't even notice outside noises, or the passing of time? One-pointedness is the ability to focus our attention. When you find something you are truly curious about, your attention can focus with great precision and unwavering energy. Some teachers say that one of these focal points in our present day is money, and that many people around the world invest most of their attentional and material resources trying to make money.

This can be a good point for inquiry.
What do you invest your energy, time and resources in?
What in your life invites a deep level of dedication?

Another way of thinking about the meaning of this sutra is that distractions result from the suspicion that other times and places are more important than the place you are in right now. The notion that other times and places are more important is, first of all, completely unrealistic because you can participate fully only in the moment that you are in. Second, the other times and places you think you could be in, are the product of your imagination (*vikalpa*), speculations based on your memories (*smrti*) from the past. Third, when you dismiss this moment, you discount the elegant synchronicity of thousands of events orchestrating this moment to be exactly as it is. Indeed, you may be ignoring that whatever it is that you notice, maybe something that is tailored to you and your situation. If you find yourself constantly distracted, you can direct your single-pointed focus to examine your inability or unwillingness to accept this moment as it is, in order to reveal the distraction that keeps pulling you away. Knowing the distraction, you can allow it to keep disrupting your commitment, or you can inquire into it, using these simple questions:
Is there anything wrong right here and now?
Is it within my power to change what is wrong?
If you can change it, just do it right there and then. If something is beyond your immediate control, then it is wise to surrender your illusion of control.

As it was mentioned in sutra 1.12, the journey towards dynamic balance requires the balanced approach of doing (*abhyasa*) and being (*vairagya*). At this point in the chapter, after listing obstacles, distractions, and their symptoms, Patañjali echoes this two-pronged strategy in this sutra and the next. This aphorism focuses on practice (*abhyasa*) or doing, and the next one can be seeing as an interpretation of freedom from attachment (*vairagya*). Notice that the characteristics of single-pointed focus include a continuous, sincere, and firmly rooted intention, which is the definition of practice (*abhyasa*). Single- pointed focus can also be interpreted as one way of engaging your mind. It is an invitation to commit with deliberate and unwavering intention. To engage consciously and deliberately you can ask yourself *What is important enough to deserve my attention, time, and energy?* To keep a single-pointed focus, it helps to concentrate on something that does not fade. So, a relevant question is:

What is permanent enough not to fade under sustained attention?

Or, what is really lasting?

1.33 Cultivating the habits of friendliness (*maitri*), compassion (*karuna*), inspiration (*mudita*) and equanimity (*upeksha*) purifies mind, body, and heart.

This sutra complements the previous one, harmonizing the effort and commitment required to maintain a single-pointed focus with the habits that purify mind, body, and heart. Since the firmness of unwavering single-pointed focus may lead some practitioners towards rigidity, this aphorism also provides ways to moderate your attitude to yourself and to the world around you by helping you notice your biases to remove judgment. If the previous sutra tried to engage your mind, this aphorism pertains to your emotions and your heart.

Biases and opinions act as filters that influence your internal environment and behavior. Your personal history and upbringing also contribute filters, while reinforcing other attitudes and inclinations. Whatever is happening around you also has an effect on your ways of being and attitudes. When you go anywhere, notice if an internal voice provides opinions and makes remarks about whatever you see, offering labels and judgments about anything that crosses your path. This sutra offers tools to clarify your internal environment, and to promote inner peace through balanced interactions with the world around you. In other words, this aphorism gives you options to turn your reactivity into responsibility, so that you can flow in harmony with life. Like with any other practice, the tools will probably expose areas where there is lack of clarity, or where there might be high reactivity. Without struggle or strain and with no self-judgment, use the tools with consistent single-pointed focus. Start by recognizing that your point of view is individual, presenting a single perspective; and that each person has her own individual perspective as well. When you reflect on your own life, you can see that your ideas, ways of thinking and behavior have changed over time, and that something you liked before may not be so important or interesting now. You have been fine-tuning your life experiment – in fact, you do it all the time – to adjust to your new levels of understanding and awareness. Sometimes you may even find that an idea that you now find powerful and exciting, escaped you completely before, because it was not on your radar or because you were not ready yet to assimilate it or apply it. Regardless of how much you adjust your ideas, chances are, that you keep adjusting them because you think and feel that this new configuration is the best you can do. *Doing what you know at the time to be the best is the guiding principle for all those changes.* That general rule is the same for each person.

As you grow and learn, you discover better ways of doing what you are doing – adjusting and transcending your previous and incomplete understanding. *This is a sign that you are evolving.* It is the same for each person. All of us are trying to find the best way of doing what we are doing to live a fulfilling life. Many times you find that what you thought was the best path of action actually wasn't, because of some restriction or limitation in your ways of seeing or thinking precluding you from seeing with clarity. At those points. rather than focusing on how wrong or misguided your actions were, you can choose to focus on a different and more beneficial way of being or doing. This sutra guides you through that process so that you can have a moderate attitude toward yourself and others. This attitude is essential to avoid the internal and external toxicity that is generated by negative criticism, bitterness, and anger directed to yourself or to others.

Consider these questions to guide your exploration:

When other people are happy (*sukha*), can you identify with them and be happy for them (*maitri*), their successes and circumstances?

When someone is suffering (*duhkha*), can you honestly wish for them to be free from pain and suffering (*karuna*)?

Can you delight in and be inspired (*mudita*) by somebody else's virtues and merits (*punya*)?

As you notice actions, words or behavior that are unkind (*apunya*), can you pause and try to remove your biases by considering the situation with equanimity (*upeksha*) from different perspectives and afford that person the benefit of the doubt?

As you see somebody doing something you disapprove of, can you remember that you are not perfect, that you have made mistakes before, and that probably you will make mistakes in the future?

What are the conditions that you place on somebody else in order to accept them, forgive them, befriend them, assist them and love them?

You can also reflect on this sentence: "Even though I may not understand their actions, every person around the world is trying to find peace, joy and love."

After reading these suggestions for exploration, you may get the feeling that you are supposed to let anybody do anything, even things you know to be unfair or harmful. However, consider what happens when somebody inadvertently steps on your toes. You probably find a way to remove your foot from under his foot, and you let the person know that they were doing something that was causing you discomfort or pain. In other words, you do what you need to do in order not to be harmed or in pain. How you choose to do that can be a conscious and life-affirming choice, or an unconscious and life-denying choice: **it is completely up to you.**

It may seem evident that cultivating these habits is working directly with your emotions. But you may ask, how does cultivating these habits purify your body and mind? You can test this out very easily. Do a simple series of movements that are familiar to you. Then, bring into your heart a memory of something that brings up mild feelings of disappointment, sadness, bitterness, or regret. Notice the effects of these feelings within you. Keep those feelings and repeat the same series of familiar movements. Then pause the movements, close your eyes, and feel. Did the movements feel different from the first time? Now, bring into your heart a memory of something or somebody that makes you feel uplifted, hopeful, or cheerful. Notice how your internal environment changes. Try once again the same series of familiar movements. Pause, relax, and close your eyes. Can your feelings affect what you are thinking, and how you move?

1.34 By exhalations and breath retentions.

After suggesting focused attention (1.32) and moderation (1.33), Patañjali offers a list of possible focal points. The first one is attending to exhalations and breath retentions. Remember that tuning into your breath is a direct portal into presence, a sure way to be in the present moment. This sutra suggests the path of mastering vital energy (*pranayama*), inviting your attention inwards and establishing an intimate connection to your breathing processes. It is important to underscore that *pranayama* is the practice of making the breath smooth, steady, and effortless. Whenever you are exploring your breath make sure that you NEVER FORCE your breath. This is very important. Abrupt breathing, headaches, gasping or getting agitated or feeling nauseous, lightheaded or dizzy are signs that you are forcing your breath. Keeping this in mind, in a comfortable position, notice what happens to your mind and internal environment when you immerse in the rhythm of your natural breath. As you observe, remember to focus on feeling without adding comments or opinions. This can be enough. However, you may also try to increase the length of your inhalations and exhalations very slowly and softly, as if you had the whole day for each single in-breath and out-breath. Try this for as long as it is comfortable, noticing what happens. Then return to your natural breath and observe once again how your body breathes on its own, as it does around 20,000 times each day, without your conscious supervision. Are there differences between the qualities of your breath when you regulate it and when you breathe consciously? As you connect to your breathing process, feel your breath, noticing if it is hurried or unhurried, smooth or choppy, free or restricted.

This aphorism talks specifically about exhalations. Chanting OM (1.27 & 1.28), making the sound smooth, fluid and long is one specific way of focusing on your exhalations. You may also explore your exhalations in other ways. In a restful and tension-free posture, you can try making your exhalations longer, softer, and effortless. What do you notice? How do sensations change? Does this change your internal climate and mood? It is important to acknowledge and underscore that in *pranayama* practices, breath retentions are traditionally considered advanced techniques requiring the supervision of a knowledgeable and experienced teacher. Another simple way to start is by noticing what happens at the intersections between each in-breath and out-breath. What do you discover? Can breathing be a useful focal point to release some of the usual distractors?

1.35 Focusing steadily on subtle sense perceptions.

The next option is sensitizing yourself to subtler sense perceptions. Some of the traditional focal points to enhance sense perception include the tip of the nose to enhance olfaction, the tip of the tongue to enhance taste, the root of the tongue to enhance hearing, the roof of the palate to enhance sight, and the surface of the tongue to enhance touch. The tip of the tongue for taste and tip of the nose for smell seem obvious to most people. One of the reasons suggested for the roof of the palate to connect with sight is because the roof of the palate is close to the optic nerve. Similarly, the reason for root of the tongue as a focal point for hearing is its proximity to the auditory system. Finally, the reason for using the surface of the tongue as a focal point to enhanced touch perception is that the tongue is the part of the body with most touch sensitivity[ii]. By focusing on the tongue, it may be possible to heighten touch sensitivity throughout the body. The only way to really know if these focal points work is to observe if there is a gradual development of the sense you are meditating on. This practice can be useful in removing distractions. However, it can potentially become a way to keep chasing after your senses. You can think about focusing on subtle sense perceptions as a sense withdrawal (*pratyahara*) practice. When you orient to your inward senses, instead of letting your mind chase after external phenomena, you can develop greater sensitivity for subtleties that currently escape your perception.

Another possible avenue is to invite external sensory stimuli to become a pathway to cultivate your inner subtle perceptions. For instance, focus on the flame of a candle for as long as possible and then close your eyes resting your attention on the resulting impressions (*trataka*). Stay with the impression for as long as possible. What do you notice? It can be valuable to pay attention to where your awareness goes to as the subtle impressions fade. This may indicate the ideas, thoughts, or ways of being that are deeply entrenched. You can do a similar practice with a specific sound, like the sound of a singing bowl. You can also use the lightest touch between your fingers, like bringing the tip of your index finger and thumb together in the softest way possible. Taking a sip of water and following the sensations of taste can also be a focal point for bringing awareness to the subtler aspects of taste and flavor. Incense is a traditional focal point for connecting with subtleties in scents.

As usual, an attitude of curiosity, the curiosity to learn more about yourself and how your systems work, can be a strong motivator to dive deeper within. In this internal journey of exploration remember that direct experience (*pratyaksha* 1.7) is the path of yoga. Thus, release predictions and expectations, and instead notice the organic changes as they develop. One further option is to follow the senses to the core of your being, so that you come to the fundamental fact about you, the "I am," your aliveness. This is a thread that continues the ideas presented in sutra 1.17. What happens in your mind, body, and emotions when you practice one of these techniques consistently?

1.36 Cultivating the inner light.

As with the previous aphorisms, this one can be interpreted in two ways. One is as a stand-alone technique to remove distractions. The other approach is to see this practice as a continuation of the process of involution. Involution is the gradual progression in exploring your inner world. As the senses turn inwards and sensitivity grows, subtler aspects of your inner world become apparent. The process is an organic enhancement of your ability to focus. This is the practice of concentration (*dharana*). The focal point in this case is your inner light. Every person has an inner light, the light of life. We see this light shining bright in babies. In fact, it is difficult not to see that brightness in them. This is one of the reasons that babies attract our attention and most often elicit an easy smile. As people get more and more established in their ways of being, internal commentary becomes an endless litany of opinions, stories, beliefs, likes, and dislikes. As it was suggested in 1.4, if those ways of being are not regulated, we tend to identify with our ways of being. In other words, the inner light at the core of our being is veiled by our ways of being. The often-used word "enlightened" refers to those whose inner light shines bright, enabling them to see everything with clarity unencumbered by who they think they are or should be.

Trataka, the practice of gazing at a candle flame, is one accessible technique to start. In a darkened room without any drafts, sit in a comfortable position two feet away from a candle placed at eye level. Focus your gaze on the center of the flame and, keeping your eyes steady, try to concentrate on the light for as long as you can without any strain. When you reach a comfortable limit, close your eyes gently and stay with the light within for as long as possible. Explore the option of trying to connect that light behind your forehead to the center of your brain and down through the center of your throat to the center of your chest. Visualize your heart enveloped in soft light, like the luminescence of the full moon. When the sensation of light fades, you can try opening your eyes and gazing at the candle again. In some traditional texts, it says to keep the gaze fixed until your eyes start watering. You may try this and notice how that feels and whether it agrees with you. Practicing with patient persistence may make it easier to just feel the impression of light behind your forehead and from there to connect to the light in your heart.

You may also bring joyful thoughts into your mind and inspiring feelings into your heart to invite this inner brightness to arise. For example, you can think of something that brings a smile to your face, or you can remember a particularly happy moment. Then, gradually let go of the details and stay with the residual feeling. One other way to access this luminescence is by aligning with the feeling of gratitude and love for your life, your partner, relatives, friends, and teachers. As usual, choose one technique, engage in the practice as best as you can, and notice its effects. Is this practice helpful or unhelpful?

1.37 Concentrating on serenity beyond desire or on the mind of someone who is beyond likes and dislikes.

There is deep calmness and tranquility within you all the time. That serenity is the ground of your being, the spaciousness and ease that you relax into at the end of your day once you let go of memories, worries, plans, and desires. In other words, when you entangle yourself in your own ways of being, it is easy to forget that deep within, there is peace, joy, awareness, and love. A simple exercise can be revealing. For one week, pay attention to the last thought you have before falling asleep. Also notice what is the first thought you have when you wake up. If there is a pattern, ask yourself if that is a habit, one of your ways of being. For instance, the last thought of the day may be a reminder of a task that needs to be accomplished the following day. These last and first thoughts indicate some of the things that you are making important enough to linger in your internal space. Notice if they are conducive to your feeling integrated, joyful, and successful. If your current tendency is not very helpful at this time, consider starting a new habit of making peace with yourself, your day and your life at the end of each day by recognizing that the day is complete. Take a few moments to reflect on your intentions, actions, and interactions. Notice what could be improved and what you did well. Then allow yourself to be relaxed and give thanks for the day. As one last thought, can you send yourself love and acceptance? Can you also send love and acceptance out to your loved ones and gradually to friends, acquaintances, and perhaps to every living being? Similarly, you can start your day with gratitude for being alive into a new day, something that was not guaranteed. Invite yourself to participate in your life today with enthusiasm, intelligence, and humility. There are similar practices from a variety of traditions that can be useful and that may resonate better with you. Try one of them for a few days and notice the effects. Do these practices contribute to creating a sense of serenity in you? Can that act as a reminder of the tranquility deep within?

When viewed in sequence with the step in the previous sutra, this aphorism can be interpreted as the path to meditation (*dhyana*). In order to meditate, you first focus your mind (*dharana*), then you allow yourself to settle, gradually loosening the intensity of your focus, while you remain witnessing what is with no effort. In other words, the transition from concentration to meditation completes the process of shifting from doing to being. Desire is helpful to set a course of action; however, desire can also be a source of internal agitation and reactivity that muddles the deep peace within you. If the deep spaciousness within you seems out of reach, you can draw inspiration from concentrating on someone who is truly beyond likes and dislikes. Although these days it may seem like there is a scarcity of people who abide in peace, these inspirational beings are all around us. Pay attention to the people in your environment and be curious about what signs indicate to you that a person lives in peace and harmony. This search can be educational and may offer surprises as well as evidence of your ways of looking. You can use the mind-heart of that inspiring person as the focal point for you. Notice if this practice offers a good anchor to dispel distractions.

1.38 Gaining insight from dreams and cultivating deep sleep.

In the timeless dream space, you witness some aspect of your mind trying to make sense of previous impressions. It is often surprising to see the fantastic scenarios and the seemingly disparate associations of events from different parts of your life. Each person is in a constant process of writing, editing, and rewriting the master narrative of life to make sense, find meaning, and create coherence in actions. There are many stimuli that are sensed but may not be processed by the conscious mind. An example is when you play a trivia game and you surprise yourself by knowing information that you didn't know you knew. In your daily activities, anything causing an emotional reaction is more likely to be noticed and stored in your memory. The dreaming process can be understood as one of the ways your mind tries to fit these impressions into your personal life story.

In sutra 1.17 the progression from gross to subtler levels of concentration was introduced, followed by aphorism 1.18, where it says that once the ways of being settle, only impressions remain. This sutra, 1.38, suggests a way of processing these impressions by focusing on the content of your dreams and the emotional impressions that they have left on you as a source of insight. As a result, you can gain a clearer understanding of your subconscious mind. As you venture on the exploration of your dreamscapes, it is important to acknowledge the value and importance of sleeping well and sleeping as much as you need. This exploration can show you how your thoughts, attitudes and behaviors during the day influence you at a deeper level. For instance, if you read something before going to sleep, or if you watch a movie before you go to sleep, do you notice some of those ideas in the book or movie blending into your dream? You can set your intention to remember your dreams and to be open to seeing your dreams as messengers traveling through channels other than deduction and inference. Like the previous exploration of your true nature, this aphorism reminds you that as you fall asleep, many of your internal activities subside, reducing distractions and giving way to a deeper calmness.

Following the thread of the previous sutras, this sutra can be understood also as the next stage in the involution process. After your mind is established in serenity, only subconscious impressions remain (as mentioned in sutra 1.18).

As your inner environment settles, what are the remaining impressions that emerge?

Are they the remnants of past desires, experiences, and interactions?

When you notice these impressions, can you allow them to fizzle out by just feeling them without trying to make them into stories to entertain yourself?

1.39 Or, by focusing on anything uplifting.

This aphorism reaffirms the fact that the Yoga Sutra is a non-dogmatic, comprehensive compendium of yoga techniques. Understanding that each person is unique and that the same path may not be the best for everybody, Patañjali offers an open invitation to remove distractions by dedicating your energy and awareness to whatever you find uplifting. This sutra also reminds you that yoga is about you making the most intelligent and appropriate choices available to you. Take a moment to consider what inspires you.

What do you find truly uplifting?

What is the direct experience that you have when you are inspired?

How does the direct experience of feeling inspired relate to other experiences like feeling friendliness, compassion, love and equanimity?

How does inspiration feel in your mind, your body, and your emotions?

How are you cultivating inspiring thoughts, intentions, actions, and interactions in your daily life?

What happens when you make the conscious choice to look for inspiration in everything that you do?

THE PROGRESSION OF INSIGHT INTO FREEDOM

The final set of sutras in Chapter One elaborates on the process introduced in sutra 1.17, moving deeper into integration after your ways of being are released and when there are no obstacles or distractions pulling you away from full presence. This is a gradual journey to move beyond the limiting beliefs and opinions that confine your mind.

1.40 Steady and focused awareness reveals insight on all aspects of the universe from the smallest to the largest.

In the coming together of life and consciousness, life is ever changing activity while consciousness is the aliveness, the knowing, the noticing, the sensing, the unmediated direct experience of being. Our ways of being are a framework, a complete set of filters, not always internally consistent, that we use to participate in life. Although useful, each framework has limitations, especially when we don't know what we don't know. Those blind spots become a source of confusion because the framework provides limited, inaccurate, or useless information when facing new, unexpected, or unpredictable situations. In those situations, the shortcomings of our framework become obstacles as well as sources of frustration. Being aware of your own framework enables you to recognize its advantages and weaknesses. Besides, having the capacity to set aside your framework for a while provides opportunities for seeing what may have been obscured by what you think you know, revealing what has been right in front of you all along. Many of the discoveries in the history of humankind have been accidental. They happened when a person noticed something that was unusual or unexpected, something that did not fit into the regular way of thinking at the time. Usually this happened when they looked at something from a different perspective or vantage point. In fact, discovery is the recognition of something that was beyond our awareness until now. The discovery is facilitated by being able to release the usual way of explaining or understanding a phenomenon, opening the door for a new way of seeing.

This aphorism reminds you of the importance of loosening your grip on the stories you have chosen to believe in. In order to see clearly, invite the possibility of seeing anew. This is like when you are trying to remember a word that you know, and the more you try, the more the word recedes. As you relax and stop struggling, then the word emerges effortlessly. When you choose to minimize all your doings to create space for just being, what happens? What happens when your attention is not pulled in many different directions? What does it take to let go of what you think you know? Then, what do you notice when you look at the world through the eyes of deep peace and calm within? Is it possible that your inner silence enables you to perceive everything around you from the smallest to the largest with the utmost clarity? A simple exploration you can try is to find a comfortable position conducive to being relaxed and alert. Then feel the outermost layer of your physical body. Notice the sensations in the places your skin is touching something. Can you feel the space around you, just beyond your skin? Can you gradually expand your receptivity to feel sensations farther and farther from you? Might it be possible for you to keep expanding your awareness? You may also try a similar exploration going inward. Start in a relaxed posture conducive to being alert. Remaining still, feel your skin from the outside. Then, notice if it is possible to feel your skin from the inside. Gradually move your attention to the adipose layer beneath your skin. Continue by feeling the superficial fascia. Keep exploring inward to feel the deep fascia and its connections with muscles, bones, nerves, and blood vessels. Can you focus on your blood vessels? Is it possible to feel your blood flowing through your body? May it be possible to feel the cells in your blood stream? Deepening your sensitivity offers you the possibility to perceive with increasing clarity. Are you developing a greater sensitivity for insight? If so, how is insight different from what you think you know?

1.41 Free from distractions, the mind and heart of the yogi become pure, like a crystal reflecting completely and without distortion whatever is in front of it (*samapatti*).

This is the entrance to meditation. The word used in this sutra is *samapatti* which means yielding, giving way, and coming together.

When you release your expectations and opinions, when you let go of who you think you are, all aspects of you come together, there is no illusion of separation between body and mind or between inside and outside. Then, there is no need for reactivity. In other words, you sense with great clarity. Rather than trying to comment on what you are experiencing; your perception becomes a clear window. Usually, all your experiences are colored by your past, including your preferences, previous events, and the impressions they left on you. For instance, for the person who was ridiculed in school, taking a class as an adult may generate anxiety because of the impressions left by early experiences. As a result, that person's perspective on the class may be clouded by past impressions. Your ways of being are all accumulations of these previous experiences that still have an effect on your attitudes, thoughts, emotions, actions, and interactions. Once the ways of being are effectively neutralized, whatever is in front of you can be perceived without distortions. As the object is removed, the mind does not cling to it. Instead, the mind remains calm and open. This is the threshold of integration (*samadhi*).

Reflect:

When you rest your mind on an object or idea, how clearly do you perceive it? If distractions emerge, how do they manifest?
Are these distractions sensations, thoughts, words, images?
What effect does the distraction have on your internal experience?
Does the distraction or obstacle generate reactivity?
To what extent are the distractions related to your expectations?
Do your distractions entangle you in an ever-growing web of stories that pull you away from your focal object and your direct experience?
Are some distractions connected to who you think you are, used to be or should be?

Can these questions be a path to releasing distractions and apprehending what is in front of you with greater accuracy and without interference?

1.42 When awareness is colored by the focal object, its name and its meaning, integration with reasoning (*savitarka samadhi*).

Continuing deeper on the meditation journey, this aphorism defines *savitarka samadhi*, the first aspect of the first stage of integration (*samadhi*) listed in the sequence in aphorism 1.17. The first stage of integration (*vitarka*) relates to what is perceptible through your senses and it is subdivided into two parts. The first, *savitarka samadhi*, goes beyond the meditation (*dhyana*) state where your mind perceives the focal object without external or internal interference. In Sanskrit, *vitarka* means argument, imagination, opinion, or reasoning. *Savitarka* means with reasoning or with deliberation. At this first level of integration, the contents of the mind include only the object, its name and its deep meaning and purpose. For instance, you can choose ॐ as your focal object. The object is ॐ, its name is *pranava*, and its meaning what you know about it and its purpose. These three aspects of the focal object are distinct. Your knowledge about it may include that it is the sound that represents Supreme Being as well as the ideas in the *Mandukya Upanishad*. However, if you didn't know anything about the *Mandukya Upanishad*, that would not affect the object itself. Even if you choose to call it OM or AUM, the focal object would not be affected. In this stage of meditation your awareness gravitates towards these three aspects of the focal object, the focal object itself, its name, and what you know about it. Your mind does not deviate from it. In other words, your meditation includes reasoning and opinion regarding your focal object. *What happens when you try to choose a focal object and meditate on it?*

1.43 When the object of meditation stands out without any thoughts or memories associated to it, integration beyond conceptualization (*nirvitarka samadhi*).

This sutra talks about the second subdivision of the first aspect of *samadhi* listed in sutra 1.17, integration beyond conceptualization (*nirvitarka samadhi*). In yoga practice there is a constant process of moving towards subtler levels of experience, which means that you continue refining your perception and becoming aware of subtler levels of perceptions as you explore subtler aspects of yourself. In the previous stage (*savitarka samadhi*), the object, its name, and your knowledge about it were useful to concentrate your attention. At this new level, those same elements become a hindrance to a deeper level of meditation because they keep your awareness at a more superficial level. Since those associated elements to the focal object are released, this stage is called integration beyond conceptualization (*nirvitarka samadhi*). The object stands out and your mind does not try to load it with meaning, thoughts, and opinions. This is a critical point to move towards being with what is, just as it is, and being with yourself just as you are. Notice that on an average day, a lot of your attentional resources are probably focused on external and perhaps surface level details of whatever you interact with. The "Am I Present?" exercise (page 38) and the ideas presented in the "Guidelines for the Journey" section (page 41) were directing your attention to the many ways that distractions emerge. It can be argued that the purpose of many yoga techniques is to help you become aware of how distractions arise. In the previous stage of *samadhi*, you can stay focused, while in this stage you are fully focused on the object alone without adding any commentary whatsoever.

During your day, choose to notice how often your attention goes to seemingly random thoughts and to memories triggered by the stimuli around you. Then inquire:

Is this a voluntary or involuntary process?

To what extent can you be so absorbed in something that your internal chatter stops?

When that happens, do you experience objects, actions, and interactions with greater vividness?

Do your memories, predictions and expectations enhance your wholehearted awareness?

What attitudes are more conducive to deeper attention?

If you remember that each moment is unique and unrepeatable, are you more attentive?

1.44 When the object of meditation is experienced in its subtle constitutive essence, contemplative integration (*savichara samadhi*). Even subtler, integration beyond contemplation (*nirvichara samadhi*) brings the yogi to experience directly the focal object.

While the previous two aphorisms, 1.42 and 1.43, explain two subdivisions of the first stage of integration (*vitarka*), this sutra refers to the two subdivisions of the second stage of integration (*vichara*) listed in 1.17. The second stage focuses on subtler objects of meditation. The meanings of *vichara* in Sanskrit include contemplation, thought, consideration, and reflection. For instance, in the "How does a smile feel?" exercise (page 52), you first tried to notice the physical sensations that took place when you smile. If you make those sensations your focal point and your experience is colored also by your knowledge about smiling, such as the names of the facial muscles involved in smiling, you would be in the integration with reasoning stage (1.42 *savitarka samadhi*). When you stay with the same focal point, your smile, and just the sensations that make up your smile without any deliberation or reasoning related to smiling, you would be moving into the integration beyond conceptualization stage (1.43 *nirvitarka samadhi*). As you remain with the same focus but go into the subtler aspects of smiling, like the emotions or memories triggered by the smile or your knowledge about this aspect of the smile, it will take you into the *savichara samadhi* stage, contemplative integration. At this level, even though there are emotions, they are not triggering any reactivity. To move beyond, to the integration beyond contemplation stage (*nirvichara samadhi*), you focus your attention on the direct experience of the emotions and feelings triggered by your smile. There is no further internal deliberation or reflection.

What focal objects are fascinating enough to invite you into these deeper stages of meditation?
What effect does it have on you to experience a focal object directly?
What effect does that have on your values, desires, and interests?

1.45 Deepening levels of subtlety reveal the undifferentiated substratum of existence.

This sutra offers a glimpse of the continuous process of yogic purification, a shedding of attachments to layers of existence from the most apparent to the subtlest until all that remains is pure awareness. In the previous four aphorisms you see this process. It starts from clarifying your mind and heart. Then you focus on one meditation object from its form, name and meaning to its subtle essence. As sutra 1.17 indicated, eventually this process leads you to connect with greater clarity with the subtler aspects of your own being. You start by feeling sensations, then you notice your thoughts and emotions until you feel the common ground were your sensations, thoughts, emotions, and experiences are taking place, your own sense of being. You feel your own aliveness directly, and without any distractions. Even deeper than your own sense of being is the foundation of life, *prakrti*. *Prakrti* is the matrix of nature. Without beginning or end, *prakrti* is the primordial and undifferentiated essence of everything that exists. *Prakrti* is the pure potential from which nature manifests in continuous and endless transformation. In sutra 1.19, the *prakrtilayas* were mentioned as those beings who identify with the subtlest aspect of nature, remaining merged in nature (*prakrti*). This is a subtler level of existence than being embodied, yet it is not the complete liberation that results from freeing oneself even from the attachment to nature.

One way to probe the meaning of this sutra is to be curious about the embodied experience of these questions:
What are the subtlest aspects of your own experiences?
What is beyond your subtlest aspect?
What is the space where all experiences take place?

Remember that you are gradually leaving behind the processes of conceptualization.
What happens when you try this?

Another option is to use the "I Am Here Now" mantra (page 53). Start chanting aloud, gradually making the sound into a very soft whisper. Then, chant silently while still moving your mouth almost imperceptibly. Keep repeating the mantra silently. Then release the word "here" so that you chant "I am now." Continue and let go of the word "now." And after a while let go of the word "I." Stay chanting "am" in the softest silent manner possible. What do you notice when you try this?

1.46 These previous states of deep meditation (integration – *samadhi*) are called with seed (*sabija*), because they use either a gross or subtle focal point.

The meditation practices up to this point have all used a focal object as a support, called a seed (*bija*). Just like scaffolding is erected during construction of a building, regardless of how useful the scaffolding was, once the building is complete, the scaffolding becomes an obstacle and, since it is no longer useful, it is removed. Similarly, the involution process of meditation keeps moving from the outside towards the innermost aspect of your being. Whatever focal point you are using to focus your awareness will eventually be released. Another reason these types of integration (*samadhi*) are called with seed (*sabija*), is because there are still some remaining impressions (*samskaras*) stored in the practitioner's subconscious memory. These impressions are the seeds of future actions and inclinations.

You can try the idea of releasing the focal point by refining the technique for chanting OM or AUM suggested in sutra 1.27. You start chanting at a comfortable level with external sound establishing a smooth flow of air and sound to invite your mind to stay with this experience. Gradually, start decreasing the volume of your chant so that the sound remains steady and fluid as it becomes softer and softer. Take your time and savor the experience. Continue making the sound softer until it becomes a barely audible whisper. Then continue moving your mouth while chanting silently, making the movements more and more subtle. Remaining focused inwardly, stop the movement of your lips and make your inner chant even more delicate so that your attention is gentle and effortless. Continue until the silent chant is as subtle as possible. Eventually release the silent chant and remain with its silent reverberation in your being. Remain with this soft yet persistent focus for as long as it is comfortable. When your mind becomes distracted return to chanting at the minimal level of effort, eventually releasing the chant again.

What happens when you try this?

What do you notice?

1.47 Integration beyond contemplation (*nirvichara*) purifies the inner self.

This sutra is a reminder that the meditation experience, like all of yoga, is a process of shedding all that is unnecessary. Going through the progression of meditation takes you from being free of distractions to refining your ability to direct your awareness towards increasingly subtle objects of meditation. Reaching the level of integration beyond contemplation (*nirvichara samadhi*) cleanses the inner self. The ways of being that used to cloud the yogi's awareness are effectively halted. The result is wisdom. This means that you perceive everything just as it is instead of seeing through the filters of your beliefs, stories, opinions, and preferences. Is it possible that the filters that color your perception are gradually becoming less dominant? Is the internal voice that comments and judges everything you perceive becoming quieter?

1.48 Then awareness dwells in absolute true wisdom (*rtambhara*).

1.49 Absolute true wisdom, arising from pure insight and discernment, differs from knowledge gained through inference and testimony.

The Sanskrit word used in sutra 1.48 is *rtambhara*, meaning to bear the truth in one's self. This is the natural outcome of the process described in sutras 1.41 to 1.47. When there are no distractions, either external or internal, your awareness can be directed with piercing accuracy. Since your inner environment is cleansed, you experience the world as it is. At this stage in the journey, you are able to master your ways of being, your senses are united, and you can focus your mind effortlessly on whatever you choose. Then, there are no extraneous threads of activity, nothing to chase after, nothing to push away. Without distractions you can clearly distinguish between knowledge and intuition or insight. You receive insights when you tap into the wisdom that informs all of life. Most people have brief glimpses of this. Has it ever happened to you that the thought or memory of somebody you know comes into your awareness and in apparent coincidence that person contacts you? Or that you feel compelled to do something and that action leads you to an unexpected – yet welcomed – encounter or experience? Or that you have been trying to resolve a problem or situation and have thought about all possible options but that you still haven't found a viable solution and, inexplicably, an idea comes into your mind suddenly delivering what feels like the perfect solution? Recognizing insight and learning to trust it as the wisdom that guides life everywhere help you acknowledge your own connectedness to the intricate web of life.

Sutra 1.49 emphasizes the important difference between what you know through inference and testimony (two of the sources of correct knowledge mentioned in sutra 1.7), and the embodied wisdom resulting from meditation. Although trustworthy sources of useful information can serve as guides along your path, your direct experience of wisdom cannot be replaced by that knowledge. As you differentiate between what you know and true wisdom, you see that wisdom does not originate in you. Thus, instead of taking credit for the insight you receive, you appreciate it with humility as the gift received when you simply listen with tranquil attention.

How are you listening for the silent whisper of wisdom in your practice?

How does this wisdom manifest in your daily activities?

Are you able to differentiate what you believe from true wisdom?

What does it take to trust this wisdom?

Do the insights you receive, when you trust them, result in greater harmony?

1.50 The impressions created by absolute true wisdom prevent other impressions (*samskaras*) from sprouting, also deactivating dormant, as well as unmanifested impressions or *karma*.

Remember that everything you do, including your thoughts, emotions, intentions, and actions, leaves an impression in your memory. The more frequently you do something, the stronger the internal web of impressions (*saṁskaras*). You can test this idea quite easily. If there is regularity in your schedule, you will notice that you will wake up at the same time every day without the need of an alarm clock. Or, if you have a routine for flossing and brushing your teeth, you do not even have to think about it to follow that routine. Many teachers suggest doing your yoga practice in the same space and at the same time every day to generate an impression that becomes a habit. Then, you do not even have to think about finding time in your schedule for practicing. You just feel the unconscious pull to practice. This is particularly so if your practice is refreshing, enjoyable and interesting. This same basic principle operates also at this higher level of practice. As you remove distractions and experience your inner calmness with diligence, your internal web of beneficial impressions grows stronger. Your organism allocates more energy and attentional resources to those helpful impressions. With less energy allocated to the less-than-helpful impressions, they dwindle and are, eventually, wiped out.

There is often an internal conflict between directing your attention to stop what is painful or harmful and cultivating more useful and beneficial attitudes and activities. **When in doubt, choose to support what is helpful and useful, and automatically what is not useful will decrease.** Remember that you will probably get distracted again and again, depending on how strong your habits are. And once again, the skill of bringing yourself back to presence without strain, struggle or self-judgment is essential. Notice if your tendencies to be distracted are becoming less pronounced. Also, pay attention to some of your unhelpful tendencies, like complaining and useless internal chatter – are they diminishing? Often, as your inner harmony grows, irritants and annoyances become more apparent. Carefully discern the difference between a new source of irritation emerging and an old unhelpful pattern becoming more noticeable. And, even when an irritant emerges, is it possible to be with the bearable discomfort and to respond as needed, without getting entangled in any drama?

1.51 When all impressions dissolve, the highest level of integration emerges (*nirbija samadhi*) when all identification ceases and only consciousness, self-contained, pure, and liberated remains.

Every step along the path leads towards liberation. This is the final step. When the remaining subconscious impressions (*samskaras*) are removed, there are no seeds for future actions. Moreover, a meditation object is no longer needed. Thus, this is the level of integration called beyond seed or beyond objects, *nirbija samadhi.* This gradual process of dissolution of all impressions does not happen overnight. It is a process that grows incrementally according to what is within reach without strain or struggle, through continuous, sincere, and uninterrupted practice (*abhyasa*) combined with increasing independence from all opinions and attachments (*vairagya*). Yogis abide in their true nature, consciousness, free from the burdens brought about by misidentification. A gentle, loving attitude to every task, every moment, and every interaction seems to be more productive than a forceful approach; the former attitude is more conducive to releasing the illusion of control, while the latter generates more impressions to be stored in memory. Perhaps this is the reason Patañjali says in Chapter Two that releasing the illusion of control (*ishvara pranidhana*) results in *samadhi* (2.45). This gradual journey of removing impurities and increasing clarity is not about bringing external elements into the self. Instead, it is a process of fine-tuning your sensitivity and cultivating your natural inner stillness and inner silence with the curiosity that might reveal the obvious yet elusive essence of existence.

You may try this approach to practice meditation: Start by giving yourself permission to let go of the world outside in order to dive into your internal world. Then, get relaxed, stable, and comfortable. Choose a focal object, internal or external, something inspiring and interesting enough to hold your attention. Continue by concentrating with gentle firmness on your focal object. Maintain your focus with patient persistence and release everything else. Refine your focus towards the subtlest aspect of the meditation object. And then, loosen the grip of your attention as much as possible while remaining focused. Eventually, allow the subtlety of the essence of the meditation object to lead you to experience the aliveness that you are. At this stage, even the sense of "I" dissolves, so that your "I am" experience merges into undifferentiated being.

What is the experience of being, when you release all extraneous activity? Does it become easier to notice subtler aspects of your experience and of your own being?

What is the experience of releasing your sense of identity?

Summary of Chapter One of The Yoga Sutra

Chapter One in the Yoga Sutra is about the *state* of being, unencumbered by our *ways* of being. The chapter reminds students that preparation and readiness are necessary to embark on the path of yoga and that yoga is regulating the habitual tendencies and patterns that manifest in body, breath, mind, and emotion. When these patterns or ways of being are mastered, the Yoga Sutra tells us, one's awareness rests in its own nature instead of becoming identified with the fluctuations of the body-mind-heart system. The ways of being can be helpful or unhelpful and may manifest as correct perception (in the form of direct experience, inference, and testimony), incorrect perception, imagination, sleep, and memory. We are called to master the fluctuations in the system with a twofold strategy: practice, tempered by freedom from attachment.

Practice is cultivated with sincerity, for a long period of time without interruptions. Freedom from attachment is a calm attitude completely unaffected by either external or internal stimuli, one which sets aside beliefs, and is further deepened by recognizing pure awareness. Complete intuitive understanding unfolds gradually through inquiry, reflection, inner peace, and the sense of being. Eventually, only the impressions left by past experiences remain. Even subtle identification will eventually be released.

Integration can be reached by releasing all identifications, however, for most practitioners progress is facilitated by trust and confidence, vitality, memory, unwavering focus, and insight. Commitment and intensity of application vary. An additional, direct path for mastering the ways of being is to realize Supreme Being, a wholehearted and unconditional acceptance of life. Supreme Being is unaffected by afflictions, actions or effects; it is the unsurpassed seed of omniscience that is unconditioned by time. Supreme Being, the unequaled teacher, can be realized through chanting OM. Awareness turns inward, and all disturbances are removed. The obstacles and disturbances along the way can be overcome by cultivating one-pointedness and by removing biases and judgment through friendliness, compassion, inspiration, and equanimity. One-pointed evenness can be directed to breathing processes, subtle sensations, the inner light, freedom from desire, insight from dreams or anything uplifting. Inner silence deepens as awareness focuses on higher levels of subtlety until there is only the unmediated experience of the focal object. Then, it is possible to experience with great clarity the primordial essence of existence and the rhythm of cosmic wisdom. Impressions of utmost clarity develop and prevent other subconscious impressions from generating internal activity.

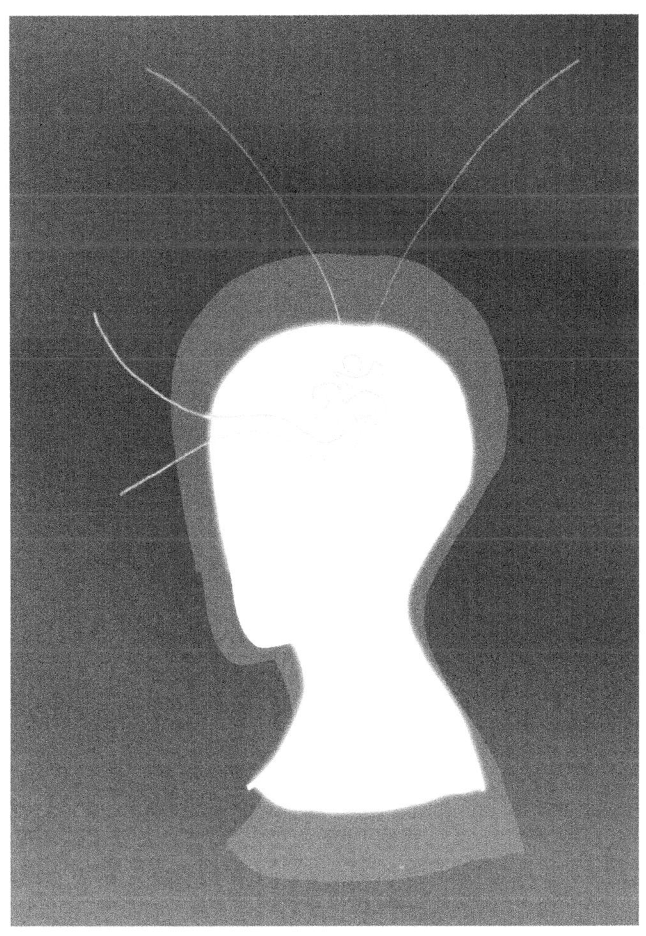

Yogic action leads effectively and efficiently towards mastering ourselves and our lives ignited by enthusiasm, guided by wisdom and participating with humility. Yoga practice is the vehicle for embodying presence in all our endeavors.

PRACTICE (*SADHANA*)

Sadhana, the title of Chapter Two of the Yoga Sutra, has numerous meanings in Sanskrit. Its definitions include *means, instrument, furthering, guiding well, efficient, effective, leading straight to a goal,* and *worship*. The overall theme of this chapter is **doing**, as articulated in seven sections:

- Yogic action [2.1-2.2]
- Afflictions [2.3-2.11]
- Effects [2.12-2.14]
- Suffering [2.15-2.17]
- Awareness and experiences [2.18-2.22]
- Discernment [2.23-2.27]
- The limbs of yoga [2.28-2.55]

YOGIC ACTION

2.1 Yogic action (*kriya yoga*) combines enthusiasm (*tapas*), intelligence (*svadhyaya*) and humility (*ishvara pranidhana*).

Consistent with the theme of this chapter, practice, Patañjali defines yogic action as an action that combines enthusiasm, intelligence, and humility. You can act only in the present. An action in the past or future is a thought about an action, not an actual action. This definition of yogic action is congruent with the definition of yoga in Chapter One. It requires enthusiasm (*tapas*) to bring your attention (*citta*) to the moment you are in. Intelligence (*svadhyaya*) helps you distinguish between the helpful and unhelpful ways of being (*vrtti*) that you have cultivated. And humility (*ishvara pranidhana*) frees you up (*nirodha*) from constant engagement in grasping, striving, judging, and resisting.

Understanding yogic action (*kriya yoga*) as an act that integrates enthusiasm, intelligence and humility conveys the richness of this idea while also making it possible to apply it in your life. *Tapas* means heat, fire, meditation, and deep concentration. To engage in any worthwhile action, you need enthusiasm, because it gives you energy and inspiration to act. That same enthusiasm motivates you to do your best. Without enthusiasm, ideas are rarely acted upon. Think about anybody you admire or would like to emulate and you will probably find that they bring passion into what they do. Moreover, as you pursue something that is important to you, you will probably find obstacles and challenges. Enthusiasm provides the determination and energy needed to remove obstacles and inefficiencies. Notice also that you will need enthusiasm to challenge your unhelpful ways of being. The process of going against those unhelpful patterns will cause friction that also generates heat. *Tapas*, enthusiasm can best be synthesized as **Do the best that you can.**

Svadhyaya means study of wisdom texts, chanting, and self-study. Intelligence is knowing yourself well so that you are aware of your ways of being, the habits you have cultivated, consciously and unconsciously throughout your life. Knowing your tendencies and habits helps you avoid usual pitfalls and shortcomings. It also guides your enthusiasm to harness your helpful habits to move in the most fruitful and beneficial direction. Since well-established patterns tend to become unconscious, *intelligence is a way to outsmart those tendencies.* Your intelligence corroborates what has been suggested for centuries by a variety of wisdom traditions as useful ways to live a meaningful life. *Svadhyaya* is embodied intelligence that can be applied by ensuring that you know why you are doing what you are doing and by confirming that you are in fact doing what you *think* you are doing.

Additionally, by knowing yourself well, you remember that you are not perfect and that there are innumerable things that are beyond your control. *Ishvara pranidhana*, as it was pointed out in aphorism 1.23, may be understood as devotion to god, relinquishing the illusion of control, or surrendering to the essence of life. When you release the illusion of control, you cultivate humility. Humility encourages you to be honest and patient while also helping you accept and appreciate yourself as you are and the world as it is. It is especially important to accept what can't be changed, so that you can allocate your energy intelligently to changing what needs to be changed. When you accept the perfection of life, then your internal objections, commentary, and predilections subside (*nirodha*). *Ishvara pranidhana* can be summed up as sincere intention coupled with wholehearted action.

This tripod of enthusiasm, intelligence, and humility provides a stable base for your explorations. When you combine enthusiasm, intelligence, and humility, your actions become vibrant, meaningful, and joyful. However, if one of the three pillars is missing, instability develops. In brief, the yogic action defined in this aphorism simply says: **Show up to every single moment of your life with your mind and heart open.**

How do you cultivate these three attitudes?
What do you do to bring aliveness into your attitude?
What motivates you?
Are you bringing enthusiasm into whatever you are doing?

Can you see yourself honestly and know your tendencies and inclinations?

Can you use your self-knowledge to guide your actions?

Are your ideas and actions logical and intelligent?

Are you doing what you think you are doing?

What are the words of wisdom that you live by?

How do you cultivate a humble attitude?

Is it helpful to remember that you did not create yourself?

To what extent are you aware of what you do not know and do not understand?

Are you acting from the wholeness of your heart?

How do you show up to your life?

Are there parts of your life that you avoid showing up for?

2.2 Yogic actions minimize afflictions (*klesha*) and bring about integration (*samadhi*).

The path of action suggested in the previous sutra focuses on removing obstacles to integration (*samadhi*). This aphorism provides a way to assess the effects of your actions. The underlying idea is that your natural state is one of integration and that your system orients towards balance and dynamic harmony. In other words, the calmness, harmony, and peace that you rest in while you are in dreamless deep sleep are always potentially available to you. In fact, that is the ground of your being, awareness. Notice, however, how your usual ways of being become active again, as soon as you wake up.

You may start your day with ways of being that are conducive to feeling centered, such as gratitude and kindness. In other cases, you may allow ways of being such as planning, worrying, and regretting to resurface. These ways of being may have the opposite effect, so that instead of supporting and enhancing your ability to be present, they end up obscuring your deep inner peace.

When you are awake and have the firm intention to be fully present, you are able to notice the distractions that keep pulling you away from having your mind and heart open and unencumbered. These distractions often take the form of patterns of tension, holding and contraction in your body, breath, mind, and emotions. Feeling these tensions is already showing you the areas where there are inefficiencies and obstructions. Acting with enthusiasm, intelligence, and humility helps you remove these tensions that disrupt the integrated harmony between body, mind, and emotion. Consistent practice of yogic actions develops helpful new habits, new ways of inhabiting yourself, gradually fostering inner harmony between being and doing. As you reduce tension, discomfort, and pain, you are better able to be present, creating a positive feedback loop – helping you feel empowered to have more agency in your life. It will also happen that some tensions and pain you have learned to ignore or sedate become more evident. Often this can be misinterpreted as an unwanted side effect of yogic practice, but the opposite is true. *Growing in sensitivity empowers you to clearly notice the irritants that distract you.* Only if you notice them will you be able to address and release them.

Learn to clarify the significant difference between uncovering existing afflictions and creating new ones. With fewer tensions and distractions, your presence grows; and when distractions happen, you can face them with less agitation, less complaining, and less drama. Attend to this process to ensure you are moving towards feeling greater calmness and evenness in your body, breath, mind, heart, and interactions.

What tensions do you experience regularly?

How do you deal with them?

Is there a growing feeling of peace and calmness within you?

What disrupts your inner peace?

Are there patterns in those disruptions?

AFFLICTIONS AND THEIR REMOVAL

2.3 The afflictions include not knowing who I am (*avidya*), misidentification (*asmita*), likes (*raga*), dislikes (*dvesha*) and fear of death (*abhinivesa*).

2.4 Ignorance of my nature (*avidya*) is the field where the other afflictions sprout. The afflictions can be dormant, weak, intermittent, or fully active.

Yogic action is focused on removing obstructions, inefficiencies, and distractions in body, mind, emotions, and interactions. Many of the obstacles each one of us faces are self-inflicted. As Sri Swami Satchidananda eloquently stated, "You are your own best friend as well as your worst enemy" (1990). Sutra 2.3 echoes the message at the beginning of Chapter One of the Yoga Sutra, that we are either abiding in the ground of our being (1.3), or erroneously misidentifying with the experiences that we have (1.4). In 2.3 Patañjali indicates that the afflictions arise from forgetting or misunderstanding who you really are. In the Who Am I? chapter, you explored the difference between who you think you are and who you truly are. From the brief summaries of the yoga sutra and from the previous chapter, you may remember that the whole practice is focused on releasing your attachment to the temporary aspects of your experience so that you can align with the lasting ground of your being, the aspect of you underlying your whole existence. **The main obstacle presented in these aphorisms is not knowing who we really are.** More precisely, this major obstacle, *avidya*, is forgetting that everything you can see and experience – including your body, your emotions, and your thoughts – is life expressing itself through your organism. As it is characteristic of life, these temporary events are changing continuously. They come and go. In contrast, the *awareness* animating your body and mind is the spark enabling you to notice. Awareness may be obscured by your constant doings, but it is always there. Awareness is what makes it possible for you to be present. Awareness is the spaciousness that you are. Awareness manifests as calmness, stillness, and oneness, and you experience it unconsciously during dreamless deep sleep, semiconsciously in the transitions into and out of sleep, and consciously during meditation. One example that can illuminate this dichotomy is looking at yourself in the mirror. If you observe your reflection in a mirror regularly, you will notice that some of the physical features are changing. This may be more evident by looking at an old photograph of you. The changes can be difficult to ignore. At the same time, there is something in the experience of being you that has remained the same. This part cannot be seen, touched, or smelled, yet it is there. It has been with you all along. *Can that unchanging aspect be the awareness that enables you to notice everything that happens internally and externally?*

Being established in true knowledge of who you are prevents you from misidentifying with the temporary phenomena you perceive (*avidya*). Identifying with those temporary phenomena you slip into self-centeredness (*asmita*) and get caught in the constant struggle of trying to bring toward you what you like (*raga*) and trying to avoid or push away what you dislike (*dvesha*). Cravings and attachments, combined with aversions and resistance, continue to feed your sense of who you think you are. *This influence is so strong that you end up believing that you are the transient experiences you go through.* This is an endless cycle in which attachment to the play of likes and dislikes grows into a sense of self-importance that feeds into the strongest instinctual aversion, the fear of dying (*abhinivesha*). This fear is strong, even in the wisest among us. These afflictions relate to the five ways of being (*vrttis*) presented at the beginning of Chapter One: correct knowledge, misunderstanding, imagination, memory, and sleep. Once you veer away from presence, when you forget who you really are and identify with the fleeting sensory stimuli, you pass from knowledge (*pramana*) to incorrect knowledge (*viparyaya*), to inhabiting the realm of your imagination (*vikalpa*), which feeds on memories (*smrti*) and plays out in your dreams (*nidra*).

Most people have a combination of afflictions, and they may be manifest and fully active or they may be in different stages of activity. Just like a seed that may take from a few days to germinate and sprout and then months or years to develop fully, afflictions can be latent, barely noticeable, sporadic, or undeniably present. In the next sutras, you can explore each one of these potential sources of suffering. As you continue, keep in mind that each one can be in any of these four states of expression.

If you reflect on how you invest your energy and time every day, can you notice clearly who you think you are?

Is who you think you are serving you, or are you serving that identity?

What do you try to attract and what do you reject?

What aspects of you keep being pulled by your likes and dislikes?

How much energy do you invest in pursuing what you desire and rejecting what you dislike?

Are your identity, likes and dislikes conducive to your conscious and deliberate participation in your life?

Is it possible for you to be at peace with the undeniable fact that one day you are going to die?

2.5 To mistake what is impermanent as permanent, impure as pure, painful as blissful, and the non-self as the Self is ignorance (*avidya*).

Ignorance (*avidya*) is the root obstacle that causes confusion and misidentification. *Avidya* is not knowing your true nature. As the previous aphorism pointed out, all the other afflictions grow in the field of ignorance. This is so important that the definition of yoga in Chapter One of the Yoga Sutra is followed by the explanation in sutras 1.3 and 1.4, which says that you either know your nature through your direct experience or you erroneously misidentify with your ways of being. That explains why earlier in the journey, in the Who Am I? chapter, you explored ways of establishing a connection to your true nature, because the quality of that connection determines the quality of every experience you have. In addition, as aphorism 1.4 suggests, when you are not aware of your ways of being, you end up believing that you are the temporary activities you engage in. In other words, *avidya*, forgetting your true nature, causes you to get entangled in stories and imagination such as who you think you should be, who you think others expect you to be, what you think other people will think if you were to do this or that, and similar nonsense. The yoga journey consists of meeting yourself where you are just as you are.

Your body, mind, emotions, thoughts, and preferences, like everything around you, keep changing, all the time. However, not recognizing this undeniable fact can lead you to think: "Since I have been on many Tuesdays before, I know what will happen today because it is Tuesday." You may also assume that you still have many Tuesdays ahead of you. These two assumptions fail to acknowledge that each day is a unique day that will not be repeated, and that nobody knows how many more days he or she may have left. Even when people are young and healthy, it is impossible to know how many more days, weeks, or years they may have. Rather than seeing this as a pessimistic perspective, it is a way to motivate yourself to make your actions matter, because today is the only day when you can act, and because as soon as you take your incorrect assumptions as correct knowledge you lose the urgency to be present in this moment. Consequently, it is easy to forget that this moment is the culmination of every moment before it, and that this moment is also the starting point for the rest of your life. These faulty assumptions also give you permission to not pay attention, opening the door for entertaining yourself with endless inner talk.

A good point of departure for contemplation is this: Every time that you meet yourself where you are, you are meeting a different version of you. Yet is there something that remains unchanged? Other useful questions to move towards the opposite of ignorance include:
What in you is permanent?

What in you is impermanent?

What is pure and what impure?

How do you know the difference?

Has it ever happened that something that used to give you great enjoyment later became a source of pain?

Is it possible that overindulging in something you love may quickly turn into a source of agitation?

At the end of each day, in order to fall asleep, what do you let go of?

What remains?

2.6 Confusing awareness with my body, mind and emotions results in self-centeredness (*asmita*).

A sense of "I" develops when the *instruments* of seeing (your body and mind) are confused with the *power* of seeing, the awareness that enables any and all perception. Your body, mind, and emotions change constantly. Your environment is also changing continuously, and all your actions are part of these endless ongoing transformations. Moreover, body, mind, and emotions have the tendency to develop habits – your ways of being. If you are not aware of those habits, opinions, and stories, you may not notice how they shape and influence your perception, actions, and interactions. If you grow up hearing that the world is a dangerous place where everybody is trying to take advantage of you, you are likely to develop a different attitude than a person who grows up hearing that cooperation and interconnectedness are what have made it possible for human beings to thrive and prosper. The ways of being that are active in your system will also influence the affliction in this sutra, *asmita* or self-centeredness. *Asmita* consists of associating your sense of being with who you think you are, with the stories that you and others have created in your head. Quite possibly, many of the distractions arising during your daily activities and yoga practice are directly related to who you think you are or should be.

To inquire into your true nature, you can re-visit the techniques in the Who Am I? chapter and in sutras 1.3, 1.4 and 1.5. You may also explore the following questions:
Are there any parts of your body that do not change?
Are there any thoughts or beliefs in your mind that never change?
Are there some emotions in you that are always present without ever changing?
Is there something in you that is not temporary?
When you look at yourself in the mirror, is there a part of you that has remained the same throughout the years?
When you are asleep, where does your awareness of body, thoughts and emotions go?
What is left then?

You may also investigate if there are some misperceptions distorting who you think you are, such as "I am not good enough," "I am not complete," "I am lacking" and "I do not deserve unconditional love."

2.7 Craving enjoyment is desire (*raga*).

2.8 Rejecting pain is aversion (*dvesha*).

Identifying with the instruments of sensation and perception (body, mind, emotions, and memories) contributes to create a sense of "I." Naturally, this "I" develops affinities for the experiences you find enjoyable and dislike for the sensations that create discomfort and pain. Therefore, you will crave enjoyable experiences and you will resist or avoid uncomfortable sensations. It is very likely that these tendencies will grow into habitual patterns. These two sutras present the two afflictions of likes (*raga*) and dislikes (*dvesha*). *They are afflictions when they get in the way of just being with what is.* In fact, likes and dislikes may become the filters through which you approach yourself, your circumstances, your experiences, and your relationships. Eventually, likes and dislikes end up deeply influencing your ideas, motivations, and actions. Your likes and dislikes may define who you think you are and can even become the conditions that preclude you from accepting this moment as it is and yourself just as you are. Confirming the notion that a sutra is a continuous conceptual thread unifying a whole text, these two aphorisms can be seen as related to the idea of *vairagya* presented in sutra 1.15, where *vairagya* is freedom from all your likes and dislikes. It is quite possible that your *thoughts* about what you like and dislike differ from your *actual experiences* of those situations and circumstances.

Consider:

Has it ever happened to you that something you worried about eventually happened, without being as devastating as you had imagined? Have you ever found that something that was "supposed to make everything ok" did not seem to have that effect?

Was there ever a time when the effect of an accomplishment may have not lasted as long as you thought it would?

Has it ever happened that something that you once considered a pleasure later became a source of suffering?

Are you in charge of your likes and dislikes, or are they driving your decisions and actions?

What is the origin of your wanting and cravings?

Are some of your actions guided by a sense of scarcity or neediness?

To what extent do fear, anger and judgment motivate your decisions and actions?

To what extent do you believe that your likes and dislikes define who you are?

Where do your likes and dislikes go when you are asleep?

Is there any time during your day when you are free from all your preferences?

2.9 Even the wise develop a sense of self-importance that causes attachment to living and fear of dying.

Based on the previous sutras, the text argues that our misunderstanding of our nature (*avidya*) leads us to mistakenly associating ourselves with our thoughts about who we think we are (*asmita*). Consequently, we develop likes and cravings (*raga*) as well as dislikes and aversions (*dvesha*). The more invested we are in our identity, with all the ideas and activities associated with it, the greater our attachment to our life. This natural survival instinct is the strongest instinct in all living beings. *The stronger our identification with our body, our mind, and our emotions, the more we cling to our life.* Regardless of how much information or knowledge we accumulate, attachment to our life remains strong. The traditional commentary on this sutra argues that fear of dying is very strong in all of us, even though we have not had the direct experience of dying. Vyasa, the author of that commentary, makes the case for reincarnation by saying our fear of dying stems from having experienced the sharp pangs of death before. This notion and its implications may be an interesting point of departure for reflection.

The concept of life is a fertile ground for contemplation.
What is your life?
Is your life the elusive energy that enables you to breathe, move, and think?
Is your life the fleeting sensory experiences that you have had?
Is your life the memories of previous moments you consider important?

Is your life the predictions you have about what you will do in the future?
Is your life your possessions?
Your ideas?
Your memories?
Your accomplishments?
Or the legacy you think you will leave behind?

As you truly ponder these questions, notice where your attachments to life come from. *Is it from ideas that you have about who you are or should be (asmita)? Do your attachments arise from your likes (raga) and dislikes (dvesha)?*

It can be useful to also explore these questions:

Do you live your life with a tacit assumption that your embodied life will last for a long time?

Does that unspoken assumption influence your attitudes and actions and how you live your life?

For instance, if you assume that you still have a long life ahead of you, does that give you permission to procrastinate?

What happens if you contemplate the fact that nobody knows how long he or she will be alive? (Some people view this question as sad and dismal. Others see it as a powerful motivation to make each moment count.)

Can you reflect on the fact that sooner or later you will die?

Can you come to terms with the inevitable decay of your physical body?

Can you also see that millions of people before you have lived and died and that life itself has continued?

Is it possible that there is no concept opposite to life and, that death instead of being the opposite of life, is the opposite of birth?

You may also consider another line of inquiry:

What is the most important moment of your life?

Is it some moment in your past that you either cling to because it was momentous (*raga*), or that you want to forget because it caused you to suffer (*dvesha*)?

Is the most important moment of your life some moment that has not happened yet?

If the most important moment in your life is in the past or the future, that moment exists only in your memory.

Keep in mind the paradox that every time you immerse in your memories and plans, you are stepping outside the ongoing flow of your life. You are ignoring the only moment where you can embody your life through your actions. *What would it take to make the present moment, every single unique here and now moment, the most important moment of your life?*

2.10 Subtle afflictions dissolve when the sense of being merges into pure awareness.

In Chapter One of the Yoga Sutra, Patañjali offered a definition of yoga followed by a list of the ways of being that keep us from embodying presence. Then, Patañjali suggested a method to regulate our ways of being. In this chapter Patañjali follows a similar logic. First, he gives the definition of yogic action with its goals, followed by a list of the sources of pain that can be removed through those actions. Aphorism 2.4 continues by saying that all these sources of suffering listed in sutra 2.3 originate in not remembering who you are and that these afflictions exist in varying levels of manifestation from dormant to fully active. The chapter continues by suggesting ways to regulate those sources of affliction. These five sources of suffering (*klesha*) in 2.3 are present throughout your day, at least to some extent. When you drop all your stories, opinions, and ideas about who you are – as well as who you used to be or who you should be – all of these afflictions dissolve. This is what happens when you are in deep sleep. In order to sleep, you must release your worries, plans, and to-do lists. Once you let go of what you do not need, you fall asleep and there is no notion of inside and outside, I and other. During sleep the grip of self-centeredness, likes, dislikes, and self-importance softens. During dreaming some of those afflictions are still active as the subconscious mind tries to make sense of all of them. In dreamless deep sleep the afflictions dissolve. At the most fundamental level, not being clear on who you are (that is, misidentification with what is temporary) is the source of the challenges that most of us face. Sutras 2.10 and 2.11 present two ways of dealing with these afflictions.

As mentioned in sutra 2.2, yogic actions decrease afflictions. Sutra 2.3 enumerated the different states of the afflictions: dormant, weak, intermittent, and active. This sutra proposes a way for removing the afflictions that have been diminished to a subtle level of manifestation. This deactivation process is called involution (*pratiprasava*). Involution refers to reversing the process of evolution of the afflictions. Combining the ideas in 1.3 and 1.4 with those in sutras 2.3 to 2.9 helps us to understand this process better. In your natural state (1.3) there is no misidentification with your sensations and perceptions (1.4). The misidentification is forgetting your own nature (*avidya* in 2.4 and 2.5). Misidentification results in developing a sense of "I" as separate from the rest of existence (*asmita* in 2.6). Consequently, the sense of "I" develops preferences in the form of likes (*raga* 2.7) and dislikes (*dvesha* 2.8). Entangled in the sense of self and its preferences, a sense of self-importance grows generating attachment to embodied experiences and fear of dying (*abhinivesha* 2.9).

Remember from the second chapter of this book that *the process of yoga is an invitation to observe yourself as clearly as possible, including observing your responses to everything that comes your way.* These observations are likely to reveal some patterns (*citta vrtti*, your ways of being) in your body, breath, mind, emotions, actions, and interactions. Then, you can choose to keep the ways of being that are supportive of being present and discard the unhelpful patterns, if even just for a few moments. Similarly, observing your patterns of thought, emotion, action, and interaction can help you notice how the five afflictions may be underlying the patterns you observe. The first step in the involution process is to turn around the development of self-importance that manifests as clinging to life (*abhinivesha*). For instance, every time that you notice your opinions, either internally or externally, you may ask yourself "Who cares about my opinions?" or "Who is asking for my opinion?" You can also reflect on the extent to which you offer your opinion to support your perceived authority and position. It was mentioned before that feeling that we are busy with many responsibilities can be one way of feeling important. Often, this can manifest as feeling that you are indispensable and that the world will stop if you are not handling or managing some situation or project. *Does that happen with you? Similarly, is it possible that believing that you can control the world outside betrays an undercurrent of self-importance?*

The second stage in this process of involution is to notice your relationship with your likes (*raga*) and dislikes (*dvesha*). By observing what you favor as well as what you avoid, you can see the deeper connections between what you grasp and some part of your sense of self linked to that grasping and holding.

What are the thoughts, emotions, movements, activities, and interactions you favor?

Which ones do you avoid or reject?

What are the roots of your preferences?

Can you clarify why you seem to like some things?

Can you notice any patterns in what you dislike?

Another effective method consists of investigating what you dislike by sitting in a comfortable and relaxed way, closing your eyes and summoning a recent event that caused you *minor* discomfort, embarrassment, or uneasiness. As you feel this tolerable discomfort, you will likely notice a tendency to generate stories, opinions and excuses or an inclination to ignore, reject or try to solve the "problem." You may choose instead to be curious about just feeling the sensations that emerge. This can be a powerful way of understanding yourself while also releasing some of the accumulated impressions and drama that most of us carry with us. This simple practice can deliver insight into your own ways of being and the triggers that generate reactivity. This insight can offer you a simple and effective way to deactivate some of those triggers.

The third stage is to gain greater clarity on who you think you are (*asmita*). The exercises "Who do you think you are?" (page 80) and "Clarify - What is important to me?" (page 113) offer you ways to explore your sense of identity. Each one of us develops an identity according to our upbringing, family, education, and society. Our identity manifests as the filters we use to interpret and relate to ourselves, to the people around us, to institutions, and to the society that we participate in. Although we may think that our identity is quite fixed, our identity, like almost everything about us, is a work in progress, with some aspects of it changing all the time. For instance, if you derive a large portion of your identity from your occupation, losing your jobs can trigger an existential crisis, partly because you will be forced to modify your sense of identity. It's the same for people who think their possessions define them: if they lose those possessions, they feel devastated. Being forced to confront these kinds of deeply held self-beliefs can generate a deep personal transformation.

A useful line of contemplation includes determining what makes you who you are. Then try to connect to who you were before, when your circumstances and situation were different. You may also imagine what would happen if your situation changed and some of the things that define you were to suddenly disappear. Notice any changes in your internal emotional environment. This inquiry can be expanded to explore the fears and anxieties that you may have. To what extent do your fears relate to who you think you are or should be? These fears and anxieties may also be connected to what you think other people expect or think of you and of your actions. Additionally, our ideas often seem to play a major role in our sense of who we are. Yet it can be an excellent opportunity for reflection to try to uncover the origin of some of those ideas. It is surprising how many of "our" ideas may not have originated in us. Finally, *is it possible that most of your sense of identity dissolves at the end of each day, with only faint traces remaining in your subconscious?*

The last stage in this involution process is best summarized in the exercise: "What is my true nature?" (page 85). In this stage you try to connect to the basic essence of your being, I AM. This approach was hinted at in the commentary on aphorism 1.35. One way of practicing is to sit in stillness with comfortable stability repeating silently, I AM, I AM, I AM, I AM, without trying to comment or generate stories, returning again and again to this most essential statement about you. During these explorations, be curious to notice how your usual distractions and internal stories may relate to your sense of identity. One more question to ponder: *What is the subtlest aspect of you?*

2.11 When the afflictions manifest as ways of being (*vrtti*), they are counteracted through meditation.

After learning about ways to deactivate the subtle forms of affliction, this sutra indicates that meditation is the tool to remove active afflictions. In other words, meditation (a complete focus and presence with what is) is used to counteract the patterns in your ways of moving, breathing, thinking, feeling, perceiving, and interacting. This is, for most people, a continual process where you try to be with what is and notice that you get distracted, over and over again. That was what Patañjali suggested in sutra 1.14 when talking about practice (*abhyasa*) as a continuous long-term endeavor. The key is to keep returning to this moment without struggle, strain, or self-judgment, until you develop a new way of being. This new and beneficial habit enables you to observe clearly, without letting self-importance (*abhiniveshα*), dislikes (*dvesha*), likes (*raga*) or your ideas about who you are (*asmita*) cause you to forget (*avidya*) that you are embodied awareness. This process of meditation was described in sutras 1.17 and 1.43-1.46. Because of being established in meditation, as indicated in aphorisms 1.47 to 1.51, unwavering awareness invites wisdom, creating a new way of being that neutralizes and deactivates all remaining impressions allowing you to be integrated, instead of fragmented by the tensions of internal conflict.

To apply aphorism 2.11, remember that meditation is the single pointedness of being with what is (1.32), or meeting yourself where you are, just as you are. When one of these five sources of pain appears, observing with clear awareness dispels the confusion generated by not really knowing your true nature. Intensity of focus is balanced through an open hearted and compassionate perspective, as suggested in sutra

1.33. Indeed, when trying to be present, in life or in formal meditation, all the distractions that arise most likely belong to one of these five categories of afflictions: confusion about your true nature, thoughts related to who you think you are, cravings for what you like, resisting what you dislike, and preoccupation about your health or even your own eventual demise. These distractions are teachers that offer you specific ways to grow in presence, despite whatever comes your way. Other fruitful avenues for counteracting these sources of suffering include cultivating gratitude, self-love and compassion. *What afflictions emerge during your meditation?*

Karma

2.12 These afflictions (*kleshas*) are the source of an accumulation of impressions (*samskaras*) that influence present and future experiences (*karma*).

2.13 Determining birth, lifespan, and quality of life experiences.

2.14 Producing pleasant and unpleasant experiences according to virtues and defects.

These three sutras explain the concept of *karma*. *Karma* in Sanskrit means action. Every action creates an echo that ripples out through the interconnectedness of all that exists. Additionally, every thought, every intention, and every action generate an impression (*samskara*) in you. The emotions that emerge as a result act as stimuli that strengthen your cravings, your resistance, your self-importance, and your sense of who you are. These impressions are stored consciously and unconsciously in the core of your being. Patañjali refers to this body of impressions as the store of *karma* (*karmashaya*). Each impression becomes a seed, influencing your future thoughts, intentions, and actions. For instance, when you are upset and have something to eat, it is likely that what you taste may be unconsciously associated with your mood; and possibly, in the future, every time that you eat the same thing, it will influence your mood, or the taste may remind you of that occasion when you were upset. Sutra 2.13 says that these afflictions (*kleshas*) and related impressions (*samskaras*) influence not only your current life but also the conditions of future embodiments. According to the originating actions, the resulting experiences will be pleasant or unpleasant (2.14). Consequently, the seeds of new impressions will be planted, perpetuating an ongoing cycle that ends up determining how your life progresses. As you consider this process, it is important to remember that when you are distracted from the present moment, by either thinking about the past or trying to predict the future, you may not even be aware of what you are doing. As a result, in addition to cultivating a tendency towards distractedness, you may be completely oblivious to some of the seeds you are planting, and you may be surprised by the effects of previous actions you were not even cognizant of.

You can gain insight into this process as you observe your life choices. For instance, recalling specific moments in your past, you can see some of the choices and decisions that influenced your identity, perspective, and circumstances. You can also notice how all those elements combined to create likes, dislikes, restrictions, and opportunities. As you contemplate the various stages of your life, aided by the perspective of time, you can see what you have made important.

Staying out of the tendency to take personally what is currently happening in your life can enable you to witness the seeds that you are planting and how they will generate similar thoughts and actions in the future. As you reflect on your life, contemplate the fact that anything that you do regularly will add to your ways of being, perceiving, and interpreting the world. If you spend a whole day saying, "I hate this, I hate that, I hate…," your own internal environment will feel quite different from when you spend your whole day saying, "I am at peace with this, I am at peace with that, I am at peace with…." As a simple experiment, you may even try these two options, each one for only a few minutes, to notice the effect of each on your attitude, outlook, and internal environment. Some other useful questions to live with include:
What motivates this intention?
What are my expectations for this action?
To what extent am I creating a new craving or new source of resistance?
Does this action increase my sense of self-importance?
How is this thought contributing to clarify who I am?
How are my current circumstances related to some of my past actions?
How am I contributing to enhance the quality of life where I am?

Suffering

2.15 The discerning person knows that all internal activities and experiences resulting from the mutability of nature (*gunas*) will eventually cause pain and suffering.

Most scholars associate Patañjali's Yoga Sutra with the ancient *Samkhya* philosophy. In the *Samkhya* system, the concept of *guna* –

attribute or feature – describes three fundamental tendencies in nature. The three *gunas* are inertia (*tamas*), energy (*rajas*), and harmony (*sattva*). When these three qualities are in balance, they exist as pure potential. Everything in nature is, at a very subtle level, the manifestation of a combination of these three tendencies. Life is an ongoing process of change resulting from the endless play between these attributes. However, each moment is unique, irreplaceable, and unrepeatable. Knowing this is a powerful reminder that *all experiences and sensations are temporary*. Strong desire for some experience or object will generate lots of emotions and expectations. The underlying assumption is that fulfilling that desire will solve your problems by making you better, more complete, and whole. But the joy of obtaining what you desire can soon turn into a new reason for anxiety, insecurity, and fear, because you may switch from trying to get what you want to trying to prevent losing what you have gained. **Becoming attached to any experience by trying to grasp it or to reject it is bound to generate suffering.** Does it ever happen to you that you keep longing for something wonderful that happened before, but that is now long gone? Does that ever bring a feeling of sadness and a desire to go back in time? Is that an example of something that was once pleasurable but has become a source of suffering? In present times, marketing and advertising seem to be almost exclusively focused on creating the illusion of fulfillment and satisfaction from objects and experiences that can be bought or sold. This is a powerful force that many of us are exposed to on a regular basis, and it leaves many impressions in our minds and hearts. *However, the wise person knows that anything that can be gained will eventually be lost and that anything that can be bought or sold is unlikely to provide lasting joy and happiness.*

Examine your own words and thoughts and notice any underlying assumptions based on the notion that once you gain something you will become a better version of you, or that your life will be somehow more fulfilling or meaningful. Is that really possible? Inquire into your desires. What do you think you will gain by what you desire? Sometimes we may want something and keep working towards it. However, it may take a long time to reach that goal, and by the time we achieve our objective we may have forgotten what we wanted or may have changed our mind and become distracted by a new desire. Has this ever happened to you? From this perspective, examine your relationship to what is part of your life now. Is there anything that you thought you wanted (like a job, title, relationship, or object) that is no longer what you want? You may also want to explore the extent to which you might be afraid of losing what you own. One more useful path of exploration is to contemplate this question: *What would it take for you to love your life exactly as it is right now?* When you decide to love your life exactly as it is, what objections arise? What do these objections reveal about you?

2.16 Future suffering can be avoided.

Confirming the famous anonymous saying "pain is inevitable, suffering is optional," in this aphorism Patañjali states that future suffering is optional because it can be avoided. In your daily life, it may sometimes feel like you are riding an emotional rollercoaster. It takes you to the heights of exhilaration, spins you around into excitement and then brings you to the lows of pain and suffering. The emotional rollercoaster keeps going all the time. It results from allowing your internal climate to be influenced by external events and circumstances. Many of us know that a turn in the weather, depending on what it is, can make us feel sad, happy, or anxious. Similarly, you may interpret somebody's words as a reason to feel happy or unhappy. But is it really possible to avoid suffering? Remember that there is a distinction between pain and suffering. Pain is discomfort, soreness or ache, a sensation that you experience. Suffering is when you charge that sensation with emotion and keep dwelling on it in ways that generate distress, hopelessness, and helplessness. The pain you feel is a sensation that offers you potentially useful information. Is it possible to choose what to do with that information? Is pain the result of an action, belief, or opinion you hold? Is it possible that suffering results from a story that you have chosen to believe? Does your suffering originate from unwillingness to be with what is, just as it is?

Recall that even what used to be a source of happiness or pleasure can become a new source of worry, anxiety, and suffering. It happens often that a person can start creating reasons to suffer just by thinking about what might happen in the future. Ask yourself:

Are you already anxious, upset or irritated by something that has not happened yet?

Are there things you worried about in the past that never happened?

To what extent are your expectations and predictions influencing your inner climate?

Could this sutra be a helpful reminder of the message in this saying: "If your problems have a solution, why worry? And if your problems have no solution, why worry?"

One important clarification to keep in mind: This aphorism **DOES NOT say to ignore pain, emotions, or sensations**. This sutra is not about becoming insensitive or unresponsive. Pain, emotions, and sensations offer useful feedback, foregrounding the interrelations between your inner world and your external world in a continuous feedback loop. As we discussed in the Validate section of the Foundations of Yoga chapter, rather than trying to manipulate your sensations, it may be more useful to start by recognizing that whatever you are feeling is valid, because you are feeling it. As a whole human being, you have a complete range of healthy emotions helping you navigate your life. Once you recognize what you are feeling as valid, then you can clarify if any action is needed. In fact, in yoga the goal is to sense and to feel in order to become aware through your direct experience of what is happening, without getting entangled in words, stories, and drama. This clarity is instrumental to determining the most effective path of action. This sutra is a reminder that anything that is alive is in constant change, and that trying to attach your sense of self, your likes and dislikes, to something that is changing will guarantee frustration and suffering. *Knowing this, is it possible to choose not to suffer?*

2.17 The cause of the suffering that can be avoided is the tendency to conflate awareness with what is experienced.

This is a key aphorism to understanding the cause of the suffering that can be avoided mentioned in the previous sutra. Suffering is the result of confusing your awareness, your sense of being, with the vehicle of awareness – your organism. Whatever you experience, whatever you can sense, is felt through your organism, through your body, mind, and emotions. The awareness that enables you to witness these processes is what brings consciousness to all that you experience. The experiences themselves, however, are temporary and ever-changing. These activities and experiences result from being alive and interacting with your environment. As was said before, in sutras 1.3 and 1.4, you either abide in your true nature, embodied awareness, or you may identify with your ways of being, meaning that you may think that you are your doing and becoming. In this aphorism, Patañjali further clarifies that it is precisely this misidentification – combining the vehicles for experiencing (your body, thoughts, and emotions) with the awareness that notices all experiencing – that generates suffering. These ideas from Chapter One and Chapter Two of the Yoga Sutra are connected to sutras 2.3 to 2.9, particularly the notions about not remembering your true nature, *avidya* (2.4).

Contemplate the fact that every night, in order to fall asleep, you let go of all that you usually have on your mind. As you drift into deep dreamless sleep you let go of worries, fears, memories, stories as well as whatever you believe in or think you know. You also let go of your name, your age, your occupation, the balance in your bank account, and everything else. *You even let go completely of who you think you are.* Despite letting go of all of this, including your own body awareness, you do not disappear. In fact, letting go of all those identifications creates for most people a sense of spaciousness and openness, because those identifications generate bindings and boundaries that manifest physically, mentally, and emotionally. This state of being unencumbered by all these temporary distractions is often called the natural state. When the identifications are released, the awareness that animates your body and that also enables you to think, feel, see, and interact, is what remains. That awareness is consciousness flowing through you. That awareness uses the body and all experiences as an instrument, yet it is not the instrument.

Yoga is a journey leading you to connect to ever increasing levels of subtlety in your own being. Try this: Every night as you prepare to sleep, consciously choose to let go of all that you will not need during your sleep. Gradually relax into feeling the subtlest aspect of you, from your body, to your breath, to your thoughts and emotions until finally you are only aware of your sensations with no internal commentary or narration. As you experience being, notice that there are sensations as well as awareness registering those sensations without having to qualify them in any way. In fact, you may notice that there are overlapping streams of sensations from sounds and noises outside your abode, to sounds and noises inside your own room, to sounds and noises inside your own body. Simultaneously there may be streams of touch sensations like the texture of whatever is touching your body. You may choose to notice each individual stream from external to internal. Try to just feel each one without describing or narrating. Then try to notice what is the vantage point from where you are witnessing all of this.

In the morning, as soon as you realize that you are awake, even before you open your eyes, notice to what extent your usual internal comments are active. Can you be interested in observing what happens if you keep a gentle connection to the calmness and silence that underlie all your thoughts, beliefs, and stories? In the process of releasing thoughts and opinions, notice what are the thoughts that keep coming back or that seem to be more deeply rooted. Explore with curiosity the possibility of choosing which beliefs, opinions, and ideas you want to turn on and which ones you want to turn off.
What do you discover?

Are some of those thoughts related to who you think you are (*asmita*), to your likes (*raga*) and dislikes (*dvesha*) and to your sense of self-importance (*abhinivesha*)?

How do these thoughts contribute to the quality of your presence?

Are these thoughts life-affirming?

Awareness & Experiences

2.18 What can be perceived has three attributes: activity (*kriya*), steadiness (*sthiti*) and illumination (*prakasha*). It manifests in the elements and sense organs in order to provide experiences leading to liberation.

As suggested in the previous aphorism, there are two different aspects interacting, your awareness, which is your sense of being, and what you experience, the actual sensations that make up everything you experience. Suffering is the result of confusing your awareness, the knowing that enables you to experience, with the experiences that you have. It is like confusing your reading glasses with your eyes. This melding causes suffering because of the human tendency to identify with fleeting experiences and their by-products, the desire to retain (*raga*) or reject (*dvesha*) them. As a result, confusing awareness with what is experienced will trigger an endless stream of emotions and feelings. Anything and everything that can be experienced is either active (*kriya*), resting (*sthiti*) or in a state of equilibrium between activity and inertia (*prakasha*). Your body is part of what can be experienced. It includes the systems that make up the body as well as the capacity to perceive the endless combinations of the tendencies in nature. When you conflate the experiences with the awareness witnessing them, you may believe that all that there is in life is to chase after experiences, because the experiences provide you with a sense of identity. On the other hand, you can choose to see all experiences as vehicles offering a pathway to deepen your clarity. This clarity leads to liberation from misidentification and its effects. This is the process of *vairagya* explained in sutras 1.15 and 1.16. This liberation happens, like all processes in yoga and in life, gradually. For instance, sutra 1.15 says that the first step is to release all cravings for externalities. Eventually, says sutra 1.16, awareness settles, not chasing after the senses and remaining anchored in pure awareness. This process happens at the pace each practitioner can handle and in accordance to her level of commitment. There are no shortcuts. You can try to start by freeing yourself from misidentifications and misperceptions, as well as by freeing yourself from adding unnecessary opinions to what is. When free from all opinions, then it is possible to see without the biases created by your opinions, beliefs, likes, and dislikes. Then you can experience everything as it is, instead of as you think it is, or should be.

Is it possible to notice how these three attributes of activity, steadiness, and balance, are present in every experience you have?

Can you notice those attributes as well in your own body?

To what extent do these variations in the attributes of experience influence your outlook and attitude?

Are your experiences creating more attachments and reactivity, or are they creating greater clarity? Do these questions have a larger underlying theme related to your life purpose?

2.19 The states of the three attributes (*gunas*) change from unmanifest to manifest to subtle to apparent.

The previous aphorism and this one can be understood as a very concise way of summarizing how nature operates. The unmanifest is a state of pure potential that cannot be apprehended through the senses. The manifest is the specific information needed for the development of that potential into something in the world not yet available to the senses. The subtle is the kernel charged with specific information needed to bring potentiality into fruition. And the apparent is the actual object that occupies space and has perceivable characteristics such as color, texture, smell, and taste. Think of a tree as an example: from the pure potential of the concept of the tree (unmanifest), to the complete genetic code of a particular tree (manifest), to one specific seed (subtle) sprouting in the right environment and circumstances conducive to developing into an actual tree (apparent). The involution process of meditation is a progression from the apparent to the subtle to the manifest to the unmanifest, as it was presented in sutra 1.17.

One way of exploring these ideas is by contemplating the process of something you have accomplished or acquired from its fruition to the very beginning of the process when the first idea about it came into your mind. As you contemplate these processes, you may gain insight into the origin of some of your wants and desires – as well as insight into the ways in which you move an idea forward into action. Similarly, contemplating the process of a project or endeavor that was not successful can offer you greater clarity into how some of your beliefs, biases, and choices may have influenced the outcome of the project.

You may also explore the meaning of this sutra by reflecting on how life can manifest in apparent ways as something that can be perceived directly through your senses. Then, you shift your focus to subtle aspects of life that may not be available to the senses but are available to your intellect and emotion (like the cellular activities taking place in any living being or the atomic and subatomic activities happening everywhere at all times). You continue by deepening your focus into the manifest aspect of life, the intricate interrelations between all aspects of life, like whatever is shared by all beings in a species. (For instance, the humanness in all human beings on the planet throughout time.) You continue diving deeper by feeling directly the unmanifest aspect of life, its essence pervading all of existence. This life essence cannot be seen, touched, or apprehended through the senses in any way. *What happens when you examine anything through these lenses of apparent, subtle, manifest, and unmanifest? What do you discover?*

2.20 The Seer is pure. It is only the power of seeing that witnesses the activities of the body-mind-emotions without being affected by them.

The first sutra in this chapter defined yogic action (*kriya yoga*) and the second sutra stated that yogic action is effective for neutralizing afflictions and for moving towards integration. Subsequently, Patañjali elaborated on the various types of afflictions and their influences and long-term effects. Then, in 2.17, Patañjali states that the cause of suffering is to confuse awareness for the experiences that you participate in. Awareness is what enables you to participate in those experiences and to notice what happens both internally and externally. In this sutra the concept of the "Seer," first introduced in sutra 1.3, is expanded upon. The "Seer" or "Witness" is awareness, the power of seeing, or the knowing that enables you to witness the changing phenomena in nature. Another word used for it is consciousness, that which enables you to be conscious.

Awareness is just the power of seeing. This is the idea discussed in the Who Am I? chapter of this book using the analogy of the sky as well as the metaphor of a movie projector. Another way of thinking about this concept is by thinking about the operating system of a computer or smart phone. The operating system is the essential software that manages the memory, processes, and resources of the computer. Although the operating system may be installed in a computer, without a source of power providing electricity, the operating system cannot control the computer. Similarly, the computer may be plugged in to an energy source, but without an operating system, the computer would not be able to start any programs. Awareness or consciousness is your operating system. The electricity running through your organism is the vital energy of life, also called *prana* in yoga. When it is working well, the operating system can run any program, including showing videos and photographs, displaying text, or playing sound files. *However, the operating system is not influenced by the content of the files that it is manipulating.* Consciousness is similarly unaffected by the constant changes of life, yet consciousness underlies every one of your states, actions, and experiences. One option to recognize this Seer is to cultivate your ability to notice space in every place that you inhabit. Instead of seeing only the objects in a room as many of us tend to do, you can choose to attend also to the space around everything. You can notice space as the foundation where everything you perceive exists. You may also notice silence as the background of every noise and sound that you can hear. Notice the silence that marks the end of one word and the beginning of the next. As you notice movement, also notice the stillness in which the movement takes place. Attending to space, silence, and stillness is one way of developing a sensitivity to perceive what is so obvious that is routinely ignored. This sensitivity helps you orient towards the awareness or consciousness pervading all of existence. You can also relax deeply, letting go of all that you do not need, including your internal commentary, so that you can pay attention to the natural rhythm of your breath. Focus on feeling as clearly as possible the slight pause between each inhalation and each exhalation. *What do you notice when you witness that pause?*

Space, stillness, and silence are the background of all activity, the bedrock of consciousness, where all change, movement and sound take place. Without space, stillness, and silence, there would be no way of knowing that something is, that it is moving or that it is making a sound. *What happens when you choose to immerse fully in the pause, the silence and stillness?*

2.21 Everything that can be experienced exists for the benefit of the Seer.

This group of sutras talks about the complementary relationship between experience and awareness. While sutras 2.18 and 2.19 explain the world of experience, the previous sutra talks about the nature of awareness. This aphorism and the two aphorisms that follow explore the relationship and interaction between awareness and experiences. All experiences are in the realm of life. Consciousness, the ability to notice the experiences, is in constant interaction with life. In this context, life is anything and everything that can be experienced, seen, felt, touched, tasted, and heard. Consciousness, as mentioned in the previous sutra, is the power of knowing, the aspect of you that witnesses your actions and your ways of being. **It is useful to think of life as doing and awareness as being.**

Returning to the analogy of a movie projector, awareness is the light that is projected, and the film is life, what can be experienced. Even if the roll of film were going through the projector, if there were no light, the movie could not be seen. Likewise, without film there would be no story to see. Arguably the ultimate goal in yoga is to abide in pure awareness without ever getting entangled in identification with any experiences. From this viewpoint, as was presented in sutra 2.18, the purpose of each experience is to lead towards liberation from all misidentification. The purpose of every single frame in the roll of film is to pass in front of the light of the projector (awareness) to provide an opportunity for awareness to witness clearly the difference between life, temporary phenomena, and pure awareness – the knowing or presence at the core of all of existence. The complete set of individual frames is dynamic, resulting from past actions and their stored impressions (2.12-2.14). All experiences provide you with feedback for growing in your capacity to distinguish between life and consciousness.

Encounters between sound and silence, movement and stillness, space and objects are the ways that awareness and life come together all the time. Energy is the catalyst facilitating the interactions between life and awareness. You may choose between two distinct options: identifying with your experiences or releasing all identification and choosing to experience directly the spaciousness, stillness, and silence of pure awareness.

To what extent can you recognize these two options in your approach to your yoga practice?

Can you notice how you choose between these two options in your everyday life?

Are there any patterns in your choices?

What are the results of your choices?

Are there some thoughts and actions more conducive to connecting to your own awareness?

Would it be possible for all your experiences to be vehicles for recognizing your own awareness?

Is there a way to embody awareness so that your connection to the spaciousness, stillness and silence pervades all your actions?

2.22 Although worldly experiences do not exist any longer for the yogi who has reached liberation, the world remains. The world is real.

In the tradition of philosophy that yoga belongs to, there are competing views on the world. Some schools maintain that the world is real and that it can be apprehended by our senses, just as it is. Other perspectives propose that the world is an illusion, pervaded by a fundamental unchanging oneness manifesting as all that there is. Still other approaches indicate that everything consists of momentary impressions that keep changing with only emptiness underlying all of existence. Each one of these options suggests a different path of action. For instance, if you see the world as a very convincing illusion under which hides true reality, your path may require you to discard everything that you experience as an illusion keeping you from experiencing the underlying reality. If emptiness is all that there is, then your focus may be on the temporariness of all internal and external phenomena.

This sutra states that the world of experience is real, it is not something to be denied. In other words, life and consciousness coexist, with life offering experiences for the benefit of consciousness. As the previous aphorism suggested, life is a vehicle for awareness. Individual awareness can either identify with the fleeting experiences (1.4) or it can abide in its own true nature (1.3), consciousness. Anything that can be experienced is not an illusion or the product of your imagination. It is real. Yet it is impermanent; it does not last. All experiences serve the purpose of providing liberation for awareness. *The yogi is the person who has chosen to abide in awareness by liberating from their attachments to experiences.* Therefore, the world, although real, does not entice the yogi any longer to identify with the temporary comings and goings of experience. In other words, yogis participate in the world without taking it personally, doing their duty without expectations or attachments. As you try to practice this sutra consider:

What are the experiences that capture your attention?

What aspects of life define who you are?

Is there something that you previously identified with, but that no longer seems to define you?

How do you see the world, your experiences and your own awareness? What are the relationships between these three ideas?

How do your views influence your thoughts, emotions, actions and interactions?

DISCERNMENT

2.23 The reason for awareness and experiences to come together is to recognize what is permanent and what isn't.

In the previous sutras Patañjali explored the complementary aspects of existence, awareness, experiences, and their relationships. This aphorism states that awareness and experiences come together to clarify the distinction between what is enduring and what is temporary. Notice the direct connection of this idea to the definition of ignorance (*avidya*) in sutra 2.5. Your experiences are in constant change. You can always choose what you identify with, and what you make important in your life. Without experiences, there would be no opportunity for human beings to participate in the endless flow of life. It would not be possible to feel the wide range of sensations that life offers and there would be no lessons to learn. As it was mentioned in sutra 2.18, all that can be experienced can be seen as an end in itself, or it can serve as a vehicle to release the misidentifications that lead to suffering. Consider the following questions to explore the usefulness of this sutra for you and your life.

How are awareness and experiences coming together in your life?

What is your objective when you approach any project?

How do you decide what is worth your attention, time, and energy?

What in you is permanent?

What in you is impermanent?

Are your experiences contributing to clarify the distinctions between what is permanent and what is impermanent?

2.24 Identifying with experiences is confusion (*avidya*).

In the previous sutras Patañjali explained that future suffering can be avoided (2.16) and that suffering results from conflating experiences with awareness (2.17). Then Patañjali contrasted the essence of experiences with the essence of awareness. Sutra 2.23, reiterating the message from sutra 2.18, says that experiences and awareness come together to give us the opportunity to distinguish experiences from awareness. The meaning of this sutra is a reminder of the message presented in sutras 2.4 and 2.5: *avidya* is forgetting your true nature. Remember how at the beginning of the thread of the Yoga Sutra, in sutras 1.3 and 1.4, misidentification is contrasted with being in your natural state, a state of abiding in inner stillness and inner silence. The importance of this idea is highlighted in this sutra once again. When you believe that you are your experiences, your stories, and your body, you live in confusion. This misconception leads you to a never-ending cycle of suffering and afflictions. Ponder the following questions to bring this aphorism into your daily life:

As you live your life, how do you clarify the difference between your experiences and your awareness?

Pay attention every time that you use the pronouns "I," "me," "mine," "we," "us," and "ours". What do you notice?

What aspect of you does the pronoun refer to?

Do you use these words to underscore an aspect of your identity, or do you use them with a sense of detachment?

Does your use of these pronouns relate to the five categories of ways of being in sutra 1.5?

Are you using those pronouns because of one of the five afflictions listed in sutra 2.3?

2.25 Freedom arises from removing confusion.

Up until this point in this chapter Patañjali has explained yogic action as a way to decrease afflictions, describing the afflictions and their effects and the relationship between awareness and experiences. Now, Patañjali presents the goal of yoga practice, liberation from afflictions and suffering.

Consciousness is the power of seeing, or the knowing that enables you to be aware. Consequently, you witness the changing phenomena in nature. Consciousness underlies every one of your states, actions, and experiences. Life is what can be experienced and perceived, as well as the continuous stream of unpredictable changes taking place. Life and consciousness are not in conflict or opposition. On the contrary, life and consciousness complement one another. One traditional example for these interactions is that of the reflection of the full moon on the surface of a still lake, when it may seem like the moon is part of the lake. When there is agitation in the water, however, you cannot see the reflection of the moon, but the moon does not disappear. Similarly, when your activities, your ways of being, occupy all your internal environment, it may seem that there is no consciousness because your awareness is completely entangled in your experiences. Yet, when the storms of internal agitation recede, the calmness within is more noticeable. Confusion and suffering arise from misidentification and when such misidentification is removed there is freedom.

One practical way of understanding the complementarity and interaction between life and consciousness is to think of life as doing and of consciousness as being. At a very basic level, you are in a constant process of negotiating between your outward orientation and your inward orientation. For example, when you notice a fragrance in the air (external) it may trigger a memory linked to that aroma (internal). You may try and smell more intently and to locate where the smell is coming from (external), by walking around and looking as you breathe deeper. This may bring your awareness to a memory (internal) of a place that you used to frequent, or a garden you visited often during your childhood. These thoughts can, in turn, bring back other memories and emotions that may have been dormant for a long time. All these activities, internal and external, are temporary experiences. You can be present in all these parts of your life thanks to awareness. Indeed, your awareness enables you to notice some aspect of you smelling, remembering, feeling, walking, and searching – internally, for memories, and externally, for the source of that fragrance. You can become so absorbed in this process that you may not even notice that you are about to step in a puddle of water. Depending on your mood, stepping in a puddle of water may make you upset or angry; or you may not care at all because you are fascinated by the scent you are trying to identify.

Life is made up of all the internal and external experiences you have, and consciousness is the space where all of it takes place – with awareness being the active aspect of consciousness, enabling you to experience it all. Confusion is the result of mistakenly identifying with your changing experiences – and forgetting that consciousness is always there for you, underlying every experience, making it possible to be present in your life. When you cannot recognize the distinction between these interrelated aspects of you, you tend to identify with experiences. Doing so leads you to suffering, resulting from the five afflictions presented at the beginning of this chapter. In your daily activities, is your tendency to identify more with the sensations, or with the witnessing awareness?

Does this vary according to what you are doing?

What can you surmise from these observations?

Do you notice patterns, tendencies, and biases?

Are they conducive to feeling free, or restricted?

Are your ways of moving and breathing restrictive, or liberating?

Are your opinions, beliefs and memories sources of restrictions, or freedom?

Are your interactions informed by your awareness or by your experiences?

2.26 The means to liberation is uninterrupted discriminative awareness (*viveka khyati*)

This sutra introduces the concept of discriminative awareness (*viveka khyati*). Discriminative awareness is noticing the fundamental difference between experience and awareness, or between being and doing. Without the ability to distinguish this difference, your ways of being will lead you to confusion, misidentification, and suffering. Uninterrupted discriminative awareness, or being established in awareness, is the way to move towards liberation. As presented in sutra 2.2, there are two basic options for living in the world: in stress (*klesha*) or in integration (*samadhi*). When you forget the fundamental truth about yourself, I AM, you tend to live in confusion (*avidya*) that causes stress and suffering. The other option is to be a discerning person living in awareness (2.15). This is what happens when you regulate the ways of being that generate misidentification, restrictions, and limitations. By modulating your tendencies, you are effectively turning off the constant generation of opinions about what is happening, about others, and about yourself. When you are established in discriminative awareness, you recognize the fundamental difference between living in harmony with the perfection of life and living in the stories in your head. Living in the perfection of life is another way of saying abiding in your true nature (1.3). The practice is simple: Every time you notice that you are attaching to some idea about who you think you are or should be, just drop it and return to just being. It is important to clarify that this is not a process of thinking or deduction: *It is not thinking about being, it is just being.* This is a gradual process.

When you are first learning a new language, for instance, any time someone speaks that language, all you hear is a sequence of unfamiliar sounds. The more you are exposed to the language, the more you start noticing brief pauses in speech that lead you to identify smaller units as words. Similarly, this process of orienting towards awareness means listening for the silence that underlies all mental processes, the formlessness in which all forms manifest and the stillness where all movements take place. It may be barely noticeable at first. But, through gentle persistence, it can grow gradually. It is important to clarify that this is not a call to inaction. Instead, it is an invitation to *harmonize your being and your doing.* So, even when you must engage in doing something, choose to do what you are doing without adding internal narration or commentary and without self-judging when you get distracted. In other words, be present in whatever you do, so that you do the best that you can (*abhyasa*), while remembering all along that your doings are temporary (*vairagya*). From this perspective, it might be easier to see all your activities, external and internal, as opportunities to know truly who you are. Can you develop the habit of aligning with the deep spaciousness, calmness, and awareness underlying all of your thoughts, emotions, and actions?

Can this practice of dropping your identification with impermanent experiences become your new "normal" way of being?

Can you set your intention to abide in awareness?

Although it may take some time for you to be established in discriminative awareness all the time, do you notice a gradual progression in that direction?

2.27 Liberation unfolds in seven stages.

After presenting uninterrupted discriminative awareness as the means to liberation, Patañjali explains how to get there in this sutra and the rest of this chapter. The seven stages mentioned in this aphorism are the steps that lead you to full integration (*samadhi*). Patañjali does not list the individual steps explicitly. However, some commentators on the text believe that the seven steps are the first seven steps included in the set of eight limbs of yoga mentioned in the following sutra. On the other hand, it is useful to know that the first complete and thorough commentary on the Yoga Sutra was composed by an author called Vyasa perhaps in the 7th or 8th century CE. (Some scholars, however, state that what we consider Vyasa's commentary may have been created by Patañjali himself.) To this day, most interpretations of the Yoga Sutra take Vyasa's perspective and examples as a fundamental companion to the Yoga Sutra. Vyasa's commentary on this sutra summarizes some of the material presented so far in the complete Yoga Sutra. According to Vyasa, the first step is noticing the suffering than can be avoided. The second step is identifying the causes of suffering in order to remove them. Third, those distractions are lessened through establishing inner peace. In the fourth step, an internal climate of clarity and discernment takes hold. As a result, in the fifth step, everything that can be experienced is seen as a pathway to liberation from the restrictions and limitations closing the heart and the mind. Then, in the sixth step, the desire to manipulate the forces of nature ceases. Finally, in the seventh step, the practitioner embodies an *effortless* harmony between life and awareness.

Liberation is a gradual process that requires acting with enthusiasm, intelligence, and humility (yogic action 2.1). Applying yourself with gentle persistence (*abhyasa* & *vairagya* 1.12), you grow in sensitivity and learn to regulate your ways of being with more finesse and fluidity. Like in any other learning endeavor, the more you practice something, the easier it is to tune into the subtle aspects of what you are doing. When you try to learn to dance to a specific rhythm, at first it is difficult to understand how the legs, arms, and body need to move from one step to the next. Then, the more you practice, the more familiar you become with different ways to make the movements more fluid and easeful. In time, you grow in your ability to match the rhythm of the music. And perhaps, after much practice, it may be possible to move in harmonious ways that seem effortless and graceful. This whole process works best when it is an enjoyable journey of learning. Otherwise, it can turn into a source of agitation or self-torture. All processes in nature are gradual. From a seed capable of sprouting to a full grown, mature tree, it takes countless weeks of gradual, often imperceptible, progress facilitated by the appropriate conditions and circumstances. Similarly, for most people, it takes a long time to free themselves from deeply ingrained ways of being. Progress moves according to your capacity and trying to handle more than you can is a sure way to regress.

It is useful to remember the notion of self-regulation, or developing the keen awareness to sense what is appropriate, relevant, and beneficial for the moment that you are in. Since each moment is unique, what used to be appropriate may no longer be appropriate or useful today. **Self-regulation necessitates awareness.** To prepare for these steps, you can establish your firm intention to commit to living your life with gracious awareness. Get good at noticing when you are calm and when you are irritated, anxious, upset, or bothered. Try to discern the causes of these irritations.

Is it possible that your annoyance at somebody's words may reflect some unfulfilled expectation or assumption on your part?

When you get frustrated by something beyond your control, could you find other, more useful mindsets and attitudes?

How are you cultivating your ability to be centered and balanced?

When you are balanced, is it easier to notice and resolve irritation and discomfort without agitation?

Does this seem to help establish a new habit of being centered?

Can you appreciate how everything you encounter offers you an opportunity to learn, and to transcend your own limitations and restrictions?

Does this attitude change your relationship to yourself, to others, and to the world around you?

How does this change your attitude and experiences?

You may have noticed that this set of questions follows the steps presented by Vyasa. Along the path towards discriminative awareness, consider if it is helpful to cultivate the qualities of yogic action listed in sutra 2.1 – enthusiasm (*tapas*), intelligence (*svadhyaya*), and humility (*ishvara pranidhana).* Since it may be a long journey, can the strategy from sutra 1.12, patient persistence (*abhyasa*) and freedom from attachment (*vairagya*) be useful? How helpful are the five attitudes from sutra 1.20 – trust and confidence (*shraddha*), vigor (*virya*), remembrance (*smriti*), evenness of mind (*samadhi*) and insight (*prajña*)?

You may also want to verify the sincerity and level of intensity of your commitment (1.21 & 1.22) and their influence on how the process is developing for you.

Limbs of Yoga

2.28 Practicing the eight limbs of yoga removes impurities, increases wisdom (*jñana*) and establishes discriminative awareness (*viveka*).

Sutra 2.2 offered clear criteria to notice if your yogic actions are working: tensions and afflictions decrease and inner harmony increases. Along the same lines, this aphorism provides ways to verify that your practice is working. This sutra says that *when you practice all aspects of yoga you are removing inefficiencies, pain, and obstructions.* In addition, you grow in wisdom (*jñana*) and in your capacity to understand yourself and the world around you. Moreover, the practice of yoga helps you become better established in discerning your true nature from who you believe you are or should be (*viveka*). The practice of the eight limbs of yoga brings about living in greater harmony, wisdom, and truth. To put this sutra into practice, notice if there are inefficiencies in your attitudes, posture, movements, breathing, thinking, feeling and interacting.
Are those obstacles similar to the ones listed in sutra 1.30?

Can you remove these obstacles using the suggestions in sutras 1.32 to 1.39? As you reduce inefficiencies and obstacles, does your body feel less pain, soreness and discomfort?

When you remove ineffective attitudes and actions, does your outlook change?

Do you feel more energized?

Are there any signs that you are growing in clarity and wisdom?

Are you better able to notice the difference between who you think you are and who you truly are? (For instance, to what extent do you believe that you are your occupation, possessions, or bank account?)

Can you see clearly if your ideas and stories are really yours?

Are you establishing more meaningful connections to others?

Is your mind more open?

Is there more love, kindness, and compassion in your heart?

2.29 The eight limbs of yoga are: opening your mind (*yama*), opening your heart (*niyama*), optimizing body function (*asana*), enhancing vital energy flow (*pranayama*), clarifying the senses (*pratyahara*), focusing the mind (*dharana*), effortless awareness (*dhyana*) and integration (*samadhi*)

The eight limbs (*ashtanga*) of yoga present a comprehensive set of practices to bring about integration and harmony within yourself. This inner integration fosters greater harmony between you and the world around you. The *yamas* are wise ways of being that remove strain and cultivate harmony to open your mind. The *niyamas* are helpful attitudes to remove struggle and cultivate balance through opening your heart. *Asana* are practices that optimize body function through postures, movements, and awareness of the interconnectedness among body systems. *Asana* results in embodied joyful equilibrium. *Pranayama* enhances vital energy flow throughout your body. It is cultivated by developing intimacy with your breathing processes. *Pratyahara* consists of practices that direct your attention inwardly, clarifying the senses and developing inner sensitivity. *Dharana* concentrates the mind and heart. *Dhyana* (meditation) practices promote effortless expansion of inner stillness and silence. *Samadhi* is the gradual and natural progression from *dhyana*. *Samadhi* happens when you set aside your opinions and inner chatter so that you are fully integrated into pure awareness rather than gravitating towards your thoughts, opinions, and beliefs.

In present times, the words *yoga* and *asana* have become virtually interchangeable. However, in Patañjali's perspective, *yoga* consists of a complete system for enhancing the quality of life for the practitioner. While some approaches to *yoga* see these eight components of *yoga* as a succession moving from *yama* towards *samadhi*, other approaches begin with meditation. Yet other practitioners see the physical practice of *asana* as the most accessible starting point. For most of us, mastering even one single branch can be a challenging and long journey. **Thus, a better approach may be to cultivate all aspects of *yoga* to the extent that is possible for each practitioner.** Since each set of practices addresses different, yet interrelated, aspects of your being, it is intelligent to combine the various limbs in order to develop a balanced, integrative and synergistic practice.

As you have seen in other parts of the Yoga Sutra, a key aspect of yoga is self-regulation. Part of the self-regulation process is to be well-aware of your tendencies. As a result, you can avoid an inclination to practice that which you are already good at, or that which exacerbates the tendencies pulling you away from balance. You can ask yourself:

What does your practice consist of?

Which limbs of yoga do you prefer to practice? Why?

Use sutras 2.1 and 2.2 (definition of yogic action and its results) as well as sutra 2.28 (effects of the practice) to guide your practice by asking:

Am I practicing with enthusiasm, intelligence, and humility (2.1)?

Is my practice creating increased harmony, integration, and greater inner peace (2.2 & 2.28)?

Other useful questions include:

Does your current practice create a balance between body, mind, and emotions?

How is your practice contributing to the quality of your participation in your life?

How does your practice influence the overall quality of your life?

YAMAS

2.30 The *yamas*, wise ways for removing strain, are: Love (*ahimsa*), Integrity (*satya*), Fairness and Generosity (*asteya*), Curiosity and Reverence for Life (*brahmacharya*) and Abundance and Simplicity (*aparigraha*).

2.31 The *yamas* are a great universal vow to appreciate and honor the interdependent nature of life in all forms and manifestations.

The *yamas* are guidelines suggesting ways to establish intelligent relationships with yourself and with the world around you. In Sanskrit, *yama* means self-control. Like any other set of guidelines, the *yamas* can be formulated in either a positive or negative way, as Dos and Don'ts. This approach, however, can lead some people to become rigid and dogmatic. Moreover, focusing on the Don'ts fails to offer constructive ways to apply these guidelines into actions. Alternatively, you may see the *yamas* as logical suggestions for opening your mind by removing strain. The *yamas* also plant seeds of wisdom that you can live by. The *yamas* are wisdom, understood as pure common sense. Therefore, they apply at all times, in all places, and to every person. As in all aspects of *yoga*, it is up to each practitioner to discover the most suitable ways of exploring these guidelines. When you are trying to apply the *yamas*, be aware of internal arguments you may have with yourself. These arguments indicate that you might be trying to find ways to not apply the *yama* fully. Please remember that the practice is to apply the *yamas* to the extent that is possible for you at the present time, without generating more reasons to judge yourself. The practice of the *yamas* is a process. It develops gradually, according to the commitment and earnestness of each person. Yet, every tiny step towards applying the *yamas* creates the opportunity to see yourself and the world around you in a new light and through a different lens.

LOVE – *AHIMSA*

Ahimsa is the Sanskrit word resulting of combining *himsa* with the prefix "a," which negates *himsa*. *Himsa* means slaying, killing, hurt, harmful act, violence, injuring. *Ahimsa* is the opposite of *himsa*. The first *yama*, *ahimsa*, can be understood as looking at yourself and the world around you through the eyes of love and compassion. *What do you see when you choose to be loving and kind? What happens inside and outside of you?* This is an idea worth exploring in your everyday actions and interactions. It is quite likely that when you try to apply this view of love and kindness in your own life, you will start to see more clearly some of your deeply entrenched assumptions. For instance, do you see the world as a hostile and dangerous place or as a friendly place? Do you prefer stories of competition or cooperation? Other times, you may find obstacles in erroneous beliefs, such as thinking that you are incomplete or not worthy of love. Contemplate the simple question: Are you worthy of unconditional love? As you ponder these questions, some of your beliefs will become more apparent. You may also see how you create stories to justify some of your beliefs. With all this experiential information available to you, you can decide if these beliefs are helpful or unhelpful by noticing if they contribute to enhance the quality of your experience as well as the quality of your participation in every moment of your life.

Another path for exploring *ahimsa* is to take time to recall an inspiring event, memory, or idea. Explore how this idea influences the sensations in your body, your breathing patterns, your ways of thinking, your decisions, and your mindset. Then, bring into your inner space a memory of something that creates some discomfort for you, such as the memory of a challenging, difficult, or embarrassing moment. Then, feel the effects in your body, mind, breathing, movement, and attitude.

What is the resulting quality on your presence and overall experience?
Which of these two options informs your general attitude and mindset more often?
Is it possible for you to choose one or the other consciously?
What happens when you choose your attitude more consciously?
How does this affect your relationship with yourself, with others and

with the world around you?

One more way of cultivating *ahimsa* is by using a mantra such as I AM LOVE, or I LOVE UNCONDITIONALLY.

INTEGRITY – *SATYA*

As is often the case in Sanskrit, *sat* has many meanings, including wise, beautiful, honest, living, being present, enduring, real, and true. Some of the meanings associated with the related word *satya* are: true, truth, sincere, valid, authentic, and pure. You can interpret *satya* as living with integrity. In other words, being whole in your thoughts, intentions, movements, words, actions, and interactions. Practicing *satya* begins with the recognition that you are already whole and complete, that your fundamental essence is peace and harmony. Recognize that at the core of your being, there is an endless reservoir of peace and calm. You retire into that peace and spaciousness at the end of each day. You emerge out of that same peace and wholeness every morning when you wake up.

Living in a world where global economies orient toward consumerism, the average person is subjected to endless messages trying to sell products, experiences, and ideas. One popular approach to marketing is to suggest that a person is incomplete or deficient and that they can become good, complete, and whole through buying a product or experience. Believing the idea that you are incomplete or deficient leads you to live in a lie, that you need something from outside to make you who you are. This fundamental lie generates all kinds of other lies, as it triggers endless processes of "self-improvement," so that you can be smarter, taller, fitter, happier, richer, etc. Believing the flawed assumption that you are not whole and complete also creates insecurities and fears that color your attitudes, thoughts, and decisions.

It is quite common to convince ourselves that we are the only ones who are not complete and that everybody else has already figured out his or her own life. This ignores the fact that nobody has been in this current moment before, and that each person is improvising, trying to do what they think will work best, even though there is no certainty that predicted outcomes will materialize. *Satya* is freeing yourself from those erroneous beliefs, so that you can start from two simple facts. First, you are complete and whole. Second, EVERYBODY is improvising. Indeed, people are trying to do what they think is best. Often, we hesitate at the prospect of trusting that we are complete. Moreover, we may be quite uncomfortable with acknowledging the fact that we are improvising. Doubts arise because we want to do what is right, and, at the very least, we want to minimize our mistakes. *Satya* is an invitation to live with integrity, improvising, doing the best you can, and being responsible for your actions. As you improvise and try to do your best, there still will be times when you will make poor choices or uninformed decisions. The feedback that lets you know that you made a poor choice helps you live with integrity because it assists you in expanding your present level of knowledge and understanding. It also prepares you to make a better choice next time.

Some questions that may guide your exploration of *satya*:

What is your true nature?

How do you honor your true nature in your thoughts, words, actions, and interactions?

What type of activities are most conducive to connecting to your

wholeness in mind, heart, and body?
How do you know that what you think is true and not a story you or somebody else has made up?

You may also remind yourself of *satya* by using the mantra, I AM WHOLE.

You can also practice *satya* by quieting your internal commentary and opinions so that you can listen for inner guidance. Inner guidance is the silent whisper of your heart offering you wisdom. *Wisdom is pure common sense.* When you pay attention, you notice that common sense may not be as common as one would think. For instance, when you are having a meal, if you are paying attention, you will notice the gentle indication from your body when you have eaten enough. You are still free to ignore that message. The message offers pure common sense. Yet your mind may start concocting excuses for overriding the message you have already received. For instance, you may say to yourself: "I can eat more because I worked really hard this week," or "Tomorrow I'll do some extra exercise." *Satya* is listening for inner guidance and choosing to follow it. When you choose to ignore your wise inner guidance, you will probably hear yourself saying something like: "I knew that this was a bad idea," or "I should have noticed...." In contrast, every single time that you align your free will to the suggestions from the truth within yourself, life flows more harmoniously. Consider if you want to test this idea out in your own life. In the process, notice that the silent whisper of your heart is different from your internal narrator. Your inner wisdom, your conscience, offers you pure common sense, something that works at more than one level. In fact, it usually works at all levels, whereas your internal narrator tries to come up with excuses or justifications to convince you to override what you know deep within to be pure common sense. Only by trying to attend to the silent whisper of your heart can you find out what happens when you do.

Fairness and Generosity – *Asteya*

In Sanskrit, the literal meaning of *asteya* is to refrain from stealing. Stealing can be understood as taking that which is not rightfully yours. In contemporary societies, belongings and fame are status symbols providing access to experiences, contacts, and opportunities that tip the scales towards inequality. When what we have becomes more important than who we are and how we act, the accumulation of possessions can seem justifiable no matter at what cost to our integrity, to others, to society and to the environment.

Isn't that mindset what perpetuates the cycles of inequality affecting the world right now?

Is it possible that some of these attitudes may be related to the assumptions mentioned earlier about the world being a place ruled by competition instead of cooperation?

What specific steps can you take to cultivate fairness?

In addition, consider that every day you benefit from the energy of the sun, the protective magnetic shield of the earth's atmosphere, the air that you breathe, the water that nourishes your body and the myriad of interrelations among the planet and all the living beings that make up the web of life. Although all of us benefit from these things, how are we embodying our thankfulness for these resources we may not be contributing to?

To what extent do your actions reflect respect for all that you are

receiving?
Is your attitude regarding the resources available to you one of entitlement or gratitude?
Which attitude is more aligned with fairness and generosity?

Besides, reflect on the fact that no human achievement has ever been the result of the actions of a single person but the accumulation of the countless actions of all human beings throughout history. *In your actions, do you honor all of these interrelations? Are your actions and interactions contributing to enrich and affirm life or do they detract from it?*

To complement these ideas, it may be beneficial to consider that at every single moment in your life you have had within reach all that you needed to navigate that moment successfully. Of course, what is within your reach may not be what you want or think you need. This idea provides a good path of inquiry into your perspective, attitude, and expectations.
What are the differences between what you want, expect and need?
How do you know the difference?
How do these ideas relate to the notion of fairness and generosity?

Furthermore, when you recognize that you are deeply embedded in the totality of life evolving from one moment to the next, you might be able to see all of these connections between what you receive, how you contribute to affirm life and how you strengthen the connections among all beings, from the most minuscule to the largest, to the whole universe. As a result, you might be better able to choose to act with fairness and generosity. Some further questions to guide you include:
How am I expressing my gratitude for my life and all that I receive?

What makes something mine?

To what extent am I honoring what I have access to?

Is what I am doing fair to others and to the environment?

What does it cost me to be generous?

You may also benefit from investigating if the actions that move you away from being generous may be a form of overcompensating for feeling that you are not enough. If that is the case, you can use the mantra, I AM ENOUGH, as a reminder.

Curiosity and Reverence for Life – *Brahmacharya*

In Sanskrit, *brahman* literally means growth, expansion, evolution, and development. *Brahman* also means absolute, divine, Supreme spirit, Universal spirit, sacred study and related to sacred knowledge. *Acharya* can mean student or follower. One meaning of *brahmacharya* is a student of the mystery of existence, or somebody who honors the absolute and follows supreme wisdom. One more meaning of the word *brahmacharya* is celibacy. In the context of the Yoga Sutras, as we have seen already in this chapter, Patañjali has pointed out that *avidya* is not knowing the difference between our essence and the aspect of ourselves that is temporary (2.4 and 2.5). In addition, in aphorism 2.17, it is stated explicitly that the cause of suffering is conflating what can be perceived with the pure awareness that makes perception possible. This pure awareness underlies all that is. This thread continues in the previous *yamas* and is emphasized once again here.

It can be argued that life itself is the manifestation of the absolute, expressed in endless multiplicity and diversity in a continuous process of unpredictable change. **Life is the greatest mystery as well as the greatest teacher**. Consequently, it seems appropriate to think of *brahmacharya* as cultivating curiosity for life, as well as honoring it with reverence and wonderment. Choosing to see *brahmacharya* in this light ignites the spark of curiosity that enables you to learn from life's constant teachings. Consequently, instead of thinking that you can predict the future accurately, you can observe how life moves gradually and gracefully, like the gentle blooming of a delicate flower. This attitude helps release the strain of trying to subdue the world around you, helping you see that every day, at every single moment, there are teachers all around you offering you lessons, setting you up to remove your misconceptions, misidentifications, and limitations. ***Brahmacharya* is an invitation to become one with the life force all around you.**

Ask yourself:
How am I cultivating life-affirming thoughts, attitudes, actions, and interactions?

You may also observe how you are honoring the uniqueness of each moment by asking yourself:
Am I participating wholeheartedly in this unique moment?
Am I cherishing the uniqueness of each breath I am taking?
Am I awake to the miracle of life in everything that surrounds me, including what I like as well as what I dislike?

One mantra that can guide your *brahmacharya* practice: I HONOR LIFE'S PERFECTION.

ABUNDANCE AND SIMPLICITY - *APARIGRAHA*

The meanings of *parigraha* in Sanskrit include taking, accepting, receiving, getting, attaining, acquisition and possession. Just as with *a-himsa*, the "a" before *parigraha* negates its meaning, so that *aparigraha* means not to accept, to renounce. We live in a world offering constant stimuli to all our senses. Moreover, the major economic systems are engineered based on consumerism, so there is relentless pressure to keep upgrading all kinds of products and experiences. It seems like the mandate of the economy is *parigraha*. *Aparigraha* is an invitation to live with simplicity. Taking, getting, acquiring, and possessing are actions that demand a good amount of energy. In addition, whatever you "own" requires maintenance. With less to keep track of, you have more energy available to invest in life affirming endeavors.

It might be helpful to realize that there is abundance in life. If you doubt this, try to grow a garden. Soon enough you will find that plants will thrive despite neglect and that many volunteer plants, including "weeds," will grow if allowed the minimum appropriate conditions. Have you ever seen a wild plant growing in a small crevice in the concrete some place in the city? The fact that you are alive is a testimony of the reality that at every point in your life, whatever you needed was within your reach so that you could move forward. However, recognizing abundance is not permission to waste. By recognizing that you live in a life-supportive world, you can choose to live with simplicity, trusting that what you need will be within your reach as you need it. Some useful questions include:
Do I really need this?
How much do I really need?
Is this something I need or something I want?

To what extent does what I have contribute to enhance the quality of my life?
What level of maintenance do my possessions require?
Do I own what I have or does what I have own me?
To what extent am I cultivating simplicity in my life?

One mantra you can use for *aparigraha* is, I AM COMPLETE or I LIVE IN ABUNDANCE.

Bringing the wisdom of the *yamas* into your life requires you to look for evidence that what you are doing is what you intend to do, and that what you are doing has the desired effects. A simple way to check if your practice of the *yamas* is working is by asking yourself *Am I noticing less strain, less complaining and perhaps a little bit more harmony within me? Is my mind less fettered by restricting misconceptions?*

Additionally, you can assess the effectiveness of your practice by noticing if you are honoring and appreciating the interdependent nature of life in all forms and manifestations.

NIYAMAS

2.32 The *niyamas*, wise ways for releasing struggle, are: Clarity (*shaucha*), Contentment (*santosha*), Enthusiasm (*tapas*), Wisdom (*svadhyaya*) and Humility (*ishvara pranidhana*).

One way of seeing the *yamas* and the *niyamas* is as complementary practices, the *yamas* presenting the Don'ts and the *niyamas* suggesting the Dos. As mentioned in the section about the *yamas*, to facilitate their practice, it makes sense to frame both *yamas* and *niyamas* in positive terms. In other words, rather than seeing the *yamas* as a command not to do something, it is easier to implement them when you see them as guidelines for mindful participation in your life. Another traditional way of seeing the *yamas* and *niyamas* is as the *yamas* being an outward practice, ways of regulating your interactions and relationships with the world around you. Conversely, the *niyamas* can be understood as an inward practice, or how you modulate your relationship to yourself to create balance within. Moreover, the *yamas* and *niyamas* can be interpreted as common-sense guidelines for managing your vital energy. These wise ways offered by the *yamas* and the *niyamas* are the foundation for yoga. They are the steppingstones for creating integrated harmony within and without. While the *yamas* offer ways to remove strain, the *niyamas* provide a path to care for your inner garden through intelligently releasing sources of struggle. Both the *yamas* and the *niyamas* are gradual processes of aligning external actions with your inner peace and harmony.

CLARITY – *SHAUCHA*

In Sanskrit, the meanings of *shaucha* include cleanliness, clarity, purification, purity of mind, integrity, and honesty. *Shaucha* is to cultivate clarity and purity in mind, body, emotions, intentions, actions and interactions. Bringing this *niyama* into practice asks you to inquire into your intentions to discern the reasons that move you to choose one option over another and to act in one way instead of another. It is fair to say that purity of intention and action sow the seeds that blossom into clarity. Remember that in sutra 1.33, Patañjali provides a path for purifying mind, body, and emotions by practicing friendliness, compassion, inspiration, and equanimity. One way to explore purity is to contemplate the notion of conscience.

Is it possible that you have an internal compass indicating with subtlety the choices leading you to act with purity?

Are your thoughts, emotions, actions, and interactions grounded in pure intentions?

Does it feel different to listen for inner guidance that is independent from your likes and dislikes?

Is the clarity to distinguish between being guided by your preferences and being guided by your conscience one way to embody the discriminative awareness (*viveka*) mentioned in aphorisms 2.15, 2.25, 2.26, and 2.27?

Can this be what Patañjali is talking about also in sutras 2.4 and 2.5 about ignorance (*avidya*) leading us to confuse what is impure for pure?

In your daily life are there any sensations, thoughts and emotions that indicate you are aligning with purity in your choices, actions, and interactions?

When you pay attention to the results of your actions is there anything in the results indicating the purity of your motivation?

You may also approach application of this aphorism by asking:

How do I know that my intentions are clear?

How do my actions embody clarity?

When you sit in silence, is your internal environment clear?

Is it possible that an uncluttered space may contribute to greater internal clarity?

To what extent do your choices of food, relationships, work, hobbies, and entertainment contribute to your clarity?

To what extent do the effects of your actions serve as testimony of your clarity, or lack thereof?

A mantra that can be helpful, I CHOOSE CLARITY.

CONTENTMENT – *SANTOSHA*

In Sanskrit, the meanings of *santosha* include delight, contentment, pleasure, joy, and satisfaction. A large part of the whole yogic process is to become aware of your tendencies. For instance, whenever you go to a new place for a few days you get opportunities to see yourself away from the routine of your daily life. Then, you can see some of the patterns in your ways of thinking and in your emotional attitudes. People who are unhappy or worried and the people who find fault in everything in their hometown will likely see those same patterns appear in the places they visit. Similarly, the people who find delight and satisfaction in the place they live will probably use those filters when visiting another location. Knowing your tendencies enables you to apply the definition of yoga (1.2) by regulating your ways of being. This *niyama* is an invitation to clarify how useful some of your tendencies may be. For instance, do you find reasons to complain, or reasons to be content?

When reflecting on contentment, it is useful to remember that *expectations are the seeds of future frustrations*. When you choose to ignore that life is always changing and, most importantly, that it is unpredictable, you may convince yourself that you are able to predict accurately what will happen. Take a moment to consider how well you could have predicted six days ago where you are right now and what you are doing. Then start going farther back in time and try to assess how well you could have predicted the twists and turns of your life. Most people quickly realize that we are not very good at predicting. Moreover, it is quite likely that some mental processes don't often reflect our inability to predict the future. Indeed, many of us act as if we were quite skilled at predicting the future. Our tendency to predict and to act like our predictions are accurate generates expectations that influence how we approach each unique moment. Often, we end up ignoring the newness of the moment because we are looking for the outcome we already predicted. This process often results in disappointment and frustration because what is happening in our life does not reflect the fiction we have created in our minds. You may ask yourself if you tend to generate predictions and expectations. Then you can assess if those attitudes and actions contribute to create contentment in your life.

Contentment can also be explored from the perspective of noticing what you complain about or what you find fault in. Pondering this can give you insight into the conditions you place on the world outside. It may even expose a tendency to let the changes happening outside influence how you feel. If this is the case, you probably invest inordinate amounts of time and energy in trying to manipulate the world outside to meet your preferences. Since everything outside of you is in a constant process of change, you will find yourself in an endless process of trying to subject the unpredictability of life to your mental models or ideals. If this is your predicament, it can be quite helpful to recognize that most of us have very limited control over our own minds, bodies, breath, and emotions. If you cannot control your own systems very well, what makes you think that you can control the world outside, including the actions and reactions of other people? Michael Singer, author of *The Untethered Soul*, eloquently encapsulates pure common sense regarding contentment when he says: "Everything will be okay as soon as you are okay with everything. And that's the only time everything will be okay." What conditions are you putting on yourself, your life and others?

What do you need in order to feel happy?
Can the practice of gratitude open a door to contentment?
What conditions and expectations would you need to drop to be okay with everything?
Can you want what you have?
What would it take for you to love your life as it is?

The mantra, I AM CONTENT, can be a useful tool to move in the direction of contentment.

ENTHUSIASM – *TAPAS*

From 2.1 remember that *tapas* can mean heat, fire, meditation, and deep concentration. From the perspective of seeing the *niyamas* as wise ways for releasing struggle, *tapas* is an invitation to show up to each moment with passion and motivation instead of avoiding being present. *Tapas* ignites the fire of your presence so that whatever you apply yourself to, you do in a wholehearted and meaningful way. If you only have a single opportunity to participate in every moment and every interaction, doesn't it seem obvious that you would want to do what you are doing fully? Even when your intention is to participate wholeheartedly, however, the natural human inclination to develop habits can become an obstacle to being fully present. Just as it happens when you visit a place for the very first time, your heart and mind open to see clearly the quality of the light, the natural beauty of the place, its colors, sounds, and scents. You explore the place with curiosity and become interested in learning more about it. Quite likely, with every visit to the same place, your experiences and impressions get blended into your perception of the place, making it into part of your own personal history. As time goes by, the place that once used to be new becomes familiar. When that happens, you automatically shift from an attitude of wonder to thinking that you already know everything about the place. Assuming you already know something causes you to take for granted what seemed fascinating before. It happens frequently that we take people, relationships, and work for granted. *Tapas* is the fire to overcome the inclination to predict and to assume that you already know what will happen.

It does require passion, fire and enthusiasm to keep showing up to your life for every single moment of every day. In other words, *tapas* is the heat resulting from the friction of going against the grain of your habits. This friction happens as a result of the tension between the comfort of your existing habit patterns and having to pay attention to the uniqueness of each experience. It does not take long to realize that you develop habits in posture, ways of moving, ways of breathing, ways of thinking, ways of feeling, and ways of interacting. Some of these habits are conscious while others are unconscious. Similarly, some habits are useful in one context and hindrances in another. It takes concentration, another meaning of *tapas*, to notice these ways of being and to determine if they are useful right at the moment you are in. Noticing an unhelpful pattern and choosing to change it will require some energy (*tapas*). Part of that energy is what is needed to persist.

How are you showing up to your life?

How do you recruit your interest for participating in your life?

How do you turn a chore into something interesting or even inspiring?

What are your sources of inspiration?

Are you more likely to respond to your own internal motivation or to external motivation?

Are you able to regulate your enthusiasm?

Would it help to remember that each moment is unique and that nothing is guaranteed?

How can you keep bringing yourself back, with gentle persistence, to this precious moment?

You may use the sentence I LIVE WITH ENTHUSIASM as a mantra to remind you of your commitment to your life.

WISDOM – *SVADHYAYA*

The meanings of the Sanskrit word *svadhyaya* include to read, to study, to recite, to study true wisdom, as well as self-study. In all the traditions of the world, there is a body of useful and practical wisdom that is transmitted down from generation to generation to ensure that new generations benefit from the discoveries of their ancestors to live a healthy, meaningful and joyful life. Since everything is in continuous change, this body of knowledge evolves over time to remain relevant for understanding ourselves and the world around us. Wisdom, understood as pure common sense, is instrumental to your most important duty: your wholehearted and open-minded participation in life's perfection. Fortunately, now it is possible to find wisdom that has been distilled over generations by different human groups. It is important to recognize that wisdom is not dogmatic. In fact, wisdom shows its usefulness in its direct application into your life. Otherwise, wisdom can become just a new story to entertain your mind.

Knowing yourself, knowing your tendencies and patterns is essential in order to recognize how those patterns influence the quality of your participation in your life. Without knowing your ways of being you are at the mercy of those patterns without really understanding why some obstacles keep appearing along your path. Similarly, it may be difficult to harness useful ways of being to enhance your experience. For instance, all of us develop postural and movement patterns. Some of those patterns compensate for the natural asymmetries of each person's body. Other patterns respond to some tendencies in us. The patterns in themselves are not necessarily good or bad. Noticing the effects of the patterns can help you decide if the pattern is currently serving a purpose. For instance, most of us will tend to use one hand to hold our toothbrush when brushing our teeth. We do not even think about it. The pattern becomes very familiar, and it may make it easier to not focus fully on the task of brushing our teeth. When you try to do the same task holding the toothbrush with your non-dominant hand you notice how unfamiliar and awkward it feels to try to brush your teeth. That awkwardness is likely the result of noticing lack of coordination or skill. However, you can train yourself to use your non-dominant hand and, over time, you will develop more familiarity and dexterity. Choosing to use your non-dominant hand can be an effective way to draw your attention to the task. It may also give you insight into the process, helping you expand your perception and awareness. Besides, by using your non-dominant hand you may expand the repertoire of options available to you.

Engaging in self-inquiry, that is, when you explore yourself with genuine curiosity, you come to recognize that you have never been in a vacuum. You have never been isolated from the world around you. In fact, you eventually realize that everything that you can perceive is connected to you either directly or indirectly, because you are deeply embedded in the universe. And, just like solar flares influence the electromagnetic fields of the earth and the moon influences ocean tides, everything that is happening around you and within you contributes to the ongoing movement of life inside and outside of you. Engaging in *svadhyaya* means cultivating a healthy curiosity about yourself so that you can see clearly how your habit patterns and tendencies may influence your thoughts, moods, motivations, breath, posture, movement, choices, actions and interactions. Keep in mind that some patterns may be useful in one context and unhelpful in another context. This healthy curiosity includes studying and trying to put into practice true wisdom. Some questions to guide your exploration:

How well do you know yourself?

What are the stories that you choose to believe and perpetuate?

How do you know if those stories are true wisdom?

What patterns do you notice in your ways of thinking, ways of breathing, ways of feeling, and ways of moving?

Which tendencies influence your decisions?

What are your tendencies in your actions?

What are your proclivities in your interactions?

Which of these patterns are helpful and which are unhelpful?

In what context is one pattern helpful and in what other contexts unhelpful? To what extent can you modulate these patterns?

You may also use the mantra, I KNOW MYSELF THOROUGHLY to maintain your commitment to self-study.

HUMILITY – *ISHVARA PRANIDHANA*

In the Sanskrit dictionary *ishvara* is defined as God, the Supreme Being, the supreme soul, king, queen, prince, and capable; and *pranidhana* as laying on, access, attention, respectful conduct, profound religious meditation, abstract contemplation of, vehement desire, vow, and prayer. *Ishvara pranidhana* can be interpreted as honoring the Supreme Being or contemplating Supreme Being with wholehearted devotion. At different points in time we may be more or less willing to contemplate notions such as God, Supreme Being and devotion because for most of us these ideas tend to be loaded with many kinds of associations. Consequently, understanding *ishvara pranidhana* as relinquishing our illusion of control, honoring the continuous flow of life, or as humility can provide a workable way to practice this *niyama*. For instance, one possible approach to contemplating *ishvara pranidhana* is to recognize that you probably do not have complete command of your own body, mind, or emotions.

If you ask your mind to stay focused on any one object or idea without ANY distractions for 5 minutes, does that happen?

Can you move your body in any of its possible range of natural joint movement without any discomfort?

Or can you regulate the flow of energy running down through the nerve on the thumb side of your arm (radial nerve)?

Can you regulate the flow of your emotions at will?

Can you control what your mind thinks?

If you find that you cannot fully control your mind, body, and emotions, what are the chances that you may be able to control the world outside of you?

If it is a challenge to control what you think, is it realistic to think that you can control what other people think about you or about anything else? Is it possible to control what other people do?

Pondering these questions may help you realize that in the grand scheme of life in the whole Universe, each individual is a very small particle with limited power and control. Recognizing this can help you develop the necessary humility to accept what cannot be changed or controlled so that you may allocate your precious energy and awareness effectively to what you can influence. The path of *ishvara pranidhana* may also be a way of appreciating the myriad of connections amongst all aspects of your life and between all that exists. You can also cherish how every moment is perfectly calibrated to provide you with an opportunity to learn and transcend beyond your current levels of understanding. Obviously, you may also engage in pondering the questions:

What is Supreme Being?

What is God?

What is my relationship to God?

Do I have wholehearted devotion for anything?

One more way of practicing *ishvara pranidhana* is by using the mantra, I SURRENDER MY ILLUSION OF CONTROL.

Like applying the *yamas*, when trying to put the *niyamas* into practice, remember to do what is possible for you at this time. Since the *yamas* and *niyamas* may uncover some well-practiced patterns in your being, it is important to learn to recognize if these practices are generating pain or if they are making you more aware of discomfort that you have learned to live with or ignore. Confusing these two outcomes can keep you from applying the *yamas* and *niyamas* in beneficial ways. Like with any other practice, you are in charge of monitoring that you are doing what you think you are doing and that what you are doing is moving you towards greater clarity and integrated harmony.

Turning Things Around

2.33 When unhelpful thoughts and emotions arise cultivate uplifting thoughts and emotions (*pratipaksha bhavana*).

After presenting the *yamas* and the *niyamas*, Patañjali introduces a useful technique for implementing them: cultivating the opposite or turning around your ways of being (*pratipaksha bhavana*). This technique is to turn our ways around to the measure that is possible for us. Remember that in sutras 1.20, 1.21, and 1.22 Patañjali offers attitudes (confidence, vitality, remembrance, evenness of mind, wisdom) for the practice and talks about levels of intensity (mild, moderate and intense) in your commitment. As with anything else in life, you turn things around in the way that is most helpful, appropriate, and viable for you. Turning things around requires that you notice unhelpful patterns of movement, breath, thinking, emotion, and behavior. You are always a complete being; all your systems work together. However, sometimes there is better integration between your different aspects while other times you may feel fragmented and out of sorts. Consider becoming familiar with the ways in which your body, mind, and emotions are deeply interconnected. For instance, you can explore how thinking about something that makes you worried or anxious most likely will have some effect on your breathing. Similarly, when you regulate your breath, by making your breathing faster or slower, your body and mind will respond in specific ways. Paying attention to these relationships and connecting to the direct experience of sensing can indicate if a change of direction may be needed. At any point you can choose what patterns to emphasize or downplay. The effects will speak for themselves.

Remember that in sutra 1.39 Patañjali offered an option for removing distractions, consisting of focusing on anything uplifting. Along the same lines, another way of thinking about *pratipaksha bhavana* is as a suggestion to uplift. *What happens when you choose uplifting and helpful ways of being?* Redirecting your attention happens in one moment. It is an easy, simple and very specific action. The well-established patterns, however, will arise again soon enough, often, without your even noticing. Becoming aware of how deeply entrenched some habits are may trigger varying levels of frustration. **The practice is to drop the unhelpful pattern as soon as you notice it and to choose an uplifting alternative.** Before you know it, the unhelpful pattern may appear again. Notice that dropping the pattern is simple and easy; its recurrence tests your patience and resolve. It makes sense that the more established a habit, the sooner it will return.

Consider that the habit you are noticing may have taken a long time to get established. Recognize that removing the habit happens by releasing it and focusing on something else that is more uplifting and useful. You will probably have to go through the cycle of actions in the Method for Presence introduced in the Foundations of Yoga chapter - pausing, feeling, validating, clarifying, choosing, and responding many times. Some part of you may ask *how many times?* The answer is: as many times as the habit keeps returning. Regardless of the claims of most advertising, it's highly unusual for anything to work instantaneously. Noticing that a pattern is appearing again is a sign that the pattern is moving from your subconscious to your conscious mind. Noticing the pattern also indicates that you are paying attention, and that the pattern is *not* who you are, because if the pattern were who you are, who is noticing the pattern? Whatever the pattern may be, it is something you have cultivated. That specific pattern may have been useful before, but once it is no longer beneficial, you choose to drop it, an intelligent choice. Once again, the four Ss are a vital skill to master to establish your new habit. Just remember to keep returning to the unique moment you are in without struggle, strain or self-judgment and with a gentle smile. By letting go of the pattern again and again, with gentle and patient persistence, you are developing a new, more helpful and uplifting pattern.

Some useful questions for exploration:

What patterns are you noticing in your posture and movements?
What patterns are you aware of in your breathing?
What patterns are prevalent in your thinking?
What emotional patterns seem to be common in you?
Are your aware of your interactional patterns?
Which of these patterns are helpful?
Which of these patterns are unhelpful?
What patterns are you turning around?
How soon do the unhelpful patterns return?
How do you feel when you turn a pattern around?

2.34 Choosing not to engage in negative and violent thoughts, emotions or actions at any level prevents never ending pain, imbalance, and suffering. (*pratipaksha bhavana*).

In the twentieth century, Gandhi, inspired by the *Bhagavad Gita* embodied non-violence in an admirable and enduring way. This sutra echoes in Gandhi's words: "If we could change ourselves, the tendencies in the world would also change. As a man changes his own nature, so does the attitude of the world change towards him. This is the divine mystery supreme. A wonderful thing it is and the source of our happiness. We need not wait to see what others do." Although it may often seem that the practice of yoga is a solitary endeavor that may lead to isolation, the contrary is true. The more you are integrated, the easier it is for you to see that you are not alone, and, indeed, that you have never been. In support of aphorism 2.33, sutra 2.34 specifically reiterates how negativity and violence plant seeds for never- ending pain and suffering. Although this may seem obvious, Patañjali categorically spells out how all violence will generate more suffering and ignorance, regardless of your role in it – as initiator, offender, or accomplice – or its cause, confusion, delusion or anger. Engaging in negativity and violence plants the seeds for future experiences that will be colored by suffering.

Observing your own internal environment, you can explore the immediate effects of negative and violent thoughts in yourself. Start by sitting or lying down in a comfortable position and relaxing any holding or tension to establish a baseline for your experiment. Then bring into your space of awareness a negative emotion. Stay with it noticing how you feel inside. Try this also with a negative thought or memory.
How are your different systems affected by this negativity?

Do you notice changes in your sensations, breath, and overall outlook?
What happens when you turn around the thought a little bit, by trying to invite a more positive angle to the emotion or thought?
You may also explore the effects of negativity in your movements by standing up in a neutral position with arms resting to your sides and with your mind in its habitual state. Then open your arms out to the sides and up and then return your arms to rest by your sides again.
Try this a few times. Then recall a negative thought or emotion and do the same movement a few times.
Does something change in the quality of your movements?
What happens when you choose an inspiring thought or emotion?
Watch for any negativity and violence in your internal commentary.

Unfortunately, for some of us, it is very common to hear our internal voice on a constant tirade berating many aspects of ourselves. It may even feel like there is ongoing hostility in our internal environment. Experiment to find out if turning around your ways of being toward uplifting and inspiring thoughts and emotions (*pratipaksha bhavana*) may contribute to create a more harmonious and integrated internal environment. Notice how these internal changes ripple out into your actions and interactions so that your participation in the world may become more mindful, compassionate, and meaningful.

Effects of the *Yamas*

These three sets of guidelines offer you ways to release strain, struggle, and self-judgement by creating harmony within you and around you through life affirming intentions, thoughts, and actions. Consider that at every moment you are reaping the harvest of your previous actions. The results tend to be of similar kind to the initiating action. In many cases, particularly when you are entangled in your relentless internal dialogue and focus on the past or future, you tend to overlook what is happening in the most important moment in your life, the moment that you are in. Thus, if you are not present, you may not be cognizant of some of your subconscious actions resulting from your deeply entrenched ways of being, and you end up surprised by experiencing the effects of these subconscious actions. From a very simple and practical perspective, the *yamas*, *niyamas* and *pratipaksha bhavana* are an efficient energy management system so that your energy is not generating more agitation but instead contributing to enhance the quality of your life.

Some of your ways of being can be deeply influenced by one fundamental assumption about the world. This assumption is revealed by your answers to these two questions: *Do you see the world and yourself as inherently good or bad?* and *Do you see the world as a dangerous place filled with hostility and ruthless competition, or do you see the world as a place of harmony and cooperation?* This fundamental assumption may also apply to the way you see yourself: *Do you see yourself as inherently good, complete, and whole as well as capable and worthy of unconditional love or do you see yourself as an incomplete and fundamentally flawed person undeserving and incapable of unconditional love?* Examining your dominant viewpoint on yourself and the world can be illuminating. As you contemplate your fundamental assumptions, you may be better able to see if your actions are motivated by fear or by trust. A similar approach is to compare what happens when you act out of fear and anger with what happens both internally and externally when you act out of friendliness, compassion, inspiration, and equanimity (as advised in sutra 1.33). This inquiry can be useful in trusting the *yamas*, *niyamas* and *pratipaksha bhavana* for bringing more conscious awareness to your everyday actions and interactions.

As usual, your experiments with these ideas validate if these sets of guidelines, *yamas*, *niyamas*, and *pratipaksha bhavana*, provide a viable and sustainable path leading you to step out of a cycle of fear and suffering. These guidelines are instrumental in resolving the emotional challenges limiting your perspective. As a result, you can allocate the energy you were investing in reactivity and suffering towards flowing gracefully with the ever-changing movement of life inside you and all around you. Just like you are not separate segments of body, mind, emotions, and breathing but a complete whole, working together with all systems integrated and interrelated, the *yamas*, the *niyamas*, and *pratipaksha bhavana* are complementary practices. Initiating any of the aspects of these practices will likely invite some of the other aspects into your life. Of course, do not take my word for it, try it out and see what happens for you. Like with anything else, try to use each one of these techniques according to your level of ability and commitment to notice what happens. One more thought, rather than trying to accelerate this process, be curious to observe its own harmonious rhythm as you apply these guidelines with patient and gentle persistence (*abhyasa* & *vairagya*) while attending to any changes that you notice to see if their effects agree with you. The next sutras list the effects of mastering each one of the *yamas* and *niyamas*. Remember that the effects of the practice move in a range encompassing a wide variation from simple and easy to extraordinary.

2.35 The person established in love and compassion (*ahimsa*), becomes a positive peaceful influence everywhere she or he goes.

Have you ever seen someone you didn't know fall on the street and you immediately felt a visceral reaction that somehow communicated some of their discomfort and pain to you? This is our nature, and perhaps, as others have pointed out before, the fact that you can relate to others' misfortunes at a visceral level may be more than just a physiological reaction. *Could it be that when you feel somebody else's pain, suffering, and discomfort you are feeling the deep connection between all living beings? Is it possible that what you feel is the oneness of all of life?* This inquiry alone is worth contemplating.

Besides, it is critical to be aware that it takes a lot of training and repetition to get us humans to dehumanize other human beings in order to be able to overrule and ignore our instinct towards empathy and connection. This relatedness is not limited to seeing somebody in distress. It also happens as you see somebody achieve something momentous causing you to feel emotional. The first of the *yamas*, to live with love and compassion, is an invitation to open your heart. When your heart opens, your mind opens, and then you can recognize that the prevalent narrative portraying the world as a hostile environment where fierce competition is the rule and only the strongest survive is not quite correct. A more accurate and useful perspective is to see that cooperation is the only way human beings have been able to survive and thrive, because nothing our species has accomplished has ever been the result of one person working in isolation. Instead, all human accomplishments are the accumulation of all kinds of contributions by many different people over time. Even people who create alone are benefitting from food, shelter, and the support of those around them.

If you are benefitting from having running water, electricity, and access to communication technologies, the list of contributors who made those comforts possible is long.

Does the practice of love and compassion feel like you are dehumanizing yourself? Or does it feel like you are reconnecting to your true human nature? The practice of *ahimsa* is one way to create a garden of love and compassion in your heart so that you can become an abode of peace, love, and compassion in body, mind, and emotions. As with any garden, this garden begins with a gradual process of preparing the terrain – identifying what thoughts, feelings, and opinions are conducive to planting love, maybe by using the suggestions from sutra 1.33. As you embody calm, peace, love, and compassion, is it possible that your presence alone already starts to communicate it to others even without words? Is this how you can become a positive influence wherever you go? Some additional questions to guide your journey towards *ahimsa*:

What enables you to open your heart?

How are you cultivating compassion and kindness towards yourself?

How are you cultivating compassion and kindness towards others?

How are you fostering a peaceful mindset and personal environment in your daily activities?

You may also invite *ahimsa* through mindful actions. For instance, for a full day, for three days or a full week, you may try to make your movements, breath, and actions smooth, gentle, and deliberate. Observe what happens inside and around you as a result.

2.36 The person established in integrity (*satya*), acts effectively and efficiently.

When you observe the purposeful movements of a sloth climbing up a liana to the forest canopy, you see that every movement and every action is effective and efficient. And although it may look like the movement is slow, if you are really paying attention you will see that the sloth moves up the liana at a steady pace that takes it as high as it needs to go rather quickly. **Having a clear purpose is one way of bringing all your different aspects together to act with integrity.** Integrity can be defined as being whole and undivided. Remembering that you are not assembled out of different separate parts but that you developed organically from one fertilized cell into a complete human being can motivate you to honor that wholeness in your life. As a result, you may be more likely to remember on a regular basis that there is nothing fundamentally wrong with you and that you are always a complete human. Indeed, your intelligence does not reside in one unique place in your body, and your emotions are not felt in only one area. All your systems interpenetrate very closely.

Integrity is also the quality of being honest and having strong moral principles. Living with integrity is feeling, thinking, acting, and interacting with wisdom, honesty, and sincerity. *Can you align with integrity by connecting to your conscience?* Each one of us has always been intimately connected to the world "outside" of us. This obvious fact – that you have never been in a vacuum – may be ignored when we choose to see ourselves as separate. At every moment in your life, you are in a context, and that context is part of you, even at the atomic level.
What happens if you choose to see you as you and everything around you from the microscopic to the macrocosmic?

What would happen if you chose to live based on that recognition?

How would knowing your deep truth influence your thoughts, words, and actions towards yourself?

Towards others?

Would that recognition help instill more meaning into your life, words, actions, and interactions?

If you embody this deep inner knowing, could you trust yourself?

Others?

The world?

Life?

If you expand your notion of yourself to include all that is around you, would it make sense to attend to the feedback you receive continuously from whatever surrounds you to enhance your participation in your life?

Would it be intelligent to use that feedback to guide your choices and actions?

Would this be one option to disentangle yourself from the ideas and stories generated by your likes and dislikes?

Would that make you both more effective and efficient?

2.37 For the person established in fairness and generosity (*asteya*), prosperity unfolds effortlessly.

In present times, consumerism is a major engine of economic activity in many countries. It's quite common to see advertisements, movies, and other media advancing the notion that a person's worth and social standing are closely related to their patterns of consumption. In such an environment, and given the growing economic disparities around the world, it may not come as a surprise that those who do not have what is so highly valued in society will try to do whatever they can to access the goods and resources that seem so important in our world. As a result of the deep influence of money in all sectors of contemporary life, it seems like many of us dedicate significant amounts of time to focusing our attention and energy on money: how to make it, how to keep it, and how to invest it. It has been suggested that because such large numbers of people dedicate so much time focused on money that money has become an idol or god and that (unconsciously) people are meditating on money and on the lack of it. A typical marketing approach is to tell you that there is something wrong with you if you do not have X product or experience. That is followed by the "call to action" you must undertake to buy it and therefore feel complete or whole. Even when you know the strategy, hearing time and time again that you are lacking something may end up becoming a message you internalize.

Do you see the world as a place of scarcity?

Or do you see the world as a place of abundance?

Does this view feed a tendency towards feeling lack or generosity?

How do you see yourself in relation to the world of material comforts?

How much of your time do you invest meditating on money?

How does that compare to the amount of time you spend cultivating genuine relationships with yourself and with others?

Does what you own you?

How do you know that what you have is truly yours?

Do you cling to what you have?

How do you cultivate fairness and generosity towards yourself?

What does it take to extend that generosity to others?

How do you determine that something is fair?

Are those decisions biased or unbiased?

What is your definition of prosperity?

2.38 For the person established in nurturing curiosity and reverence for life (*brahmacharya*), great vitality and enthusiasm develop.

The essential difference in attitude between young people and old people, regardless of age, is that old people think they have already seen everything and know everything. That attitude tends to give you permission not to pay attention to the moment you are in. Thinking that way may also lead you to think that there is nothing left for you to live for. Furthermore, you may also become arrogant. On the other hand, one of the most refreshing things about little children is how they are curious about their surroundings, wanting to find out what makes things tick and how things work. This curiosity is energizing. Developing curiosity for the mystery of life can generate plenty of enthusiasm to engage in living your life to the best of your abilities. Moreover, when you cultivate reverence for life, your heart and mind open.

Has it ever happened to you that something you thought you knew may have revealed some unexpected and useful insight?

Or, is it possible that life is constantly offering you proof that you are not very good at predicting?

Can that be a reminder to witness the miracle of life directly in your own being and in your surroundings?

How do you know if you are living in harmony with life?

How do you gauge moderation in your actions?

Is there balance in your life between work, play, personal development, and relationships?
Is there balance in the attention you give to your body, your mind, and your emotions?
Is there balance between the vital energy you spend and the vital energy you replenish?
How are you learning from the essence of life?
How does learning influence your choices and actions?
If you find yourself with low energy, which of your ways of being are contributing to deplete your energy?
Which ways of being contribute to refreshing and restoring you?
Is there anything that sparks the light of vitality and enthusiasm in you?
What thoughts, emotions and actions are life-affirming?

2.39 The person anchored in freedom from cravings and appreciation of abundance (*aparigraha*) recognizes impermanence, clarifies life's purpose, and gains insight into past and future.

When you were born, you arrived with no personal possessions. During your life you have probably seen times when you had access to fewer things as well as other times when you had access to more. If you were able to adapt and be content with more and with less, your adaptability has made it possible for you to find contentment in many situations and changing circumstances. If, on the other hand, you are constantly craving what you don't have, you have probably found yourself frustrated and disempowered by feeling that you can't be at peace with what you have. This sutra invites you to reflect on the role of material possessions in your life.

Do you see your life and yourself in terms of what you have acquired?

What will happen when some of those things you have are no longer satisfactory?

How much time, energy and resources do you allocate to maintaining what you own?

Traditionally, one interpretation of this aphorism suggests that a successful *aparigraha* practice will uncover the secrets of past and future lives. Another way of interpreting this same sutra is that clarifying our relationship to the material world will give us insights into our own personal past – because our relationship to our possessions can have a strong influence on our beliefs, ideas, and actions. In addition, how we have connected to our cravings and possessions in the past has influenced our current life situation. Moreover, our attachment to what we have and what we want will also determine many of our choices. To what extent can you see this playing out in your life? You may use the following questions to guide your *aparigraha* practice:

Do you live in abundance, scarcity or craving?

How do you embody gratitude?

How much is enough?

Are you immersed in the game of winning and losing?

Do you derive your sense of self from your material possessions, appearance, and circumstances?

How do your actions align with your life purpose?

Furthermore, do not discount that there may be other forms of craving, like craving for acceptance or recognition.

EFFECTS OF THE *NIYAMAS*

2.40 Developing and refining mental, physical, and emotional clarity (*shaucha*), results in releasing blockages that inhibit optimal function, including habits and attitudes towards yourself and interactions with others.

By paying attention to physical, mental, and emotional processes, it becomes clear that most of us have blockages restricting the optimal flow of vital energy in body, mind and emotions. These blockages manifest as patterns of tension in the body, as unhelpful beliefs, and as unkind emotions. The first step is to become aware of these patterns, which is another way of saying *know your tendencies*. Then, determine if those patterns are helpful or unhelpful by asking *Is this supporting my intention and purpose?* Whatever is keeping you from dedicating your awareness and energy to your purpose can be released. Repeatedly bumping up against the same obstacle will eventually prompt you to make the decision to release it. Often the question that comes up is: How many times will I have to drop the obstacle? The answer is that you will keep doing what is unhelpful until the pain, discomfort, or agitation that it creates is greater than you are willing to endure. If you are attached to a belief or attitude, especially when you think that it makes you who you are, it will seem hard, maybe even impossible to release it. When the discomfort caused by the belief is unbearable, you will be put in the position of deciding between staying with a belief or attitude that causes you pain and letting go of your identification with it. The practice of gradually turning your attitude around can be useful in this process (*pratipaksha bhavana* in 2.33 and 2.34). Progressively, a different attitude becomes established leading you to see yourself, body, mind and emotions with greater clarity and less identification.

When you sit in silence for meditation, just to be with what is as it is, notice what distracts you from your natural clarity. The internal distractors are usually mental, physical, or emotional, or a combination of the three. Choosing to be still helps you notice where there is movement. Similarly, making the decision to be silent will make all sounds, external and internal, more evident. As you remain focused on being present, it becomes easier to notice if these internal activities are helpful or unhelpful. You become aware of patterns in the distractions as well as of your own reactivity patterns. Some of the reactivity may emerge as irritation, frustration, or annoyance. However, reactivity may also arise in the form of trying to fix or sedate the symptoms of irritation.

When you are engaged in a mindful physical activity, you can notice the portions of your movements that are smooth and effortless, which will betray the movements that are erratic and fitful. Bringing more clarity into one movement will offer insight into ways of smoothing out the irregular movements. Further questions for exploration include:

How do you cultivate clarity in your own life?

Are there areas of your mental, physical, or emotional life that you choose to ignore?

What is the nature of the blockages that you find?

Is it possible that some of those blockages result from your own beliefs?

Is there a relationship between who you think you should be and those blockages?

How do you deal with the obstacles on your path?

Do you see the obstacles as nuisances or as teachers?

What contributes to cleansing your senses?

How can you cleanse yourself mentally, physically, and emotionally?

How are you refining your present level of clarity?

In the next aphorism you can see the results of practicing *shaucha.*

2.41 [As a result of *shaucha*] increased evenness of mind and heart, joyful attitude, focused one-pointedness, mastery over the senses and insight into one's true nature.

This sutra lists the symptoms of practicing *shaucha* successfully: evenness of mind, ability to focus, capacity to regulate your senses, and seeing yourself accurately. It presents a stark contrast to sutra 1.31 where symptoms of distractions – distress, despair, suffering, trembling, and abruptness of breathing – are enumerated. Clarity or purity (*shaucha*), like the other guidelines, is a process; as clarity expands it creates stability and steadiness in your mind and heart. As you see yourself more clearly, your attachments to who you think you are, who you think you should be and who you think you are expected to be soften. Then your mind and heart gain steadiness because you let go of all the distractions that these unhelpful thoughts generate. Seeing yourself clearly and removing obstacles keeping you from presence and from conscious participation will have an impact on your attitude. By releasing limitations and restrictions, you are also letting go of rigidity. Your attitude becomes more easeful, gradually cheerful and, eventually, joyful. Maybe it begins by having fewer reasons to get annoyed and fewer complaints. Clarity also makes it easier to notice your tendencies to allow sensory stimuli to pull your attention away from presence. *As a result, what used to be an easy distraction gradually loses its appeal.* When your attentional energy is not chasing after sensory fluctuations, you notice glimmers of that aspect of you that does not change. As you commit to establishing clarity within, what do you notice?

Remember that gaining clarity will make more apparent the areas where there is still confusion, just like cleaning and organizing one closet or room in your home will make the disorderliness in other rooms more evident. This is a sign that the process is working. Thus, instead of feeling disturbed by noticing the areas where there is lack of clarity, you may favor recognizing that some harmony is developing at the pace and to the extent that is feasible for you, at this time. Consider checking in with yourself on a regular basis:
Is there more evenness in your mind?
In your heart? Is your attitude more pleasant?
Are you more focused?
Is it easier for you to attend to your priorities?
Is it easier to discern what contributes to enhance the quality of your life?

2.42 By cultivating contentment and inner peace (*santosha*), supreme joy unfolds.

When you ask yourself if you live in contentment, what do you find? Sometimes you may start the day with the firm intention to invite the peace and calmness from your yoga practice into the rest of your day. However, sometimes it may seem that your intention may have invited the opposite. For instance, somebody cuts you off in traffic, someone you know says something to you that you find offensive, or you are confronted by something you have been trying to avoid. Your intention to embody peace and contentment is a sign of commitment to living in wisdom. As a result, you get feedback that helps you test your commitment. Sometimes, your ease and calm may be challenged by what you encounter. Rather than interpreting this as a sign of failure, recognize that you are being set up to let go completely of the reasons you create for not being content. Creating contentment from within is a smart and very practical choice. Thinking that contentment comes from outside will lead you to try to manipulate the world around you to avoid anything that goes against your preferences. This latter option is not only impractical, it is exhausting and, frankly, impossible to achieve. As suggested before, you can nurture your contentment by becoming aware of your complaints, both explicit and veiled, so that you can remove their causes. You may also contemplate if there is a relationship between your expectations and your ability to feel content. Another viable way of promoting contentment is by exploring how your judgments and opinions may reveal the internal filters that cause dissatisfaction.

What happens if you ponder the fact that every single situation and experience is the result of countless factors and elements coming together in a specific way that is perfectly calibrated just for you and nobody else?

Are all these things coming together to annoy you, or are they a lesson to help you release attitudes and beliefs that no longer serve you?

What needs to happen for you to find joy deep within?

2.43 Cultivating enthusiasm through removing inefficient patterns in body, mind, and emotion (*tapas*) heightens all senses and abilities.

Being aware of your patterns is one of the main skills in yoga. All your ways of being are filters that color your experiences. All of them influence the quality of your participation in your life. Some of those tendencies contribute to enhance your participation, while others may preclude your conscious and deliberate participation in the present moment. Noticing the difference between helpful and unhelpful ways of being empowers you to make intelligent decisions. Because the pull of well-established patterns is quite strong, bringing your awareness to the moment you are in is already an act that requires energy, commitment, and enthusiasm (*tapas*). In fact, most of us get distracted constantly. Exercising your skill of returning to the present moment with no struggle, no strain and no judgment also demands enthusiasm, especially when frustration arises as you notice how frequently you get distracted. This process of self-regulation of personal propensities offers several benefits. First, you develop the habit of presence by redirecting physical, mental, and emotional energy from distractions to conscious participation in the moment you are in. Second, the more you turn an unhelpful pattern around, the more sensitive you become to its symptoms, which enables you to catch the tendency before it distracts you fully. Besides, that sensitivity enhances the quality of your awareness. As a result, you are already present and receptive to noticing what is happening in your life. Being awake to your life enables you to discern the difference between discarding an unhelpful pattern and taking the pattern into a different area of your life. For example, if my tendency is to exaggerate in some behavior, like overeating, when I try to stop that tendency it may happen that I shift that tendency to a different area, like over-exercising or over-working. Awareness of that tendency can help me keep it in check. Something else you may find is that the ways of being that were useful before may stop being useful. This is like training wheels in a bicycle helping you learn to ride by providing stability. Once you know how to ride, the same training wheels will get in your way. At that point, it makes sense to discard them.

For this sutra, the Sanskrit word used to indicate the results of bringing enthusiasm into life is *siddhis*. This word, like with so many other words in Sanskrit, has a variety of meanings including, accomplishment, performance, fulfillment, complete attainment (of any object), success, solution of a problem, readiness, prosperity, personal success, fortune, good luck, advantage, bliss, perfection, and the acquisition of supernatural powers by magical means. This last meaning has been historically one of the trademarks of a true yogi. However, supernatural powers may not crystallize for every practitioner. It may be a good option to withhold judgment and be open to observe what happens. At a more practical level for most of us, it may be more useful to consider that attending to life and its always arising newness can become a source of energy that sparks your enthusiasm enabling you to participate in the dance of life with sensitivity and exquisite responsiveness.

Taking responsibility for your life despite distractions, interferences, and disruptions also requires enthusiasm. Moreover, commitment to the goal of being present for every moment of your life demands passion as well. It is that enthusiasm, balanced by intelligence and humility (sutra 2.1), that can make the difference between seeing a project to completion and giving up along the way. Although, as you will find in Chapter Three of the Yoga Sutra, the idea of *siddhis* is traditionally interpreted as being able to perform extraordinary feats and magic, it may be helpful to start by thinking about how exceptional it is to meet people committed to being fully present in their own lives. In fact, it is remarkable to find people participating in life with commitment and enthusiasm, particularly in the face of obstacles and challenges. The etymological meaning of the word enthusiasm in Greek is to be in the essence of God. Another way of understanding enthusiasm is to gather inspiration and support from life.

What are your sources of enthusiasm?

Are you aware of your patterns in movement, posture, breathing, thought, and emotions?

What are your tendencies in attitude, actions and interactions?

Which patterns contribute to enliven your outlook and the overall tone of your feelings?

Which don't?

How does it feel when you bring enthusiasm into your attitude, actions, and duties?

Do you notice any changes in your sensitivity and level of energy when you act with inspiration?

How do you invigorate yourself?

2.44 Deepening your understanding of yourself and embodying wisdom (*svadhyaya*) results in communion with Supreme Being.

Knowing yourself, your tendencies and patterns in body, mind, emotion, and breathing empowers you to participate mindfully and wholeheartedly in your own life. This meaningful engagement with life offers you many opportunities to witness the complex interrelationships between your ideas, emotions, breath, and actions. It also affords you the perspective to notice the elegant interconnections between all of life. This nuanced orchestration of all the forces of life is an adaptive and responsive dance that influences how everything moves. Life is the manifold manifestation of Supreme Being, the whole, complete, most exalted, and all-encompassing expression of being. Some people would call it life's perfection, others may call it the ineffable, Source, Spirit or God.

Is your study of true wisdom and your study of yourself leading you into a comprehensive understanding of yourself, your relationships, human nature, all of nature and the universe?

How are you embodying a deeper understanding of yourself and of life?

To what extent are you honoring the forces of nature?

How do you enter communion with life's wisdom in your personal yoga practice?

Are you aligning with life's wisdom in your everyday decisions and actions?

How are you honoring life in your interactions?

2.45 Humility, relinquishing the illusion of control (*ishvara pranidhana*), enables integration into deep inner stillness and silence (*samadhi*) that facilitates extraordinary insight and effectiveness.

It is important to recognize that deep integration (*samadhi*) is a central concept in the Yoga Sutra. This is the reason Patañjali dedicated all of Chapter One to this idea. Here, sage Patañjali reminds us that the objective is modulating our inner life (sutra 1.3) and that we can accomplish it by practicing humility (*ishvara pranidhana* in sutras 1.23, 2.1 and 2.32); in other words, acknowledging that we are not in charge of life or the Universe. This sutra may contribute to the notion that *samadhi*, the exalted state of becoming a receptacle for wholeness and fullness, cannot be accomplished by effort, that it results only from grace. Through recognizing the pervading magnificence of life and of the expanse of the cosmos you gain an all-encompassing perspective that informs your understanding and your attitude. As a result, you can see your internal activities, including the storms brewing within, in their appropriate proportion so that you can adjust your tendencies away from personal drama. Noticing that there are thousands of factors that come together to create the circumstances you are in offers you insight to step outside your internal story to act decisively and effectively when and where is appropriate and needed. This same perspective of seeing yourself and your life in the wider context of life in space and time invites you to modulate your internal reactivity to fittingly appreciate life in its full magnificence. **Expanding your perspective beyond the confines of your immediate field of vision opens a window that invites you to be in harmony with the miracle of life.**

This same humility helps you recognize that many, if not all of your best ideas, quite likely have been the result of inspiration arising when you are not preoccupied with your personal stories. Inspiration has always been there, but many times being entangled in our own internal dialogue and reactivity precludes us from noticing the beauty and elegance of life As with any of the other *yamas* and *niyamas*, it is helpful to give up expectations for potential results and instead it is more productive to focus on cultivating the guidelines fully. In this case, some guiding questions include:

How do you relate to what is beyond your control?

Are you aware of the limits of your understanding?

What do you consider your power?

How are you cultivating humility in your daily activities?

How do you invite inspiration into your life?

Can gratitude for everything, including what you dislike, open a door to see the magnificence of life?

Where does your inspiration come from?

How does it feel?

What attitudes are more conducive to attracting insight?

Do you take credit for the insights you have received?

What does it really mean to take something personally?

What happens when you apply intuition in your life?

How do you feel?

What are the results?

LIVING THE *YAMAS* & *NIYAMAS*

The *yamas* and *niyamas* are very similar to guidelines for living from other wisdom traditions around the world. These guidelines encompass the common sense of a person who lives according to the dictates of conscience. Living with conscience removes the inefficiencies that result from trying to serve your likes and dislikes. Notice how these guidelines work together. They do not contradict one another. Instead, practicing one of the *yamas* or *niyamas* may invite you to incorporate the others into your daily life. As you consider these guidelines, you may think that putting them into practice will require a lot of effort. It may be helpful to notice that practicing each one of these guidelines helps you reconnect to the deep calmness and ease at the core of your being. In fact, since practicing the *yamas* and *niyamas* is one way of embodying common sense, your practice facilitates effortlessness. As with anything else in life, the value of the *yamas* and *niyamas* emerges from their application into your life. At first, the *yamas* and *niyamas* will make your well-established ways of being more apparent. Gradually, you start to turn around the less helpful patterns (*pratipaksha bhavana*). This process of reconnecting to the stillness and ease at the core of your being will expose the conflicts between your mind and the silent whisper of your heart. Contemplate the idea that the voice of insight always offers a suggestion that moves you towards presence and integrated harmony. The *yamas* and *niyamas* are tools for putting into practice sutras 2.10 and 2.11 to release the afflictions that obstruct your clear vision. In addition, the *yamas* and *niyamas* are conducive to steadily releasing your sense of self-importance (*abhinivesha*), your likes (*raga*) and dislikes (*dvesha*), and who you think you are or should be (*asmita*). You know that the practice is working when there is less dis-ease, discomfort, and dissatisfaction in your mind and emotions.

ASANA, JOYFUL POSTURE.

Certainly, the physical aspect of yoga has become the most popular expression of yoga nowadays. In fact, when people say yoga, the implied meaning is most often the practice of postures and movements with very little, if any, regard for an integrated and balanced articulation of all the practice guidelines compiled by Patañjali. Some of the meanings of *asana* in Sanskrit include abiding, stool, dwelling, place, seat, stopping, sitting, sitting down, and posture. When *asana* is broken down into separate sounds, the Sanskrit dictionary offers the following meanings for the particle "*as*": to be present, to exist, to inhabit, to celebrate and to make one's abode in. The particle "*sa*" means knowledge and meditation. And "*na*" means vacant, empty. Thus, *asana* can be interpreted as living in knowledge and meditation, empty of distractions, free of likes and dislikes. The three aphorisms about *asana* in the Yoga Sutra, make up only 1.5% of the total 196 sutras. The practice of postures, just like the practice of the *yamas* and the *niyamas*, provides one opening for exploring with playful curiosity how to abide in a state of presence, free of distractions. In the Yoga Sutra, the *yamas*, the *niyamas,* and favoring uplifting thoughts and actions (*pratipaksha bhavana*) are presented before *asana* to provide a framework for the conscious exploration of *asana* to optimize the functioning of all physical and physiological systems without strain or struggle. Consider that *pranayama* is the next limb along the journey, so *asana* can be practiced as a way to optimize the flow of vital energy and intelligence through your whole being.

2.46 Steady and joyful posture.

The importance of balance between being and doing reappears here. *Asana* consists of striking a balance between steadiness and joy. Steadiness is an expression of consistent practice (*abhyasa* 1.12, 1.13 and 1.14) facilitated by single pointed focus (*ekagrata* 1.32). Joy results from cultivating peace of mind through wise attitudes (1.33), practicing purity and clarity (*shaucha* 2.32, 2.40 and 2.41), and developing contentment (*santosha* 2.32 and 2.42). Moreover, releasing attachments and expectations (*vairagya* 1.15 and 1.16) leads to being deeply at ease within. *Asana* is joyful abiding through creating a steady body that is completely at ease. Just like you adjust the firmness of your grip depending on what you are holding in your hand – a flower, an apple, a heavy book, or a baby's hand – this sutra asks practitioners to become skillful in adjusting posture and movement in a graceful articulation of strength, flexibility, and relaxation.

Does the definition of *asana* as present abiding in meditative emptiness describe your *yogasana* practice?

Do you have a tendency towards more firmness or more ease?

Is there any strain, struggle or self-judgement in your physical yoga practice? How do you ensure that you are balancing your strength, flexibility, and relaxation?

Are your movements and posture fostering a sense of steady and enduring joy?

Is that a sustainable state for you?

If the steady joy is intermittent, what are the distractions pulling you away from that centeredness? (Remember that feeling tired, sleepy, agitated, very thirsty and hungry after *asana* practice may be symptoms that you are trying too hard.)

Can balance between steadiness and joy be extended to the rest of your daily activities?

Take a posture that is easy for you and make it firmer during your inhalations and more comfortable during your exhalations. Then try to modulate the right amount of firmness and comfort and notice what changes. Repeat the previous suggestion with a posture that is challenging for you. What do you notice?

When you move from one posture to another can you try to make your movements as slow, fluid, and smooth as possible?

How do you feel when you move in this way?

Does this give you any insight into how you work and how efficient you can be?

Observe your usual actions, such as walking, talking, moving, carrying things, folding your clothes.
Do you find that you achieve a balance between steadiness and ease in your actions?
What are your tendencies?
Are those tendencies similar to what you find when you are practicing *yoga* postures?

2.47 Releasing struggle and endlessly integrated.

The previous aphorism is often quoted as the guideline for *asana.* Yet for some reason this sutra is not cited so frequently, although it is an equally important guideline addressing how *asana* is practiced. Once again there are two ideas combined. The first one is letting go of all struggles, and the second is to remove all distractions. This brief instruction can be interpreted as a call for high efficiency. Struggle and distractedness will squander physical and mental energy, becoming an obstacle to the meditative nature of your posture and actions. "Endlessly integrated" describes all resources articulating harmoniously. In practicing *asana* (posture) and *vinyasa* (transition between postures), all systems and all aspects of yourself are coming together, supporting and enhancing one another. Endlessly integrated also means to weave together your physical, mental, emotional, and respiratory aspects seamlessly and effortlessly. Releasing all struggle is a suggestion helping to prevent the common action of increasing force when something is not working, just like a person who is not understood by a speaker of a different language will tend to increase the volume of speech to bring the message across, or the person trying to fit a piece into another may try to push a little bit harder to accomplish the task. Releasing struggle is common sense to remind you that struggle is not only ineffectual, it is also a waste of your precious energy. The converse side of this idea is that you can tell a seasoned craftsperson by the elegance and economy in his actions. From the purely physical perspective, a sign of physical fitness is a body that maintains a low heartbeat and easeful breathing even when engaged in challenging physical activity.

From the vantage point of "endlessly integrated," consider what happens when you observe a consummate performance in any field. It seems like time stands still. An attitude that contributes to timelessness is the attitude of having infinite time. Then there is no rush, no hurry, and no struggle so that everything can articulate effortlessly. One way to embody this guideline is by letting go of your agenda and by choosing instead to explore with playful curiosity so that you may experience directly what it feels like to do what you are doing. This seems like a healthy approach conducive to experiencing *asana* according to the comment on the previous sutra, becoming a steady meditative abode of emptiness. This aphorism echoes the sentiment expressed in sutras 1.3 and 1.4, abiding in one's true nature and free from misidentification with one's temporary ways of being. Releasing of struggle is stepping into being with what is, as it is, and being with yourself just as you are. Many of the struggles and distractions result from trying to be something that you are not, like when you try to be as you think you should be or as you think others expect you to be.

As you practice *asana*, what are the struggles that emerge?
What are the sources of those struggles?
Are your struggles a symptom of your assumptions and expectations?

Can you notice mental, physical, or emotional agitation?
Is your breath continuous, smooth, and fluid?
Are you in a rush?
Is there a hidden agenda?
Is your practice a way to meet yourself, to make yourself into somebody different or to avoid meeting yourself?
What is your relationship to time in your practice?
Can your *asana* and *vinyasa* practice be a timeless abiding in contemplative presence?
What happens if you take several rounds of breath ensuring that your inhalations and exhalations are smooth, continuous, and long?

Try a few rounds of a sequence of postures that is quite familiar for you.
Observe your breath as closely as possible.
What do you notice?
Is your breath easeful?
If it isn't, when do these qualities change?
What happens?
Do you hold your breath?
Does your breath get jerky or jagged?
Does your breath get short and labored?
How are the transitions between your inhalations and your exhalations?
Can you balance the length and quality of your inhalation and your exhalation?
You may also want to observe if your practice feels different when you match your movements to your breath.

What is your attitude when you practice?
Can you be fully focused on what you are doing?
Is your practice a tool to integrate your body, mind, emotions, and breathing?

2.48 As a result, evenness beyond dualities.

The third sutra related to asana indicates the results of the practice, leaving behind the play of opposites. Once again, the Yoga Sutra offers a twofold approach combining being with doing, resulting in joyful ease. This approach, when presented in Chapter One as the combination of practice (*abhyasa* 1.12) with detachment (*vairagya* 1.15) was said to bring about stillness to one's ways of being. Sutra 2.46 invites you to consider a specific way of doing that integrates firmness and ease into either firm gentleness or gentle firmness. Sutra 2.47 contributes a way of being combining a release of all struggle with continuous focus. This sutra presents the results of combining these ways of doing and being, you free yourself from gravitating toward the endless play of opposites like good-bad, hot-cold and like-dislike. In addition to connecting to the notion of yoga as being (1.2) and yoga as doing (2.1), this aphorism connects to the threads related to likes and dislikes at the beginning of this chapter (2.3, 2.7 and 2.8). Likes and dislikes play a major role in generating reactivity and agitation. When you are endlessly unified, you transcend your limited sense of self defined by the temporary ebbs and flows of your preferences. You move your fundamental sense of identity beyond the major duality between I am this and I am not this. This happens when you are in meditation or dreamless deep sleep and your physical boundaries become blurred so that there is no sense of inside and outside. Even the need to try to make that distinction at all vanishes. There is only being, everywhere.

Notice how you may be engaged in a constant process of creating distinct categories. For instance, to understand ourselves better, we divide ourselves from whole beings into body and mind, body and spirit, into a whole set of systems like musculoskeletal, neurological, respiratory, digestive, endocrine, etc. These separations are useful in understanding some aspects of ourselves, yet your experience is always whole, complete, and indivisible. Even the distinction between life and awareness is only useful as an analytical tool because life and awareness are in constant interpenetration. Thus, it is instrumental to remember to reconnect to your wholeness and completeness. What are the dualities that influence your understanding?

To what extent are I and not I useful categories for enhancing the quality of your life?

Is it possible that there are areas in your life where attachment to your sense of self spins you into an endless rollercoaster of dualities?

What is the relationship between dualities and preferences in your life?

Are there some dualities that trigger your actions and reactions?

What dualities emerge as you practice your yoga postures and movements? Do dualities serve as a filter that colors your interactions?

Could it be that some of the struggles you face come from being caught in the game of opposites?

PRANAYAMA

While the Yoga Sutra includes only three aphorisms about asana, the following section about *Pranayama* consists of five sutras. Sutra 1.34 alluded also to *Pranayama* as a method for eliminating distractions. *Pranayama* is the practice of enhancing the flow of life energy (*prana*) through your being by regulating your respiration in a variety of conscious and deliberate ways.

2.49 Once unified and free from struggle, *pranayama*, regulating inhalation, exhalation, air flow and retention.

After establishing a friendly and helpful attitude towards your circumstances (*yamas*) and yourself (*niyamas*), *asana* practice serves as a tool for removing inefficient patterns in posture and movement to enhance your adaptability and resilience. One major goal of *asana* practice is to promote optimal body function by enhancing the flow of vital energy (*prana*) throughout your system. This goal is closely related to the quality of breathing during postures (*asana*) and movements (*vinyasa*).

Although the air you breathe is not exactly the life energy that keeps you alive, in the yoga tradition, yogis have observed through personal experimentation that the breath is an accessible vehicle for life energy to keep the body alive, to enhance vitality and to promote health and well-being. Seeing *asana* as preparation for *pranayama* suggests, following sutra 2.47, that it is always intelligent to ensure that during *asana* practice the breath is smooth, fluid, and free from all abruptness. In other words, *asana* practice contributes to create stability in your breathing patterns by ensuring that your breath is conscious and deliberate throughout. At the same time, practicing in such a way also assists you in developing a greater sensitivity to the subtle qualities of your breath. This sutra defines *pranayama* as attending to the movement of air through our system by regulating inhalations, exhalations, and retention of inhalations and exhalations. All reputable sources advise practitioners to explore *pranayama* under the supervision of a knowledgeable teacher.

The human respiratory system is highly integrated into different aspects of your nervous system and metabolic functions. It may be obvious to point out that the quality of your breathing can have a strong influence on your health, mood, and awareness. Moreover, breathing in specific ways has been used by some human groups as tools for triggering specific body reactions as well as for accessing different states of awareness. It does make sense to connect to a teacher who can provide useful advice and feedback on your breathing processes. The suggestions about pranayama offered here are at the simplest level that can be considered safe.

To put this sutra into practice, find a comfortable position and observe your inhalations, exhalations, and air flow. Rather than trying to control your in-breath and out-breath focus on feeling the sensations accompanying your natural inspirations and expirations. Notice what moves when your body is breathing at its own rhythm. Notice as best as you can the different qualities of the air that you are breathing, its taste, smell, texture, humidity, and temperature. Try to feel as clearly as possible where you feel sensations indicating that an inhalation is happening. *Are there specific sensations that indicate the beginning of your inhalations?*

Do the same with your exhalations.

Are the sensations arising towards the end of your inhalations different from the sensations towards the end of your exhalations?
Is the flow of air more noticeable in some areas than others?
Is there a difference between the volumes of air flowing through each nostril? Are there differences in your ways of breathing when you are standing, sitting, and lying down?
If you think of something uncomfortable or embarrassing does your respiration change?
Is your respiration different when you think of something uplifting?
Can you identify some patterns in what you observe?
Do you hold your breath involuntarily?
When?
Does your body automatically adjust its breathing rhythm to your level of activity?

2.50 The breath becomes long and subtle when inflow (*puraka*), outflow (*rechaka*), and retentions (*kumbhaka*) are observed precisely according to location, count, and duration.

Upon birth, your first inhalation marks the beginning of your life as an individual. Your breath also marks your last embodied action when your final exhalation closes the cycle that started at birth. Life is what happens between your first inhalation and your last exhalation. Attending to breathing is a simple, practical, and effective way to foster presence, because the breathing process only happens in the moment you are. Besides, each inspiration and expiration are unique, irreplaceable, and unrepeatable. **Paying close attention to your breath invites you to be aware of what is happening at the most important moment of your life, the moment that you are in.** Cherishing each breath ensures that you make each inhalation and exhalation count. You can choose consciously to be inspired with each inhale so that you prepare to receive all that is life affirming and life supporting. Conversely, you can choose to make each exhalation the perfect vehicle to allow whatever doesn't serve you any longer to expire for good.

This aphorism lists the breathing processes of inhalation, exhalation, and retention. The simplest expression of the retention is the brief transition between each in-breath and out-breath, and between each exhalation and inhalation. Patañjali also notes that *pranayama* consists of a systematic observation of the breathing processes according to the parts of the body involved, the duration of each one of the aspects of the breath, and the count or number of repetitions for each cycle. The number of possible combinations of these elements is practically infinite. If you choose to see *pranayama* as falling in love with your breath, you can take time to appreciate and explore all the subtle intricacies of your respiration. This inquiry is done with love, curiosity, and great care. Recognize that you can create a lot of internal mental and physiological agitation by hyperventilating and that you can also make yourself unconscious through manipulating your breath. These are some of the reasons every single *pranayama* treatise warns practitioners about the power and risks of this practice.

It is also useful to recognize that Patañjali includes in this sutra the idea that *pranayama* inquiry is directed towards making the breath long

and subtle. You may investigate this by observing the qualities of your natural breath when you are relaxed. Notice if observing the breathing processes already starts a process of lengthening each inhalation, exhalation, and the transitions between them. Recruit your attention to find out if you tend to hold your breath unconsciously.
Do you tend to breathe with your mouth open or closed?
What happens if you favor breathing through your nose only?
What is the duration of your natural, involuntary inhalation?
How does it compare to the duration of your natural exhalation?
Is there a brief pause during the transitions between exhalation and inhalation?
What happens when you lengthen your inhalations very gently and gradually while also keeping them smooth and fluid?
Is it possible for you to breathe creating movements in your lower torso, the lower abdomen and lower back?
How is it different to breathe creating movements mostly in the ribcage area? Could it be possible to breathe directing your breathing movements toward your collarbones, shoulder blades and armpits?
What are some similarities and differences when you breathe with movements in these three areas (lower torso, mid torso, upper torso)?
If you breathe with longer, conscious, inhalations and exhalations, what is the duration of the inhalation and the exhalation?
Are they very similar or different?
With voluntary breathing, breathing that you regulate, do the qualities of your inhalation and exhalation change when you keep the same duration constant for a specific number of breathing cycles?

In all *pranayama* practices remember the suggestion to release all strain, all struggle, and all self-judgment. If you are interested in embarking on a systematic journey of *pranayama* practice, remember the traditional recommendation of finding a qualified teacher you can trust to ensure a fruitful and beneficial practice.

2.51 The fourth type of breath is beyond internal and external regulation.

The whole yoga project is a journey that moves you from the gross, outermost level of experience to subtler and deeper levels of internal experience. That is one reason for practicing *asana*, to gain enhanced awareness of bodily processes and then to deepen the practice with *pranayama* in order to explore and feel the breath and the vital force that it carries. After presenting the definition of *pranayama* in sutra 2.49 and the variables that are observed and manipulated in sutra 2.50, this aphorism introduces another type of breathing. This fourth type of breath is known as *kevala kumbhaka*, a pure and effortless state of breath retention. However, it is important to notice that this sutra also says that it is beyond regulation. In other words, this is a special kind of breath that happens spontaneously without any forcing or manipulation. In Sanskrit, meanings of *kevala* include alone, isolated, simple, pure, entire, whole, and the doctrine of the absolute unity of spirit. Some sources suggest that this fourth type of breath is the result of the mind being still, while others indicate that it is an experience of connecting to the subtlest aspects of respiration. Yoga lore suggests that this type of breath may be related to the legendary ability of master yogis to stop their own heart for brief periods of time. This may have been a result of the close relationship between breathing and heart function. This highest form of breath retention points to a deeper connection to the subtlety of the breath and of the life force. As author Gregor Maehle suggests, it is not coincidental that Patanjali calls *kevala kumbhaka* the fourth, linking it to the fourth state of consciousness, *turiya*, described in the *Mandukya Upanishad* as the ever-present all-encompassing consciousness (Maehle, 2012, p. 311).

One way to make sense of this aphorism is to notice what happens when you develop the capacity to observe your breath in its full spectrum of options according to the guidelines offered in sutra 2.50. As a result, all inefficiencies in the breathing process may be removed. Along with expanding your breathing abilities, you are also developing your capacity to pay close attention to subtle processes. Then, notice what happens when you are fully absorbed in something that draws all your attention, like a fascinating reading or story. Quite likely your inhalations and exhalations are so subtle that they are hardly noticeable, and it seems like you are barely breathing. Therefore, one avenue of exploration of this aphorism is to find something that is truly fascinating to you. Perhaps, a question that you are willing to contemplate with deep interest and motivation, like *who am I really?* Or *where in my physical body do I feel love and compassion?* It can be anything else that you find powerfully intriguing or anything that you find inspiring and uplifting (as suggested in sutra 1.39). Then, see what happens as you contemplate your point of focus for a while:
Does your breath change?
Does it become subtler, slower, and gentler?

Another approach is to continue the journey from the previous sutra to make your inhalations and exhalations as long as possible. Notice that in order to make your breath longer, by necessity it will become subtler. This requires your body and your mind to be very relaxed and at ease.

What happens when you try lengthening your breath with consistency? What are the limits of subtlety that can be experienced?

Yet one more option for inquiry of this fourth type of breathing is to decrease gradually the length of your inhalations and exhalations. Remember that any gasping or abruptness might be warning signs to protect the integrity of your organism, so take agitation in your breath as useful feedback that invites intelligent action. Notice what changes as you gradually make your breath shorter and shorter, eventually, letting go of all control over your breath and simply witnessing what develops.

2.52 As a result, the inner light of awareness becomes brighter.

After presenting a definition of *pranayama* and its features, now you find the results. Following the incremental path of the limbs of yoga produces specific effects. Just like practicing *asana* delivers freedom from the play of opposites, practicing *pranayama* develops sensitivity to the flow of life energy and removes the veil that obscures the light of awareness. This sutra weaves the thread from Chapter One, when Patañjali offered ways to overcome the distractions listed in sutra 1.30 by practicing single pointed focus (1.32) with a relaxed mind and heart (1.33), attending to exhalations and breath retentions (1.34), feeling subtle sensations (1.35) and cultivating the inner light (1.36). It is not uncommon to feel fluctuations in the flow of your vital energy. Sometimes you feel more awake or more enthusiastic while other times you feel down, confused, or slower to react to what is happening around you. *Does it ever happen that you feel very sharp and with great clarity and other times it seems like it is hard to focus?*

Remember that at the very beginning of Chapter One, Patañjali already stated that regulating your ways of being – releasing your opinions and internal commentary – provides access to your true nature (1.3). The yogic process consists of removing the obstacles that lead you to misidentify with your internal stories and reactivity so that you can align with awareness. *Pranayama* practices act as bellows that remove inefficiencies and enhance your connection to your inner light, producing greater clarity and awareness. As usual, to find out if this is the case for you, you can establish your own baseline of current levels of awareness and clarity. Maybe each morning you can make note of how awake and clear your mind is. Try this for a few days. Then practice *pranayama* consistently for some time. If a qualified teacher is not available, you can try exploring some of the ideas in the comments to sutras 2.49, 2.50 and 2.51. Of course, be mindful and ensure that what you are doing does not generate any strain, struggle, or self-judgment, and notice if regular practice influences your mood, perception, and general outlook. It is quite possible that practicing conscious breathing consistently can help you find clarity about other factors influencing your current level of energy and awareness. As a side effect, just paying attention to these subtle processes may also sharpen your perception. If you practice conscious and easeful breathing every morning or every night, are you better able to tell how some of your activities and diet influence the quality of your breath?

Are you developing greater sensitivity to your own vital energy?

Is your consistent *pranayama* practice offering you a greater feeling of clarity or brightness?

2.53 Subsequently, the mind is fit for concentration.

Engaging in the life experiment of yoga is a gradual progression of waking up to your life and living wholeheartedly by following the *yamas, niyamas, asana,* and *pranayama* with regularity. This process is already training your ability to focus. This is a two-pronged approach: Each limb is asking you to strengthen your capacity to focus by giving your attention to some aspect of your life. In this way you are shining the light of awareness on your life. At the same time, each one of these practices efficiently decreases sources of agitation and reactivity, effectively diminishing distractions. It is a feedback loop that keeps enhancing your ability to concentrate. Removing strain (*yamas*), releasing struggle (*niyamas*), favoring uplifting thoughts (*pratipaksha bhavana*), creating joyful steadiness in your body (*asana*), and enhancing the flow of vital energy through conscious and deliberate breathing (*pranayama*), all effectively contribute to focusing your awareness.

This sutra provides a simple way to assess if your *pranayama* practice is working:
How steady is your mind?
Once you choose a point of focus can you stay with it?
In your own practice and life, do you have clear intentions and goals?

Are you clear on your priorities?
Are you moving in the direction you intend?
Are there fewer distractions?
Can you neutralize arising distractions? (Most often the distractions are related to your likes (*raga* 2.7), dislikes (*dvesha* 2.8) and who you think you are or should be (*asmita* 2.6).

Is this the case for you? If you are noticing a calmer and more focused mind, how does it influence your outlook, perspective, choices, and interactions?

Is your ability to focus influenced by choosing a meaningful focal point?

PRATYAHARA

2.54 *Pratyahara*, cultivating inner sensitivity to bring awareness into its own form.

The previous limbs of the yogic process are an invitation to focus internally. Generally, your senses are alert to the changing external phenomena. This is helpful so that you can orient to what is happening around you in order to respond intelligently to the changing circumstances in your immediate surroundings. However, to create internal harmony, it is also beneficial to be able to turn your attention inwards, to the ground of your being. Our human minds are highly responsive to sensory input, generally chasing after the stimuli gathered by the senses. Now that more than half of the population of the globe lives in urban environments, many of us find countless sources of sensory stimulation. Moreover, our technologies compound this situation by constantly delivering more stimuli in a variety of forms and media. In fact, it is fair to say that most of us are training our attention unconsciously to be highly responsive to external stimuli, shifting from one to another in rapid succession. This is not necessarily negative, if we are also able to disengage voluntarily from external stimuli. This is important. *If we can't focus our attention inwardly, we are training only one half of our full range of ability.* The previous limbs of yoga have set up a solid foundation offering techniques to initiate the process of internal exploration. Just like it is possible to cultivate your olfactory sensitivity by training yourself to distinguish among different scents, it is also possible to train your ability to sense yourself from within. The practice of both *asana* and *pranayama* enhances awareness of the body, the respiratory processes, and their interrelations. *Pratyahara* is an organic continuation of this process.

Pratyahara requires a conscious decision to change the focal point for your senses from outside to inside. In a way, *pratyahara* is the process of redirecting your usual external activity, your doings, to merge into the state of being, just witnessing. Or, to switch from doing and thinking to being and feeling. *Pratyahara* leads you to research systematically your internal landscapes. One approach to deepening your sensitivity is to transition from outer orientation to inner orientation. You may start by consciously recruiting awareness into each sensory process so that you move from tasting to savoring, from hearing to listening, from seeing to observing, from touching to feeling and from awareness of smell to awareness of scent. In other words, you pay close attention to your sensations while withholding opinion and commentary by witnessing with curiosity and without expectations. Then, you remain focused on the subtler aspect of the perceptive process you are attending to in order to experience all possible nuances. As with all natural processes, this takes time, yet it can be an enlightening way of uncovering a whole range of experiences that were not within your awareness before.

You can continue this journey by following the path of any sensory stimulus from outside to inside as was suggested in sutra 1.35. Then you move further inward by developing sensitivity of your internal sensations. Curiosity about the myriad sensations making up your inner life provides the motivation and drive to continue along the inward journey. Some questions to guide you along the way:

How does it feel inside of you?

How are the sensations in your skin different on the outside and inside?

Can you follow a sound from outside to inside of you?

What are the natural sounds that are happening inside of you?

To what extent is it possible to feel your inhalations and exhalations from within?

Is it possible to feel your own blood flowing through your body?

What are all the places you can feel your own heartbeat?

What are the sensations inside your joints?

Can you feel your bones and the marrow within them?

What are the sensations in your eyes as light filters in through your closed eyelids?

Where do these subtler experiences lead you?

2.55 Then, the senses are mastered and at the service of the highest goal.

The objective of *pratyahara* is to expand your repertoire of options for your senses, so that you can feel both what is outside of you and what is inside. In other words, you develop a mastery over your senses so that they are at the service of your awareness. As a result, you can direct your senses to serve the most important objective: to be with what is without distractions. All the yoga practices so far provide ways to optimize the flow of vital energy and to direct it with single pointed focus. As you turn your senses inward, you set the conditions to gain true knowledge of yourself through your direct experience (*pratyaksha* 1.7). *Without commentary, what is the direct experience of being you?* Notice that it is not a fixed or static experience. It is a constant flow of multiple streams of sensory information. This is an experience like no other. It cannot be captured, recorded, or expressed accurately in its entirety in any medium. Moreover, nobody else can experience what it feels to be you. One clarification is necessary at this point. The whole project of yoga is not about isolating ourselves from other human beings. **The goal is not to escape from your life**. On the contrary, all yoga practices offer you opportunities to see how your beliefs and inaccurate sense of who you are may be limiting your wholehearted participation in the eternal dance between life and consciousness. The more you experience yourself clearly, the more you notice that you were never separate. You directly experience that in every single moment you are deeply embedded in the all-encompassing interconnectedness of the matrix of life. *As you experience yourself as whole and complete, it becomes more evident and eventually undeniable that the differences between you and other beings are rather superficial.* Mastering your senses and regulating your ways of being foster your open hearted and open-minded participation in life with kindness, compassion, and joy. In fact, yoga helps you become a life-affirming presence in the world. *Can you articulate your senses to support your single pointed focus? Can you merge your sensations and thoughts into the direct experience of your vital energy? What is important enough to you to deserve your wholehearted engagement?*

Summary of Chapter Two of the Yoga Sutra

Enthusiasm, intelligence, and humility are the components of yogic action. Yogic action reduces tensions and increases harmonious unity. Afflictions result from not distinguishing the fundamental difference between who you are and who you think you are, which leads you to mistake joy for suffering and the temporary for the permanent. This confusion results in misidentification. The mistaken sense of self generates attachments and aversions, which create a sense of self-importance. Subsequently, attachments and identification with what is temporary strengthen, obstructing clear perspective and understanding. These sources of tension can manifest in different degrees. Once afflictions are diminished by yogic actions, the afflictions can be neutralized through releasing all identification. When active, afflictions are neutralized through meditation. Afflictions store impressions in memory. These impressions become seeds of future actions that will generate pleasure and pain in an endless cycle.

The wise person understands that all experiences will eventually bring about suffering. Thus, future pain can be avoided. Conflating the seen and the seer is the source of suffering. The seen is nature, life. In constant change and manifesting in various stages, the seen is what can be experienced. The seer, on the other hand, is pure awareness, the consciousness using the body, mind, and emotions as instruments for experiencing. When the seen and the seer come together, experiences take place with potentiality for recognizing the role of each. Discernment – knowing the difference between seen and seer – is the path to liberation. Discernment develops gradually by practicing the limbs of yoga to remove inefficiencies, increase knowledge, and eventually embody true wisdom. The first five limbs of yoga are introduced. First, living with intelligence that removes all strain (*yamas*). Second, acting with contentment that removes all struggle (*niyamas*). Third, cultivating integration among all body systems by removing physical inefficiencies and enhancing circulation of energy and intelligence through the body (*asana*). Fourth, deepening awareness of the embodied vital force (*pranayama*). The fifth step fosters mastering the senses by turning them inward (*pratyahara*).

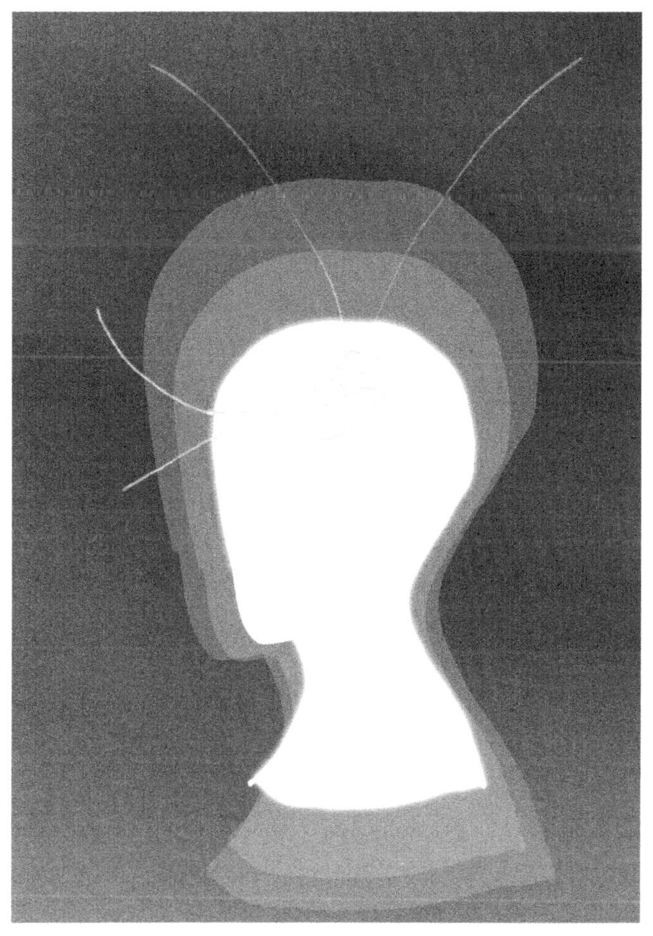

Chasing after power wastes energy and attention. Yoga is empowering when it leads you to your natural state. Then, you are more likely to become supernatural by seeing everything with impeccable clarity.

MAGNIFICENCE (VIBHUTI)

The title of Chapter Three of the Yoga Sutra, *vibhuti,* may be translated as *penetrating, abundance, welfare, wealth, magnificence, great power, prosperity, splendor, greatness,* and *fortune.* The overall theme in this chapter is the advanced meditation practices and how they reveal the subtle aspects of reality. The sutras in this chapter can be organized in the following groups:

- Concentration, meditation & integration [3.1-3.8]
- Transformation [3.9-3.15]
- Meditative integration & its effects [3.16-3.37]
- Warning [3.38]
- Subtle energy [3.39-3.44]
- Highest attainments [3.45-3.50]
- Freedom [3.51-3.52]
- Purpose [3.53-3.56]

Regarding Extraordinary Powers

Some interpretations of the Yoga Sutra cover Chapters One and Two and the first dozen or so aphorisms in Chapter Three, choosing to set aside comment on the rest of the original work by Patañjali. In this third chapter, out of a total of 56 aphorisms, 24 sutras talk about the extraordinary effects of applying a meditation technique called *samyama* defined at the beginning of the chapter. This means that 12% of the Yoga Sutra deals with some sort of extraordinary or supernatural powers. In fact, there are more sutras dedicated to these powers than to *asana* and *pranayama* combined.

It has often been said that the legendary 20th century teacher, T. Krishnamacharya, used public demonstrations of extraordinary powers such as complex asanas and feats of force (like lifting heavy objects with his teeth and stopping his pulse) in order to revive interest in *yoga* during the 1920s and 1930s. Krishnamacharya's son Desikachar told the story of asking his father to teach him how to stop his own heart, only to receive a negative response explicitly indicating that such feats were not useful to society and that they could become ways for self-aggrandizement. This is but one example of this topic in more recent times. There are numerous accounts of supernatural powers (*siddhis*) in the South Asian subcontinent. Many of these accounts present these powers as the result of practicing high levels of meditation. Indeed, in the Monier-Williams Sanskrit-English dictionary, the definitions of *yoga* include *supernatural means, charm, incantation, and magical art*; and the definition of a practitioner of *yoga*, a *yogin*, includes *magician, conjurer, and someone possessed of superhuman powers* (1899). Some scholars suggest that the long history of yoga is related to early shamanic practices as well as to practices directed to gain occult and supernatural powers.

Perhaps a useful approach is to consider the objective of your yoga practice. For instance, practicing the *yamas* and *niyamas* are effective ways of creating harmony within and around you. Engaging in *asana* practice can be a way to facilitate optimal body function by removing inefficiencies and obstructions so that energy, nutrients, oxygen, and information flow efficiently. Of course, some people may choose to regard *asana* as a goal in itself and thus may prefer to practice postures and movements to find the limits of what their bodies can do. *Pranayama* can be practiced with the goal of expanding one's capacity to inhale, exhale, and withhold inhalation and exhalation to find the complete range of function of the respiratory system. In addition, it is also possible to practice *pranayama* as a way of purifying one's body, to heighten perception of subtle energy flow in one's body and/or to grow in one's ability to concentrate. Similarly, *pratyahara* can be practiced as a way to orient one's attention inward. *Pratyahara* may also be practiced with the goal of developing the ability to feel the internal vibration of specific organs to the level of being able to notice differences among organs, such as distinguishing the sensations between one kidney and the other. Similarly, concentration may be practiced as ways to deepen one's capacity to focus one's mind so that all extraneous thoughts – including thoughts related to one's perceived identity – do not interfere with one's presence in any way.

Taking any one of the limbs of yoga to its limits will likely result in extraordinary abilities. For instance, some *pranayama* practitioners can demonstrate a capacity to inhale for more than 40 seconds and to exhale for more than 40 seconds without any gasping or tension. It has been suggested that Krishnamacharya's approach to reducing his pulse at will was directly related to his capacity to regulate his breath. It is fair to say that the average person may not be able to control his or her breath to that extent. Moreover, at a time when many people are unconsciously training their minds to keep jumping from one focal point to another all the time, it may be extraordinary to be able to stay focused on a single idea or object for an extended period.

At deeper levels of practice, it may be possible to reach even more extraordinary abilities. *Patañjali warns about these supernatural powers as potential distractions.* Some people may choose to see supernatural abilities as a way to participate more effectively in life and the world while others may see supernormal capacities as a way to improve their lot in life. On this point some teachers suggest that perhaps not every extraordinary ability may be available to every practitioner and that the abilities within your reach will manifest only in support of your specific life purpose.

When thinking about extraordinary powers, it may be helpful to consider that we live in a world where humans have created truly remarkable technologies that only one or two centuries ago would have seemed akin to magic. For instance, many people participate daily in the incredible event of flying across the sky on an airplane. Current technologies enable us to communicate wirelessly with people across the world; we can transfer the contents of a complete book from a digital file to a printed page in a matter of minutes or seconds; we can also listen to music or watch movies streamed through the internet. These and many other current technologies that would be deemed the stuff of fantasy, illusion, or fiction are so common to many of us that we may even take them for granted.

Yet, even with all these technological achievements, science cannot explain fully the mystery of life as it manifests in the complexity of our human bodies. As usual, in the interest of following the yogic approach, the exercise below can help you recognize some of the things that can be perceived when we focus with clear intention. Although we may not be able to explain exactly what is happening or how it's happening, we can use the experience to help us keep our minds open as we read about extraordinary powers.

The unfolding of the first 5 limbs of yoga – the *yamas*, *niyamas*, *asana*, *pranayama* and *pratyahara* – requires continued, wholehearted, and uninterrupted practice (*abhyasa*) balanced by detachment from the outcomes and goals of the practice (*vairagya*) as suggested by Patañjali in sutras 1.12 to 1.16. Yoga practice, as defined in 2.1, is the threefold combination of effort (*tapas*), insight (*svadhyaya*) and surrender (*ishvara pranidhana*). This practice of removing inefficiencies in attitude, movement and posture, breathing, and attention prepares the dedicated practitioner to develop single-pointed focus over years and decades. **Yoga practices cannot be forced or rushed.** Consequently, the capacity to apply the meditative integration defined in this chapter, *samyama,* requires the ability to focus with loving awareness and gentle attitude while allowing you to decouple from your identity. For most people, the practice develops gradually according to each practitioner's motivation and application over a long period of time (1.21-22). It is helpful to remember that the resulting experiences will proceed according to their usefulness to fulfilling your life purpose. Even more important is to remember that practice with detachment IS the most important part and is the aspect that is completely within your control.

In a comfortable sitting position close your eyes and invite a feeling of relaxation and ease. Take several rounds of fluid and effortless inhalations and exhalations. Bring the palms of your hands together in front of your chest or solar plexus area. Press the palms of the hands firmly against each other and feel as clearly as possible the sensations in the palms of the hands and fingers. Gradually ease the pressure until your hands are not pressing against each other. Again, feel the sensations in hands and fingers. Ensure that your shoulders are relaxed and bring your attention to your hands again. Make the contact between your hands as subtle as possible attending to how the sensations are changing.

As you keep feeling the sensations in your hands, start to separate your hands as slowly as you can while continuing to pay close attention to the changes in those sensations. With the hands close to each other without touching, notice the sensations and try to feel the air in the space between your hands. If you move your hands very slightly towards each other and away from each other, how do the sensations in your fingers and palms of hands change? Is it possible to feel the "cushion" of air between your hands and how it responds to the subtle movements of your hands feeling like there is a puffiness or stickiness? It is OK if you do not feel anything at all. Just stay open to the possibility of feeling some connection between the hands even when they are not touching. If you feel some stickiness or magnetic attraction between your hands, consider moving the hands gradually away from each other to explore the subtle sensations of connectedness between your hands even when they are not close to each other at all. You may even point the tips of your fingers towards the palm of the opposite hand and notice if there are any sensations in the palm of your hand indicating what your fingers in the opposite hand are doing. After a few minutes of exploring this, bring the palms of your hands close to your navel without touching your body, then close to your chest, then in front of your face. At each point feel if any sensations change in your hands and in the area your hands are close to. Then rest your hands on your thighs and just feel whatever is happening.

Can this exploration bring your attention to the fact that you can feel things that may be outside of your regular way of being and feeling? If you feel something outside of what you normally experience, can you explain it accurately? Similarly, you probably feel sensations of boredom, elation, love, or anger that are difficult to measure objectively in any way. However, the fact that you cannot measure how much love or anger you feel does not mean that those emotions do not exist.

As you traverse through this chapter, keep the recommended yogic attitude, open mind, and open heart to discover with curiosity what may be possible. *As part of keeping your mind open, it might be possible that there is no single correct answer.* The comments to these sutras use mostly previous testimony from trustworthy sources (*agama* 1.7). Since direct experience is the preferred yogic approach (*pratyaksha* 1.7), the practices suggested follow a logical and non-dogmatic perspective. As usual, you are in charge of investigating these practices and how they contribute to enhancing the quality of your participation in your life.

Concentration, Meditation, Integration and Integrative Meditation

3.1 Concentration (*dharana*) is directing the mind to a specific point.

Chapter Three of the Yoga Sutra continues the journey along the eight limbs of yoga. The preparatory steps have been completed, the seeds of unconditional love have been planted (*yamas*), contentment is setting the stage for the journey (*niyamas*), body function has been optimized (*asana*), improved vital energy flow contributes to enhancing sensitivity of the subtler aspects of your being (*pranayama*), and your senses have been directed inwardly for internal exploration (*pratyahara*). Following these steps has strengthened your capacity to direct your mind. It is evident that whatever you practice establishes a pattern that grows stronger over time. Throughout your exploration you have become more familiar with your ways of being and their effects as well as with effective ways for regulating them to improve the quality of your participation in your daily activities and interactions. In Sanskrit, *dharana* means to hold, to bear, to keep in remembrance, to assume the shape of. The exercises in the earlier portion of this journey guided you to explore what you make important enough to dedicate your time, energy, and attention to. This sutra invites you to direct your awareness to that same question. What is important enough to deserve your attention? Have you noticed how focusing mostly on temporary experiences and goals often results in riding an emotional rollercoaster from success to defeat, from dissatisfaction to feeling accomplished? Remember that Patañjali suggested single-pointed focus in sutra 1.32 as an effective way of reducing distractions. In addition, sutra 1.16 indicated that awareness centered on truth is beyond distractedness. Sutra 1.23 may also be interpreted as a way to release distractedness by relinquishing the illusion of control and accepting life unconditionally, exactly as it is. Then, all worries and tendencies to manipulate the world are removed.

Currently, the word meditation is used to talk about a wide range of practices. For instance, setting intentions and visualizations are often considered meditation. However, from the perspective presented in this aphorism, it is more accurate to think of intention setting and visualizations as concentration practices directed to set a meaningful path facilitative of wholehearted action. This interpretation articulates with the idea of *dharma*. *Dharma* is a Sanskrit word that can be interpreted as duty, life purpose, and living according to one's conscience. Moreover, this interpretation complements the call for single-pointed focus suggested in aphorism 1.32 as the way to remove distractions on the path to self-realization (1.30 & 1.31).

As you attempt to focus, notice what draws your attention away from your goal. Remember from the section on afflictions in Chapter Two of the Yoga Sutra that quite likely, who you think you are or should be will keep interfering with your goal. In the yoga tradition, there are very simple and specific focal points for concentration including the center of the pelvis, the solar plexus at the top of the upper abdomen just below the lower tip of the breastbone, the center of the chest, the center of the throat, the base of the tongue, the tip of the tongue, and the middle point between the eyebrows. *When focusing your attention on any of these points, remember the basic guideline: There will be distractions.* Just keep bringing your attention to your focal point without strain, struggle, or self-judgment, and with a gentle smile. To set yourself up for concentration you can apply the previous five limbs of yoga practice: First, invite gratitude and love for yourself and your life (*yamas*). Second, make peace with yourself and choose to be content with yourself and your life (*niyamas*). Third, find a steady and enjoyable posture, free of struggle and conducive to being endlessly focused (*asana*). Fourth, connect with your natural breath, feeling the sensations that arise with each easeful inhalation and exhalation, until your breath feels quite subtle and effortless (*pranayama*). Fifth, be curious to experience the aliveness in your body directly, by sensing the internal experience of being (*pratyahara*).

For concentration (*dharana*), rest your attention on one of the focal points listed above and witness whatever is happening without attaching opinions, stories, or expectations to what you are experiencing. *Be with what is as it is and with yourself as you are.* It can be useful to recognize that no number of words can ever encapsulate the immersive richness of being you. Welcome whatever arises and remain attentive to your focal point. Keep the technique simple by remembering that the experiences that come and go, regardless of how enjoyable or uncomfortable they may be, are not what you are concentrating on. They are the byproducts of your concentration, so stay with your focal point. After you are finished, reflect on how you felt before, during and after your concentration practice.

Are there any patterns in the distractions that you notice?

Are there some expectations interfering with your intention to concentrate?

Are some of those expectations tied to your sense of identity, like who you should be or are expected to be?

3.2 Meditation (*dhyana*) is to maintain the focus effortlessly.

Meditation is the natural progression resulting from concentration. Once again, the suggestion of complementing doing with letting go (being) appears in this aphorism. Concentration is a doing, inviting your attention to stay on a single point. As you remain in concentration, you gradually ease the amount of effort to staying focused so that you progressively let go of all tension and unnecessary doing to remain present without wasting any physical, mental, or emotional energy (being). It is like riding a bicycle. At the beginning, staying on your bike requires a lot of your energy and attentional resources. The more adept you become at riding, the more efficient the process becomes. At some point it may be possible to use the minimum amount of energy to hold the handlebars to determine your course with great ease. It may even happen that eventually you can let go of the handlebars and continue to ride your bike, changing direction by just shifting your body weight. Meditation is like any other skill; it improves through deliberate practice. Expectations may be the most frequent source of frustration in meditation, and in life. Some expectations include not getting distracted at all or being able to empty your mind completely. In addition, common accounts of extraordinary experiences or insight are often a hindrance rather than a catalyst for meditation. For instance, if you read that advanced meditators see lights akin to fireworks or feel this or that, you may expect to have those experiences, or you may try to emulate them. When your meditation practice does not produce the expected results, you will likely feel disappointed in yourself, maybe even coming to think that there must be something wrong with you because you cannot see the purple iridescent light you read about in some book, or when you cannot levitate as it says in some other text. Meditation is the highest of yogic practices especially when seen as **just being with what is as it is and with yourself just as you are**. Developing this attitude is very useful for all of yoga and very practical in all aspects of life.

Beware of any inclination to generate more opinions, comments, and preferences to what you are experiencing, as this is often an easy way to get entangled in your own stories. It is more productive to practice detaching (*vairagya*) and releasing physical, mental, and emotional gripping in order to sense with diminishing reactivity. In other words, you keep honing the skill of tuning in, feeling, and witnessing the richness of your inner universe. Remembering that your inner life is ineffable can assist you in releasing your tendencies to add labels, opinions, and explanations to what can only be experienced directly.

One of the traditional meditation techniques is called *japa*, which means muttering, whispering, or repeating a prayer, passages from sacred texts, or the name of a deity. In sutras 1.27 and 1.28, one way of practicing *japa* was introduced when talking about the syllable OM (ॐ) as a key to align with Supreme Being. One way of practicing *japa* with OM, or with any other meditational mantra, such as the seed (*bija*) sounds lam, vam, ram, yam, ham and ksham, is to start chanting aloud and gradually decreasing the volume of the sound so that the chant eventually becomes a whisper that finally turns into an internal silent chant. Even after the chant is silent it may be possible to change the level of intensity of the silent chant to make it increasingly subtler. Attention remains focused on the subtlest version of the chant until it may be possible to have the faintest connection to the silent whispering within. When the chant becomes an effortless echo it is called *ajapa japa*. At this level of practice, the goal is to maintain that subtle unconscious repetition. However, when distractions emerge, it may be necessary to return to a louder silent chant or to audible chanting to re-focus. As usual, noticing your distractedness indicates that you are growing in your capacity to recognize how some of your ways of being pull you away from presence. Just return to the subtlest version of chanting possible gently letting go of all unnecessary effort. Remember that staying with any practice can be facilitated by telling yourself *I want to do this, I need to do this, I can do this,* and *I will do this.* As expectations arise, recognize that it is important not to confuse the practice with the resulting experience (sensations, thoughts, emotions). With patient persistence keep returning effortlessly to your focal point, as many times as you need to.

What happens when you try to practice meditation?

What do you notice?

What are the sources of distraction?

How do you feel?

3.3 *Samadhi* is the ensuing dynamic integration empty of separateness.

In the Sanskrit language some of the meanings of the word *sama* include even, level, equable, complete, and whole. *Dhi* means to hold, to possess. *Samadhi* can be defined as becoming a receptacle for wholeness or possessing equanimity and fullness. The journey through the preceding seven steps leads incrementally into a state characterized by the release of any remaining attachment to your preferences, likes, dislikes, and objections that results in being with what is as it is. *Samadhi* is the result of the dynamic process of letting go of everything that generates the idea of being separate, alone, and disconnected. Growing evidence from research on meditation seems to confirm what Patañjali is saying about removal of separateness. Brain activity of consistent meditators shows a reduction of activity in areas of the brain involved in self-centeredness and rumination (Wolkin) as well as an increase in positive emotions like generosity, compassion, and loving kindness (Lutz, Brefczynski-Lewis, Johnstone, & Davidson, 2008). In the yoga tradition, this is the process initiated by practicing the *yamas* to create harmony in one's life and complemented by the *niyamas* to establish internal harmony.

As you grow in your ability to focus, it becomes apparent that most of what you consider you and your life consists of changing phenomena, your body, your thoughts, your memories, and your preferences.

Consequently, your attachment to your ideas about who you are or should be weakens because it no longer makes sense to try to "hold yourself together." As a result, the practice of letting go of the illusion of control (*ishvara pranidhana* 1.23, 2.1, 2.45) grows organically. It is not surprising that Patañjali says in aphorism 2.45 that being established in humility brings about *samadhi.* The ability to let go of the filters used to process all perceptions creates the possibility of experiencing life as it is, without having to pass everything through the filter of "I." This has tremendous implications because it compels you to experience directly the deep interconnectedness between you, your life and all of life as it is manifesting everywhere.

As you recognize your connection to all of life, it becomes more evident that your participation is needed and that it has effects on whatever is happening. The effectiveness and efficiency of your participation depends on the clarity of your intentions, which are predicated on your internal harmony. Thus, rather than seeing *ishvara pranidhana*, releasing the illusion of control, as a way to abdicate your agency, you recognize that it is important and necessary for you to participate in life with enthusiasm, wisdom and humility (2.1). In other words, instead of choosing to give up and to isolate yourself, you decide to contribute to enhance the expression of life in the best ways available to you. *Remember, do not allow other people to make choices for you.* Instead, choose to act from your internal harmony and from the direct experience of deep interconnectedness with all that exists.

The deep integration of *samadhi* is not a static state but a dynamic and wholehearted participation in the endless interaction between life and awareness. Integration (*samadhi*) is the result of articulating all your internal aspects at the physical, physiological, mental, and emotional levels by dropping obstacles, restrictions, inefficiencies, and all misidentifications. The complementary integration contributing to *samadhi* is the effortless articulation between you and the rest of you, the world that you are embedded in. By freeing yourself from the ideas and preferences that generate and perpetuate the notion of being disconnected from yourself, from other people, from the environment and from all of life, you create the necessary mental and emotional space to recognize that *you have never been isolated.* Similarly, you realize that you are the locus where life is manifesting in ever changing, unique, unrepeatable, and unpredictable ways. Therefore, the Yoga Sutra reminds you that the greatest obstacle is to forget your true nature (*avidya* 2.4 & 2.17), because you end up confusing who you think you are with who you actually are, the direct ineffable experience of life and embodied awareness in a unique manifestation, you. The desire to become evinces this fundamental misidentification.

Samadhi is integration understood as a symbiotic, synergistic, and comprehensive articulation between inside and outside. *Samadhi* cannot be forced into happening. It blossoms by removing the obstacles along the way.

Is it possible for you to notice your own interpretive frames and to be able to regulate them?

Is your experience different when you choose to witness life instead of trying to control it?

Can your distractions reveal the obstacles that need to be removed?

Is the desire to become one of these obstacles?

Can you shift from reactivity to responsiveness by releasing attachment to identity and outcomes?

What contributes to deepening your inner silence and stillness?

Is it possible to let go of your individual identity during your meditation?

Is the ground of your experience separateness or connectedness?

What is the difference between the two?

Which one feels better for you?

Does one feel more like you are coming home?

3.4 *Samyama* (meditative integration) combines concentration (*dharana*), meditation (*dhyana*) and integration (*samadhi*).

Some of the meanings of *Samyama* include whole self-control, being equable, and neutrality. *Samyama* is a natural progression from concentration to meditation and then into the deep integration of *samadhi*. This meditative integration, *samyama*, is a process of concentrating on a meaningful focal point which can be a heartfelt intention, a mantra, an inspiring idea, a physical point in your own body, your breath, or anything uplifting as mentioned in sutras 1.34 to 1.39. Gradually you soften your grip of the focal point until your connection to it is as subtle as possible (*dhyana* – meditation). As you remain in that effortless focus, you eventually release the focal point into the wholeness, stillness and silence of pure awareness (*samadhi* – integration). This gradual process obviously requires the capacity to concentrate first without distractions, which will lead into the ability to remain focused with minimal effort. Once again, notice that many of the distractions disrupting the concentration process might be related to your opinions, your desire to become and sense of identity. If you are sitting watching as the sun sets, there is nothing you need to add to make that moment more beautiful, inspiring, or fulfilling. *This is because there is no conflict in what is.* Whatever is happening is a manifestation of the perpetual interaction between life and consciousness resulting from the confluence of a multitude of factors and previous events, most of them beyond your control and awareness. Similarly, there is no inherent conflict in the colors that you see, the scents you smell, or the flavors you taste. For instance, if you are used to drinking coffee every morning and for some reason you decide to stop drinking coffee for a few days, the same familiar aroma of coffee brewing that you welcome every morning can become a source of conflict in your own mind. Now that aroma of coffee feels inviting as it always does for you, but since you created a reason not to drink coffee this week, conflict arises, generating internal opinions and arguments between one aspect of you that wants to drink coffee and another aspect of you that wants to stick to your decision not to drink coffee at this time. These opposing perspectives within create a conflict that manifests as internal commentary, doubt, questioning, and perhaps even self-blame.

The same theme from aphorism 1.4 characterizes this process, when your ways of being are not modulated you tend to misidentify with the internal activities. This is a reminder that integration (*samadhi*) happens when your sense of identity dissolves by releasing opinions and preferences. Aphorism 3.4 reminds you also of sutra 2.2, yogic actions minimize afflictions, which are the fruit of misidentification. Attenuating those afflictions brings about integration (*samadhi*). Sutra 3.4 echoes also another theme in the Yoga Sutra, the complementarity of doing and being. *Samyama* is the transition between the doing of concentration (*dharana*), which gradually becomes subtler as meditation (*dhyana*), to lead into the result of just being, integration (*samadhi*). The basic premise is that the yogic process leads you from a superficial identification and understanding of who you are into presence, embodied awareness. This does not mean that you should give up on doing. Instead, it is an invitation to align with the conflict-free peace and clarity pervading your being and all that exists. As you participate in your life, you choose to maintain a clear connection to that conflict-free consciousness during all your actions. This is what sutra 2.1 suggests when it directs you to act with enthusiasm, wisdom, and humility.

The practice of meditative integration (*samyama*) develops naturally through the progression from concentration to meditation to integration (*samadhi*). Find a comfortable and sustainable position conducive to being relaxed, awake and aware. Connect to your natural breath. Choose a focal object that uplifts you and inspires you to contribute your best to your life and to the world. Hold that intention in your heart and mind with care and love. Focus on the sensations generated by your intention and gradually let go of your thoughts and stories about that object. Remain focused on the direct wordless experience of holding your intention in mind and heart, and keep returning to it after every single distraction. As you stay focused on sensations, be curious about the subtler sensations. Relaxed and aware, gradually soften your hold on your intention while still being curious about directly feeling the subtle sensations that arise. Let yourself be open, free of effort, and just *be*. Once you feel it is time to return to the boundaries of your physical body, lie down and relax for a few minutes.
What do you notice when you try this practice?
Are there any patterns in the distractors that emerge?
Can you practice without any expectations?
Does a regular practice make clarity more familiar and accessible?

3.5 Meditative integration (*samyama*) results in direct insight into higher wisdom.

This sutra echoes sutras 1.17, 1.18 and 1.49, where Patañjali enumerated the steps leading to integration (*samadhi*) and the culmination into connecting to wisdom that does not result from inference or somebody else's testimony. The parallel between these sutras also reiterates that yoga is a dynamic process that develops at the natural pace that each practitioner can handle. This process begins by modulating your ways of being (1.3) to remove the obstacles that obstruct your natural awareness, love, and clarity. In other words, when awareness illuminates your understanding, extraordinary clarity results.

Meditative integration (*samyama*) is not a process of analysis or deduction. In fact, *samyama* is the release of all that you think you know so that you can gain undiluted insight into the constant interpenetration of life and consciousness. Rather than competing against your rational mind, insight complements it. *It is important to recognize that in yoga you are not in conflict with your mind.* Your mind is very useful and essential to your life. Fighting your mind wastes your valuable life energy. In fact, concentration starts by inviting the mind to focus, and it continues by softening the focus. Your mind helps you notice distractions and it also helps you return to your focal point. A useful strategy is to leverage your mind's curiosity to lead you into exploring the subtler level of phenomena. As the previous sutra stated, it is a gradual process because it is quite difficult to perceive what is subtler if you cannot clearly perceive what is more apparent. You may use your curiosity to remain focused on something so that it reveals its subtler aspects. In addition to sharpening your concentration, there is another practical benefit to developing higher sensitivity: you become better able to notice insight.

Practicing the limbs of yoga presented in sutra 2.29 fosters the development of inner silence and stillness by decreasing reactivity and by removing obstructions at the mental, emotional, physical, and physiological level. The combination of inner silence and higher sensitivity facilitates perceiving insight. In fact, you are constantly receiving an unending stream of stimuli, both external and internal. For instance, when you are walking on the street, you learn to attend to what is most important while ignoring what seems unnecessary. That is a reason you do not remember all the people that were walking in the opposite direction or the cars that were on the road. Similarly, in your mind you are constantly ignoring many thoughts and other stimuli while favoring others. Insights are among the many stimuli that you perceive. Insights tend to be subtle and may be triggered by something somebody said, a sign on the street, a license plate, the shape of a cloud, a sound, the song playing on the radio, a scent, or some other sensation. *Your yoga practice helps you recognize insight by distinguishing it from thoughts, opinions and stories.* The mind is a vehicle for insight. Awareness yokes mind and insight together. When you perceive insight, you experience a knowing that resonates with you, even when the knowing is quite different from your usual ways of thinking. Although insight may appear unusual, it never contradicts common sense. **Remember that wisdom is pure common sense.** You can use your mind to verify each insight, because it is pure common sense that sparks a connection with a deeper source of truth. However, sometimes insight offers a subtle suggestion to move in a direction different from your preference or agenda. In those cases, it is key to clarify the distinction between intuition and your own preferences. Gaining access into greater insight opens a door into re-cognizing the world and all of existence through a transparent lens (*samapatti* 1.41). As a result, you may be able to relate to the world from a perspective of connectedness. Obviously, if there are still traces of reactivity and tendencies towards seeing yourself as separate, the insights gained could be used to advance those traits leading you to think and act motivated by personal gain and with complete disregard for others. So even at this level of practice, a firm foundation on the *yamas* and *niyamas* is essential.

As you become more practiced in connecting to your inner spaciousness, stillness, and silence, what do you discover?
How is your yoga practice fostering your receptivity?
Some people say that a flash of insight comes to them as images.
Other people say that they just get a subtle hint or gentle knowing.
How does insight manifest in you?
Is it possible that your daily interactions and activities expose you to insight and wisdom on a regular basis?

3.6 Meditative integration (*samyama*) unfolds gradually.

When you are learning to ride a bicycle, you often start with somebody guiding you, with training wheels attached to your bike, practicing in a space with no traffic and minimal distractions and obstacles. Once you can keep your balance, you may remove the training wheels and gradually you start venturing out into different areas and terrains. It is common sense to start under conditions that will enable you to succeed. However, this is not an invitation to be complacent. This sutra is a reminder to practitioners that all of yoga is a process resulting from consistent practice (*abhyasa* & *sthira*) balanced by easefulness and moderation (*vairagya* & *sukha*). *There are no shortcuts in yoga*. Attachment to outcomes often results in trying to skip steps. This is a major cause of frustrations, distractions (1.30), injury and suffering. Thinking that yoga is a practice to transform you into something different from who you really are is the cause of suffering that can be avoided (2.15 & 2.16). Yoga is not trying to add something to you. In fact, the Yoga Sutra has been saying from the very beginning (1.3 & 1.4) that modulating and eventually releasing your ways of being will lead you into experiencing your true nature.

In this journey towards embodying awareness, you take one step at a time with patient persistence (1.12) and with the appropriate intensity (1.22). To be successful, it is most helpful for you to know your tendencies and your abilities so that you can choose intelligently the tasks that will help you grow in your abilities without causing strain or injury. The skill of concentration can be honed through consistent practice, so that meditation starts to happen organically. Your motivation is fundamental to keep you returning to your goal, especially when you get distracted. The general approach is to do the best that you can as consistently as you can, while setting aside your expectations (*vairagya*). As you keep doing the best that you can, your dedication causes your best to change incrementally. To soften the grip on expectations it may be helpful to consider that the results of *samyama*, just like the results of any other meaningful action, are not immediate. Moreover, the process of *samyama* itself is a gradual distilling of attention from a gross object towards increasing levels of subtlety (1.40 to 1.51). As you try to practice, notice if your sensitivity is growing so that your attention goes from the superficial features of your focal point towards its subtle aspects and eventually into its essence. Similarly, pay

attention to noticing if insight and intuition are growing.
Is there a sense of flashes of clarity delivering suggestions for action?

Do you feel like you are receiving subtle guidance during your day?

Are you letting go of your desire to become?
How are you keeping your expectations in check?

3.7 *Dharana, Dhyana* and *Samadhi* are more internal than the previous five limbs.

3.8 Yet, *Dharana, Dhyana* and *Samadhi* are still external to the subtlest state of pure awareness (*nirbija samadhi*).

Just as a skilled scribe expertly modulates the pressure and movement of a stylus to create shapes and forms with pleasing proportions and harmonious coherence, a yoga practitioner grows in sensitivity to attend to the inner world with ever-growing skill and subtlety. The natural process initiated by the first five limbs of yoga develops into the capacity to be effortlessly focused (*dhyana*), becoming a receptacle for equanimity and fullness (*samadhi*) that results in the capacity to abide in neutrality and self-control (*samyama*). These final three limbs of the eight-limbed path of yoga require great dedication and a consistent uninterrupted practice over a long period of time (*abhyasa*). They continue the process of removal of obstructions, limitations and inefficiencies initiated with the first five limbs. Although reaching the high levels of meditative integration presented in the previous sutras represents a significant achievement, these two aphorisms indicate that there are still lingering traces of separateness preventing the practitioner from fully embodying pure awareness. These traces are either past impressions or the remnants of subtle identification with externalities (1.18). Although more internal than the previous five limbs, these final three limbs are not the peak of the complete integration that has been mentioned before, the seedless integration known as *nirbija samadhi.* In seedless integration, all remaining labels of identity cease to define you and your life, thus facilitating the direct experience of utter connectedness with the awareness that pervades all aspects of life everywhere. This progression through the levels of *samadhi* was presented towards the end of Chapter One from sutra 1.40 onward.

It has been said by many teachers before that integration (*samadhi*) can be received only by grace and that there is no formula for it other than the full surrender of the illusion of control (2.45), because only by forgetting your individual identity can you embrace the perfection of life in all its myriad of unique, diverse, and ever-changing manifestations.

As you cultivate spaciousness, stillness, and silence within, can you soften your grip on anything and everything?

In other words, can you do consciously what you do every night unconsciously when you go to sleep?

Would it be possible to relinquish ownership of your beliefs?

Can you choose to let go of the filters coloring your perceptions so that your mind and intellect can be a clear and streak-free window into life?

TRANSFORMATION

3.9 Increased tendency to inner stillness and away from outward attention. Growing inner awareness transforms the body, mind, and senses (*nirodha parinama*).

The practice of yoga is a journey to regulating our tendencies. The overall process can be understood as an application of sutras 1.39 and 2.33. The former aphorism invites you to focus on anything that inspires you, while the latter echoes that message, encouraging you to redirect your tendencies from unhelpful to uplifting (*pratipaksha bhavana*). The first seven limbs of yoga promote ways to remove inefficiencies and to establish tendencies conducive to living in harmony with yourself and the world. As a result, all your different aspects articulate together seamlessly. In this sutra the word *parinama* indicates change or transformation. At this stage of the practice, all emotional, physical, respiratory, and mental obstacles have been removed, and the practice transforms the body, mind, and senses so that instead of being at the mercy of innumerable distracting tendencies pulling you away from presence, you now gravitate towards embodied awareness. Instead of entertaining yourself with irrelevant internal chatter, you align effortlessly with your inner stillness and silence. That inner stillness is the result of the suppression, restraint, or control (*nirodha*) of the wayward ways of being. Hence, this stage of the process is called *nirodha parinama*, the transformation of your inner world because of the practices that control, restrain and eventually remove your unhelpful ways.

Current science seems to confirm what early yogis learned through using their bodies and minds as a laboratory of inner exploration.

Recent research indicates that regular meditation practice seems to cause physical and physiological changes to the brain. These changes appear to contribute to enhanced performance in processing information, making decisions, forming memories, and improving attention, as well as enabling improved learning and emotional regulation, reduction of fear, anxiety and stress, increase in positive emotions, emotional stability, and mindful behavior. Some other changes include enhanced capacity to choose between automatic habits and thoughts and meaningful choices as well as deep feelings of well-being and oneness.[iii] As you practice with patient persistence, notice if there is a change in your attitude, mood, distractedness and overall experience. *Are you currently complaining more or less than before? Are you more willing to participate in all aspects of your life with kindness and compassion?*

3.10 Effortless inner silence is established through peaceful impressions.

The message in sutra 1.50 is reiterated in this aphorism. For most practitioners, the process of establishing greater inner peace results from sustained practice over time. Notice that many of the obstacles along the way are self-created. **Therefore, it is instrumental to shift from being your own worst enemy to becoming your greatest friend and supporter.** At first your tendencies rule your body, mind, breathing, and emotions, and you may not even be aware of them. Often, you may even think that your tendencies are who you are and you may end up identifying with the continuous stream of thoughts distracting your attention (1.4). As you practice the limbs of yoga you become more aware of your tendencies, choosing to cultivate helpful tendencies instead of investing energy and attention on the tendencies that create confusion and suffering. The gradual process of turning your attention towards uplifting thoughts, intentions, and actions creates new tendencies (2.33 & 2.34). Sustained practice over time generates impressions (*samskaras*) that overcome the previous, less helpful tendencies in you. Similarly, by meditating on whatever is uplifting to you, you create impressions that overpower existing impressions (1.39). Notice how the content of your internal dialogue has changed as a result of your practice and how your practices influence your internal environment as well as your actions and interactions. Obviously, your actions and interactions also influence your inner state. For instance, when there is conflict between what you know and what you feel, whatever you focus your attention on may appear to be in conflict. Conversely, if you behave in an adversarial manner your internal environment will be filled with conflict. As you gradually modulate your ways of being, the energy that you were investing in it becomes available and the tension your ways of being was generating gives way to increasing peace and stillness.

How are you cultivating greater peace in your external and internal life?
What are the effects of your practice, a tendency towards greater harmony or disharmony?
Are you organically becoming an abode of peace?
Is the garden of your heart filled with peace and kindness?

3.11 Releasing internal commentary and identification with externalities brings about a transformation toward integration (*samadhi parinama*).

The transition from the previous two sutras to this one moves along a similar process to the change from concentration (*dhyana*) to meditation (*dharana*). Your tendency towards inner stillness shifts gradually from intermittent to steady. Inner silence becomes established once all opinions dwindle and identification with changing external phenomena ceases. This aphorism contains the echo of sutra 1.4 that suggested that identification with your ways of being resulted from not being aware of and not regulating your ways of being. As you effectively neutralize your temporary ways of being, you release tension, and your awareness moves from being focused on the gross aspects of perception toward the subtlety of the perceptual process itself. This is the change known as the transformation of deep integration (*samadhi parinama*). For instance, notice what happens when you change from being entangled by your perceptions and reactivity to what you perceive, to being aware of your own perceptual processes. Does this shift generate a different experience of being? Another question to apply this sutra: Are you in greater harmony with life regardless of whatever happens? Because it is always easier to be at peace with life when everything goes according to your plans, desires, and expectations. What happens when life brings you something different from what you prefer or like? You may want to pay attention to any inclinations to generate opinions and judgments about anything that crosses your path. Notice if the internal voices offering commentary on everything you perceive are quieting down. *In other words, are you being with what is happening without placing conditions? What is the actual experience of awareness of your own perceptions? When you have less judgments and opinions, what is the quality of your participation in your own life? Are you more present?*

3.12 Single pointedness (*ekagrata parinama*) is the transformation when subsiding and arising perceptions are identical from one moment to the next. Then the illusion of fragmentation and separateness subsides.

In Chapter One, sutra 1.32, single-pointed focus (*ekagrata*) was offered as the way to eliminate distractions of all kinds. The transformation of oneness (*ekagrata parinama*) is the ability to direct attention to a single point without attention being scattered. Such single-pointedness facilitates the transition from *nirodha parinama* (3.9) to *samadhi parinama* (3.11). This single- pointedness is the foundation of all the yoga practices, and it is cultivated through sustained wholehearted practice (*abhyasa*) as well as by being disinterested in anything and everything that is not conducive to the experience of Truth (*vairagya*). One-pointedness changes your perspective so that, rather than seeing or thinking of yourself as made up of different fragments, you experience your own wholeness directly. Moreover, this level of internal integration makes it more evident that you have never been isolated and that there is a profound unity between everything that exists. **You can no longer be your own enemy or be at conflict with yourself.** At the same time, you are better able to relate to the world outside through kindness and compassion.
Is it possible for you to stop self-judgment altogether?
Can you indeed be your best friend?
Can you also let go of judgment of whatever you perceive?

Can you start seeing everybody as your brother or sister?
Can you relate to life as something you are deeply embedded in?
Can you recognize that you are an individual manifestation of awareness in life?

As the illusion of separateness dissolves and the feeling of oneness pervades, distractions are removed. Then your awareness remains focused, because the tendency to generate an opinion over everything you perceive becomes unnecessary. As a result, you are better able to direct your awareness with greater clarity to what is actually happening from one moment to the next instead of creating stories to entertain yourself. This single-pointed focus makes it possible for you to stay on the same focal point from one instant to another. Whatever you are meditating on remains, without being displaced by anything else. This is a reminder that in order to get to the level of practice when there are no distractions, the key skill is the capacity to keep returning to your focal point without strain, struggle, or self-judgement and with a gentle smile in your heart. Eventually your ability to remain focused grows. Applying the *yamas* and *niyamas* in your life contributes to removing sources of distraction. Notice if your ability to focus has increased not only in meditation but also in your personal activities and interactions. There are many sources of distractions in everyday life, and many of the technological tools prevalent in contemporary life seem to keep offering more sources of distractions. Notice what distractions get a hold of you. Pay attention also to where your distractions lead you.
What are these distractions offering you?
How are they contributing to your sense of wholeness and inner connectedness?
Is it possible that your inner connectedness is the path to grow in your inter-connectedness?

3.13 Consequently, awareness attunes to changes in the senses and in the natural world. These changes manifest as variations of properties (*dharma*), characteristics (*lakshana*) and states (*avastha*) and include changes in one's own being.

Your capacity to maintain your single-focused attention enables you to direct your awareness so that you can notice the changing nature of all phenomena, including the external world as well as the changes in your own body, mind, and emotions. Patañjali and the traditional commentators indicate that something that exists manifests with specific properties (*dharma*). Those properties are different for a horse, a cow, and a dog. Although they are all animals, their properties make them different from one another in height, weight, appearance, strength, and speed. Each one of those animals will display its own set of specific characteristics (*lakshana*). For instance, a calf's characteristics are different from another calf of the same age born to a different mother and different from those of a calf belonging to a different breed. The state or condition (*avasthana*) will change over time. At some point a dog may be young and another time it will be old; similarly it can be happy, unhappy, clean or dirty, healthy or unhealthy. Everything that exists, including you and your internal world, manifests along those three dimensions: properties, characteristics, and condition.

The canonical example offered by Vyasa is clay. Clay has some properties. When you shape it into a bowl its characteristics will change. If you made several bowls from the same clay but you choose to keep some unfired, others bisque fired, and others glazed fired, their characteristics will change. These varying characteristics will influence the state of each bowl. As time goes by, you will notice that they will age differently, so even when they are all old, their characteristics will be different. Paying attention to those three dimensions enables you to notice changes.

You are a unique manifestation of the properties of a human being, with specific characteristics that change over time. Your state or condition also changes. Focusing your awareness on these changes makes it possible for you to notice all in you that is in constant change as well as the vantage point from where you are observing. Being aware of what changes reveals if there is anything in you that is not subject to change.

Can you notice the changes in the characteristics of your physical body over time?

Can you tell that your ideas and thoughts have changed?

(For instance, is what you consider important now the same as what was important to you five or ten years ago?)

Are you aware of how your emotions change as well as why?

Are the stories you tell yourself the same as they were some years ago?

Among all these changes is there anything that has remained the same?

For instance, if you celebrate your birthday every year, is there anything that remains the same despite the physical changes your body is undergoing?

3.14 The characteristics of an object can be dormant, active, or potential, yet there is an essence underlying the object.

Yoga philosophy is one perspective among many views developed over centuries in the region currently known as India. Some views maintain that the world we experience is a very convincing illusion that covers an unchanging reality that is eternal, while other viewpoints argue that there is no real enduring essence but a confluence of ever-changing streams of stimuli coming together at each moment. This sutra can be interpreted as saying that the world is real instead of being an illusion, and that there is an essence to any object in existence. That essence is independent from whoever perceives that object. Each essence has inherent characteristics that can be in three states. In the first state, inert or dormant, some characteristics of the object are at rest and thus not manifesting. In the second state the characteristics are active, so they are manifest and therefore can be perceived by an outside observer. The third state consists of latent or potential characteristics that are yet to manifest.

One way to illustrate this is by thinking of a mango. The fruit hanging from the tree no longer shows the characteristics of the pollinated flower from which the mango developed. That same fruit does not show the characteristics of the mango trees that are directly linked to this particular mango over centuries. The mango fruit hanging from the tree presents the characteristics active at the time in its color, fragrance, and shape. If the fruit is not ripe yet, it will not have its typical sweetness, so the sweetness is potential. Also potential in the seed at the core of the fruit is a full mango tree that, if planted under the right conditions, will take several years to produce new mangoes. Also potential in this mango fruit are all the mango trees that could be planted from the mango seeds produced by the mango trees resulting from the seed of this mango. Thus, each mango fruit has a dormant set of characteristics, a past. It also has a set of potentialities that have not manifested yet, a future. Its current characteristics are its present. Comparing this mango to other mangos on the same branch of the tree may show that, despite all their shared characteristics each mango is slightly different.

This sutra suggests that beneath all the subtly changing characteristics there is an essence, something that makes each mango unique. This underlying essence makes all the characteristics of the mango come together in a particular way, yet its characteristics manifest at different times in a variety of ways. This is another concept where there may be various perspectives:

Does the essence of the mango exist as a pure idea somewhere beyond physical reality?

Or, is that essence purely physical? In that case, does the essence of something relate to its DNA?

Or, is the essence of every mango connected to a virtual network of information connecting all mangoes of that species overlapping in turn with a similar network encompassing all mangoes, which is embedded in a larger network of fruits and so on?

Or, does the essence of a mango manifest as a result of the interaction between awareness and the natural world?

Is it possible that the essence of each object is part of what some people call consciousness, a distributed, dynamic, multi-dimensional matrix connecting all of existence, with the myriad of manifestation of objects in space and time being only the tiny fraction available through our senses?

Can that consciousness be what is called God, the Absolute, Supreme Being, the Source?

These large questions can offer you a point of departure for contemplation. Remember that whatever response you arrive at consists only of thoughts, ideas, or words, it is only a pointer to that ineffable wholeness. If *samyama* is one way of tapping into that deep interconnectedness, then it makes sense that the following sutras present specific ways of accessing that matrix of existence.

At a more personal and concrete level, you may explore your ways of being – physical, mental, and emotional – to find out if they are dormant, active, or latent.

If your ways of being change continually, consciously and unconsciously, who is noticing these changes?

Can the observer of your ways of being be observed?

You may also choose to contemplate these questions about whatever you experience:

Is there an essence to it?

Is it an illusion?

Is it a temporary confluence of sensory input and awareness?

You may also inquire into your own ways of being, such as how the characteristics of your body have changed over time.

Are there areas of your body that now (active) seem stronger/weaker or more rigid/flexible than they were before (dormant)?

Are some of your thoughts and beliefs different (active/dormant) depending on the context or company you are in?

Do your feelings and emotions regarding yourself change during your day with feelings of self-acceptance being active at some points while feelings of self-criticism are dormant?

Do these and other feelings change or are they always the same?

Are some of your feelings towards your loved ones varied as well?

Is it possible that there is an underlying essence to all these changing ways of being?

3.15 Awareness of the sequence of manifestation of these states causes the perception of change.

The process of attuning to the subtler aspects of you through the practice of the eight limbs of yoga results in increasing clarity. As a result, you become aware of the interpretive filters you use to make sense of the world. You also recognize that you acquired those ways of being, thinking, and feeling through your upbringing, education, interactions, and overall participation in society. You become better able to discern (*viveka* in 2.26) between your essence and the aspects of you that change. Once you choose not to entertain yourself with the stories and opinions vying for your attention, you create the possibility of witnessing reality unencumbered by your assumptions and expectations. Then, instead of taking everything personally, you can see how the characteristics of any perception shift between the three states mentioned in the previous aphorism. Whatever was active but is now dormant becomes something you label as past. Whatever is currently active is perceived as present. And whatever has not yet manifested is thought of as future.

Noticing variations in the sequence of manifestation of these characteristics registers in your awareness as change. For instance, your presence is always at the core of every one of the experiences you have. As a result, when you act centered on your presence, like when you are having a genuine interaction with somebody else or when you are laughing wholeheartedly, time seems to dissolve. Similarly, when you truly look at yourself in the mirror focusing in on your eyes, you may be able to see yourself in timelessness. However, when you focus on the characteristics of your physical form, or on the evolution of your beliefs or on the changes in your emotions, those changes create the notion of time. That may be one way of explaining what happens when somebody shows you a picture of yourself from a decade ago and you go from the feeling of presence, just being you, to focusing on the noticeable differences in the observable characteristics of your body. As a result, you think in terms of time with some characteristics associated with your past, others to the present, and some other changes not manifesting yet.

What happens when you choose to focus on the perceptual characteristics of whatever is around and within you?
At what levels in your being (physical, physiological, conceptual and emotional) are there discernible changes?
Are there sequences in the manifestation of these changes?
How do those changes influence the ways you think and the stories you create about you, about life and about the world?

RESULTS OF MEDITATIVE INTEGRATION (*SAMYAMA*)

When it is possible to regulate your ways of being, you stop trying to accommodate what you perceive to what you think you know, your predictions and assumptions. Then you are centered on presence. Presence becomes the unfiltered window through which you experience the world. Consequently, you gain insight into existence, perceiving the world, your ways of being, your own presence as well as the intricate web of interconnections among all that is. This is a radical transformation that orients your ways of being towards experiencing life as an integrated human being, responding intelligently and wholeheartedly to the endless fluctuations of life. The goal of the practice is not to escape from the world, your life, or your circumstances. On the contrary, your practice is most effective when it harnesses your presence and insight as the compass for your participation in your life. This can be one of the meanings of sutra 1.26 when it suggests that pure being is the greatest teacher.

Like other sections in the Yoga Sutra, after explaining a concept, Patañjali continues by specifying the effects of the practice as when he introduced the practices to overcome distractions in 1.30 – 1.39 and their effects starting at aphorism 1.40. In Chapter Two Patañjali also presented a path of practice, the eight limbs of yoga in sutra 2.28, defining them (2.29 – 2.34) and then presenting the results in aphorism 2.35. Sutra 3.16 begins the list of results that can be accomplished by applying the combined trio of meditative practices (*samyama*). This is an extensive list that takes up most of this chapter. There is ongoing debate regarding the appropriateness, usefulness, need, and potential misuse of these results. *Is it possible that meditative integration (samyama) is a self-regulating process that, just like any other tool can be used to grow in awareness, connectedness and compassion? Is the progression that starts with the yamas one way of fostering a movement towards unconditional empathy, compassion, love and joy?*

3.16 Meditative integration (*samyama*) on the three dimensions of change (properties, characteristics, and condition) reveals past and future.

At the most obvious level, when you look closely at one of the cups you use regularly to drink your favorite beverage, you can probably see some signs of wear including tiny scratches, some stains, and perhaps some other subtle discolorations. These are marks that tell the story of that cup, they are signs from its past. At the same time, there are potential changes in the future of the cup that are most likely beyond what you can ascertain. This aphorism continues the previous discussion about meditative integration, the technique for directing your awareness with laser-like precision towards any focal point. Through meditative integration you can discover the properties (*dharma*), characteristics (*lakshana*), and condition (*avastha*) (3.13) of anything you focus on. You can also apprehend its essence (3.14). Becoming aware of the sequence in the manifestations of those states you can know the various changes that object undergoes (3.15). This sutra continues that line of thought by saying that *samyama* on the changes along the three dimensions (properties, characteristics, state) can show you the changes that an object has undergone as well as the potential changes to happen in the future. So you may be able to know the composition and origin of the clay used to make the cups, as well as where the cup has been and where it will be in the future. You may even be able to learn what will happen to the cup once it is broken and becomes shards. Of course, it is possible to test these ideas by meditating on any object and trying to notice what information may be revealed.

As you reflect on this and the preceding sutras, consider that it took more than a thousand years for the idea of an atom to be tested empirically. For more than 200 years this idea of an atom has evolved based on technological advances that have prompted discoveries that have continued up until recent years. Every discovery can corroborate some assumptions about the universe and refute previous ways of understanding. All these discoveries are related to something that is present in our everyday life yet beyond our sensory perception.

When we think about accessing information about the past and future of a certain object, is it possible that there is an all-encompassing timeless awareness that pervades all of existence, yet cannot be fully apprehended through our senses only?

Could it be that whatever manifests in the world of the senses enters the dimension of time?

Can it be that, in awareness, time collapses just like it does in our subconscious mind where memories from events that happened at different times come together regardless of the order of their occurrence?

Is it possible that you can learn to regulate your internal levels of activity and reactivity so that you can turn your senses inward (*pratyahara* 2.54) to explore the timelessness of your being? (And, perhaps, in that timelessness there are cues to seeing beyond the boundaries of time?)

What happens when you try to relax yourself deeply into the spaciousness, silence and timelessness within?

Possibly, another avenue of application for this sutra would be in order to gain a deeper intuition about some of the patterns in your physical, mental, and emotional composition. *Would samyama on your inclinations, preferences and actions shed light on some previous actions that were unclear to you? Can it reveal potentially fruitful avenues for your actions and interactions? Can it indicate future suffering that can be avoided (2.16)?* Remember, this is not a process of convincing yourself of something. It is an invitation to let the mystery of your own life offer some clues to guide you in making intelligent and sensible decisions and choices.

3.17 Meditative integration (*samyama*) on the difference between word, object and concept offers insight into the language of all beings, enabling deep communication with all beings.

This sutra presents the effects of practicing *samyama* on communication and it can be related to the thread started with sutra 1.42 (*savitarka samadhi*). As humans, we use words to refer to objects in the world. The word is not the actual object. The word apple is not something that has a color, texture, fragrance, and taste that can be eaten. The word is a sign pointing to a class of objects agreed upon. As you are reading the word apple, you may immediately think of a specific type of apple, maybe it is a gala, fuji, pink lady or granny smith. Each one of these types of apples has some overlapping properties with the others, while at the same time each one has its own unique characteristics. The word apple triggers a recall for the concept in your mind associated with it. That concept is different from the actual object and from the word. The concept is likely influenced by your own personal history. So, if you grew up eating apple pie baked at home, it is likely that the concept of apple may be related to the smell of apple pie baking and of the person who used to make it. A person who grew up in a subtropical region where apples did not grow may think of different images or memories when seeing or hearing the word apple. The concepts each person carries are influenced by that person's life experiences and personal history. Those concepts may become an obstacle to apprehending something fully, especially when what is perceived goes against what is assumed or expected. In those cases, perception tends to be biased by unchecked assumptions.

At the simplest level, this sutra can be interpreted as meaning that *samyama*, because it happens once internal chatter has been removed, provides greater clarity of mind, enabling you to communicate deeply and genuinely without misunderstandings resulting from biases and assumptions. Then, when you are listening to any message, you are truly listening and not trying to respond or defend an opinion or belief. This is the simplest level of meaning in this sutra, yet arguably it is extraordinary to find a person who is capable of listening without confusing word, object, and concept and thus able to understand with an open mind and an open heart. Is this an avenue you'd like to explore?

This sutra may also mean that *samyama* can make it possible for the practitioner to understand all languages and all forms of communication. If you have a pet, can you notice the different ways they use to communicate with you? Might it be possible that communication with all beings can be deepened?
Is it possible that all humans know a language that is deep at the core of our beings – a language that is expressed through laughter, gratitude, love and compassion?

3.18 Meditative integration (*samyama*) on impressions (*samskaras*) offers insight into previous births.

Samskaras are the impressions recorded in you because of the experiences you have. Some of those impressions are conscious, while others are unconscious. It appears as if emotion is one of the most powerful catalysts to embed the impressions into your space of awareness. As you reflect on your memories, notice how emotion contributed to deepen the hold of some of those memories. Emotion is expressed and felt in close connection to awareness, because emotion is energy that is active in the present moment. Emotion captures your attention. If the experience you are having comes to a balanced resolution, its emotional charge travels through you leaving an imprint as a memory that can bring that same feeling of buoyancy, spaciousness, and clarity. On the other hand, if the experience leaves an unresolved emotional residue, the energy that feeds that emotion attaches to you, triggering a similar feeling every time you remember that event. This emotional residue is stored regardless of it being positive or negative. This phenomenon may explain why sometimes there are some feelings that seem difficult to shed even though we consciously may try to convince ourselves that we do not want to keep ruminating about a past event that is long gone.

One very useful practice to try to turn these well-established habits is sitting with tolerable discomfort as it was mentioned briefly in the commentary about sutra 2.10. You may choose a recent event that seemed to trigger some tolerable discomfort, such as something that made you feel slightly embarrassed, anxious, or frustrated. Rather than focusing on the surface aspects of the experience choose to focus your attention on the actual sensations that you felt. This is easiest by recalling the event and its effects on your body, mind, and emotions. Instead of trying to come up with opinions, explanations, or solutions to the situation, use the sensations triggered by the event as your focal point. Concentrate upon those sensations and stay focused on them choosing to travel along the emotional dimension. Recall a previous event that generated the same overall feeling and reactivity, feel the tolerable discomfort without trying to figure it out, without attempting to numb it, medicate it or ignore it. This is important. Stay with your focal point and continue finding past experiences that cause you to feel this way. It may not be difficult to keep traveling to earlier and earlier parts of your life. Is it possible to find the earliest memory of feeling this way? Notice that this concentrated focus on emotion may be revealing that dissimilar situations tend to resonate emotionally in very similar ways within you. Could it be that the earliest memory is still somehow trapped within you, creating a sore spot that is quite sensitive because it has not been resolved? What happens if you sit with this tolerable discomfort and let it flow through you without trying to suffocate it or to ignore it? Can you allow this emotional energy to be used up instead of keeping it trapped within you? It may be necessary to make peace with the feelings within that trigger this response. Those feelings may include inadequacy, scarcity, fear, worry, anxiety as well as numerous others. Most likely the majority, if not all these feelings, conflict with the fundamental truth that you are complete and whole. The conflicting feeling may deny or obstruct your deep connection with the embrace of all-pervasive love, compassion and awareness that makes up all that exists. Can you surrender to this fundamental truth instead of believing in the inaccurate notion that you are isolated and in need of justification for your existence?

This practice can have profound effects on your relationship with yourself, and it is just a simple practice that asks you to confront deep-seated fears about your true nature. This practice is a productive way to harness the powers of *samskaras* to offer you insight into both your past and your present so that you are no longer at the mercy of past impressions controlling your thoughts, reactions and interactions now and in your future. If this is possible, might it also be feasible that practicing *samyama* into your deep-seated impressions may uncover even deeper connections to events beyond your current embodiment? In case that it might be possible to learn about your previous lives, rather than seeing what you find as a source of entertainment, the information you discover may provide you with useful insight into your current life and life purpose. *For instance, if you realize that you have been alive before in a different body and different circumstances, what effect would that have on how you currently invest your awareness, energy and time?*

3.19 Meditative integration (*samyama*) on somebody's gestures, actions and demeanor indicates his/her state of mind.

3.20. However, the cause of that state of mind is not revealed.

Meditative integration is a high state of receptivity enabling you to apprehend information instantaneously through intuition. This heightened perception is directed toward a specific focal object. This is one reason *samyama* is thought of as integration with seed (*sabija samadhi*), because the focal object is the seed around which your awareness gravitates. This perceptivity is cultivated through time. It is like the gradual development of NASA's Deep Space Network over decades to become an international array of powerful radio antennas capable of sending and receiving information to and from distant spacecraft like Voyager I and Voyager II for over four decades. By adjusting the Deep Space Network over time, NASA is still capable of communicating with these spacecrafts travelling beyond our solar system, even though capturing their signals is like seeing a refrigerator light bulb that is more than sixteen billion kilometers away. The focal point for these two sutras is the demeanor, gestures, and actions of a person. It stands to reason that paying close attention to a person may give you a fair indication of that person's state of mind. The more acute your concentration and perception, the more likely it is that you can learn something about the person you are directing your attention to.

Aphorism 3.20 clarifies that since the focal object of *samyama* is the external features of the person observed, his or her state of mind would be revealed but the cause of that state of mind would not be known because the cause is not the focal point. Even without applying *samyama* you can make some inferences about a person by observing gestures, actions, and demeanor attentively. Observing a person with sustained focus is a viable stepping stone towards practicing the technique in this sutra. What do you find when you try it?

To what extent are your inferences accurate or inaccurate? To what extent are you distracted by your own thoughts and unrelated ideas? Are your opinions of this person helpful or unhelpful in ascertaining their state of mind? Since *samyama* is a technique that goes beyond the mental processes of inference and testimony, what happens if you focus on the person while remaining centered and completely calm? Whatever you perceive, it may be interesting to investigate if the information you receive provides a hint or invitation for mindful, compassionate and life affirming actions on your part.

3.21 Meditative integration (*samyama*) on the relationship between form, light and the eyes enables the yogi to become invisible.

3.22* Similarly with sound and other stimuli.

**Some versions of the Yoga Sutra include aphorism 3.22 while other versions don't; this explains why some sources say that there are 195 sutras and others say 196.*

Yoga is a practical experiment for participating in life fully guided by your conscience, your open mind, and open heart. The experiment consists of removing all obstructions and inefficiencies that prevent you from graciously embodying the flow of awareness through all of life processes. As with any other process, patient persistence gradually reveals subtler aspects of anything you attend to. For instance, as you start practicing the postures and movements in yoga, it may be difficult for you to regulate effectively how far you can move an arm or leg or move into a squat while maintaining a desired level of muscular engagement. Over time it may become second nature to move in and out of each posture with finesse and elegance. Similarly, the thought of lengthening your inhalations and exhalations so that each one lasts for more than 30 seconds may seem impossible. However, as you apply yourself with gentle persistence, you may notice how lengthening your in breaths and out breaths requires a combination of actions in your abdomen and thorax, while making your inhalations and exhalations quite subtle.

Moving into the realm of meditation continues that journey towards exploring the innermost depths of your being. These aphorisms may be seen as a continuation of the practice in sutra 1.35 related to focusing on subtle sense perceptions. Sutra 3.21 suggests a *samyama* practice focused on the interaction between a form, light, and the eyes. A form or object with light shining upon it will absorb, reflect, or refract that light. This interaction between light and objects is what makes objects visible to you. Your eyes capture the changes to the light according to how each object absorbs, refracts, and reflects light. In the way that advanced yoga practitioners can make their breath so subtle that it may be imperceptible to an outside observer, this sutra indicates that it may be possible to arrange the atomic structure of the body so that it does not absorb, reflect, or refract any light. In other words, the body of the yogi becomes completely neutral and light travels through it without being distorted in any way. Sutra 3.22 suggests the same would be true of other sense stimuli, like sound, touch and taste.

One way of understanding this phenomenon is that yoga is literally a practice of being unconditionally with what is. *The yogin does not create interference in the world and is in complete harmony with the perfection of life.* One way of trying to put this aphorism into practice is to notice the imprint that you leave – in yourself, others, and in the world – through your actions and interactions.

To what extent do your actions generate more turbulence in the world?

Are your actions motivated by being seen and by recognition?

To what extent are your actions enhancing life in the world?

Is it possible to act without drawing attention to yourself?

Of course, should you find it meaningful and life affirming, you may also explore practicing *samyama* on the relationship between form, light and sight to make yourself invisible, on the relationship between sound, air and ear to make yourself outwardly and inwardly silent.

3.23 Meditative integration (*samyama*) on active (*prarabdha*) and dormant (*sanchita*) karma, or on the omens of death, discloses the time of death.

Consistent with the notion that a sutra is a thread of related concepts brought together, this sutra is another place where Patañjali connects to previously presented ideas, like the general idea of *karma* in sutras 2.12, 2.13 and 2.14. *Karma* means action, and every action has consequences, if only because everything in existence is deeply interconnected. The five afflictions you carry with you (2.2 to 2.9) cause you to act in certain ways that leave a mark (*samskara*). Those impressions accumulate in the store of *karma* (*karmashaya*) (2.12), determining the characteristics of your life as well as pleasant or unpleasant experiences, depending on your original intention and action (2.13-2.14).

Those impressions manifest in one of the three states listed in aphorism 3.14. They can be dormant, active, or potential. Dormant *karma* is called *sanchita karma*, consisting of impressions that await the appropriate conditions to manifest. The second type of *karma* is known as *prarabdha karma*, the karma that is currently active. The third kind of *karma* is *agami karma*, the karma that is currently accumulating because of your current intentions, actions, and interactions. This future *karma* will manifest at a later point in this or a future lifetime. According to this perspective, your actions will keep generating your future experiences unless you act without any expectations whatsoever; or you surrender fully to life's perfection; or you have reached integration (*samadhi*) and your actions are filled with wisdom and in harmony with the ongoing flow of life.

In sum, if you practice *samyama* on your dormant or active *karma*, you will eventually learn when your current life will come to an end. Hence, this sutra also connects to the concept presented as the fifth of the afflictions in 2.3 and more explicitly in 2.9, fear of dying, *abhinivesha*. Rather than seeing death as something to be afraid of, you can choose to see your own death as both the culmination of the life process initiated at your birth as well as a strong motivation to participate consciously and deliberately in all aspects of your life. *To what extent are you aware of the connections between the events emerging in your daily life and your previous actions? Is it possible that you can gain insight on the repercussions of your current actions and interactions?*

This sutra also mentions the omens or portents. In the earliest commentary to the Yoga Sutra, Vyasa indicates that there are three types of portents that announce impending death: personal (*adhyatmika*), elemental (*adhibhautika*), and divine (*adhidaivika*). According to Vyasa, the personal omens include not perceiving any light with one's eyes closed and not hearing any bodily sounds when one closes one's ears. The elemental or impersonal omens consist of suddenly seeing one's dead ancestors or the messengers of death. The third kind of omen is seeing deities or heavenly beings. A fruitful avenue of exploration is to contemplate your relationship to the notion of death. Also, what can you learn by meditating on your own eventual demise? As usual, if you choose to explore this sutra, ensure that you are doing it in a life-affirming way that does not generate agitation or reactivity.

3.24 Meditative integration (*samyama*) on friendliness (*maitri*) and the other qualities (compassion-*karuna*, inspiration-*mudita*, and equanimity-*upeksha*) brings about their powers and effects.

While some people tend to think about the chapters in the Yoga Sutra as independent paths for practitioners at different levels, it is also possible to notice that there is indeed a thread connecting the sutras so that each aphorism provides support, explanation or reinforcement for effective application into life. Similarly, it can be argued that Patañjali created a compendium of yoga practices coming from a variety of approaches and traditions. If that is your position on the Yoga Sutra, you may feel inclined to focus mostly on the parts of the Sutra that resonate with you, your opinions, and beliefs. On the other hand, you could be open to the possibility that yoga is an integrated approach to living that addresses the needs of your body, mind, and emotions as well as your own social nature and your role in the world at large. This aphorism expands on sutra 1.33, the invitation to cultivate friendliness, compassion, inspiration, and equanimity towards yourself and others. *Samyama* acts as a catalyst that accelerates the power of these qualities.

What happens when you focus fully on becoming an abode of friendliness (*maitri*)?
What do you notice when you meditate on compassion (*karuna*) by sending wholehearted wishes for freedom from suffering and for the well-being of all living beings without exception or condition?
What develops when you meditate on feeling inspired by the accomplishments of those who are making the world a more just and fairer place?
What happens when you meditate on equanimity, openness to give others the benefit of the doubt?

A simple approach to bringing these questions into application is by bringing into your mind an image or memory that triggers the desired feeling. Notice the resulting sensations and emotions. Gradually release the contents of your mind that triggered the sensations and emotions. Remain with sensations and emotions only. Stay with the subtle sensations, gradually softening your hold on the sensations. Witness whatever unfolds.

3.25 Meditative integration (*samyama*) on the strength of an elephant and similar qualities, delivers them.

Whenever you want to achieve something, the first step is to imagine that goal clearly in your mind. This is true, for instance, with the practice of *asana*, yoga postures. To be able to practice a posture it is most helpful to imagine clearly what the posture looks like and from there you begin your journey. In most spiritual traditions, there are archetypes representing a variety of virtues. Whenever people want to cultivate a certain virtue, they are advised to invite the archetype of that virtue to assist and support them in moving towards the desired objective by engaging in prayer or ritual with that archetype in mind. This sutra presents a similar idea by using meditative integration on whatever archetype represents the qualities one desires in order to embody those qualities. Although this notion may not seem realistic, consider that recent research has found that it is possible to gain muscle strength by imagining that one is exercising even when the muscles don't move[iv]. Thus, is it possible that Patañjali and the ancient yogis may have already established those connections through their own research using their own bodies and minds as their laboratories? You can empirically research the question *Can I embody strength, kindness, intelligence, prosperity, compassion?* It stands to reason that you are more likely to dedicate the necessary time and energy to this endeavor if the question is meaningful and relevant to you and your life. Otherwise, it may become a short-term project with less probability of success. Whatever quality you desire will be most valuable if it contributes to enhance your internal harmony. Usually, when something enhances your internal harmony, it will probably be uplifting for other beings and for life in general. Thus, if you choose to embark on the journey of bringing this sutra into your life, it will be wise to begin by clarifying your reasons for cultivating those qualities as well as by assessing the usefulness of the desired effects.

3.26 Meditative integration (*samyama*) on the inner light reveals the subtle, hidden, and distant.

This aphorism echoes the idea of focusing your attention on the light of awareness at the core of your being presented in sutra 1.36. It is also related to the effects of *pranayama*, uncovering the effulgent light of awareness at the center of your chest (2.52). *Samyama* on your own internal light provides a way to find answers to questions that seem to escape your reasoning, inference, and existing testimony from bona fide sources. By attuning to your inner light, you gain greater clarity that enables you to see people, situations, and interactions without interference from your opinions and beliefs. As it was mentioned in the comment on sutra 1.40, many discoveries in human history arose when our way of perceiving became clearer, often when we let go of our preconceived ideas about what we should find or how things "should" work. To apply this sutra, you can begin by noticing, when you feel worried, upset, or frustrated how does your internal environment feel?

Do you feel the clarity and evenness known as *sattva*?
Or do you feel the internal agitation and reactivity called *rajas*?
Or, perhaps you feel the torpidity and heaviness named *tamas*?
Which emotional state is most conducive to revealing the answers that are more life affirming and supportive of your life experiment?
Does it ever happen to you that you are trying to solve a problem and you keep thinking about it or making lists of pros and cons and you seem to get more confused?
Does it ever happen that right after you have been brainstorming and you shift activity then an insight seems to suddenly illuminate your awareness delivering an unexpected, simple and effective solution that was beyond your reach before?

This sutra is an invitation to cultivate the clarity of *sattva* to guide your participation in life. The first step is to relax deeply by releasing worries and tension. The second step is to focus on the inner light, either in the space behind your forehead or at the center of your chest. The third step is to formulate a meaningful question to reveal something relevant to you and your life. Focus on the question with gentle firmness and gradually soften your grip on the question until you eventually release it. As you release it, release all expectations. This is where the practice of *vairagya* comes in handy. Then stay with the clarity, spaciousness, and silence inside. *What happens when you give this a try?*

3.27 Meditative integration (*samyama*) on the sun results in knowledge of the universe (the 7 realms).

An underlying theme in these sutras is that there is a pervasive interconnectedness among all of existence. The fabric of life is woven with threads of awareness. Life manifests in an infinite and ever-changing variety of ways. Focusing your awareness on any phenomenon with gentle firmness pierces through the superficial levels of appearance and reveals the subtle aspects of the phenomenon meditated upon. As it was explained in the latter section of Chapter One of the Yoga Sutra starting with aphorism 1.40, **through deep meditation you gain access to the true wisdom present everywhere**, in the shape of every leaf, the magnificent color gradations in any flower, the rhythms of animal migrations, and all the astonishing complexities and simplicities that come together in every ecosystem. This sutra can be interpreted as offering a way of understanding the physical universe through practicing *samyama* on the sun at the center of our solar system. On the other hand, following the ancient notion that there is a correspondence between the macrocosm and the microcosm, "As Above, So Below," this aphorism offers the avenue of research adopted by yogis for millennia, to look within to learn about the Universe. In its extensive commentary on this brief sutra, Vyasa offers a complete description of the seven regions – the earth, the sky, the planets, the *Mahaloka*, the *Janaloka*, the *Tapoloka* and the *Satyaloka* – and their divisions and sub-divisions, dimensions, arrangement, and characteristics. For this second approach, Vyasa suggests that to access the hidden regions of the Universe the yogi needs to practice *samyama* on the solar entrance, the *sushumna.*

The *sushumna*, literally the very gracious or kind channel, is described as a subtle channel at the central axis of the human body through which the vital force of *prana* flows, connecting the center of the pelvic floor to the crown of the head. According to Swami Hariharananda Aranya in his commentary to the Yoga Sutra, rather than a channel running along the spinal cord, the *sushumna* is a nerve that goes up from the heart.

Is it possible that applying samyama to the central axis of your body may reveal what ancient yogis call the sushumna? May this focus on the subtle aspects of your body reveal hidden universes in their full splendor? One approach to exploring this question is to focus on the sensations along a thin thread starting at the center of your pelvic floor and moving along your spinal cord all the way up to the crown of your head. You may visualize the thread as a thin thread of light flowing up as you inhale and flowing down as you exhale. Alternatively, you can focus on the subtle connection between your heart and the crown of your head. *What happens when you start with this?*

3.28 Meditative integration (*samyama*) on the moon results in knowledge of the constellations.

For this sutra, most commentators indicate that the focal point is the moon that orbits our planet, and that by practicing meditative integration on the moon you can learn about celestial bodies. Indeed, scientists have used the moon as a subject of study to understand astronomical events. For instance, by observing the moon, the notion that the craters on its surface were remnants of volcanoes eventually gave way to a more accurate theory, that the craters where formed by thousands of impacts of meteorites or other celestial bodies. Then, it became more evident that the earth has been, and is hit by tens of thousands of meteorites ranging in weight from dust particles to more than ten grams on a regular basis.

What happens when you choose the moon as your focal object for meditative integration?

What do you learn?

How does learning about constellations influence your perspective on you and your life?

3.29 Meditative integration (*samyama*) on the polestar unveils the movements of the stars.

By being virtually fixed, the pole star has been a dependable bright indicator of the location of the north pole for navigation for centuries. It makes sense to use it also as a reference to see more clearly how other stars seem to trail around the pole star.

If you choose to focus your attention fully on the pole star, can you learn about the movement of other stars?

Does retreating to an area where there is no light pollution, where stars are more easily visible, contribute to helping you feel more integrated with nature and the universe at large?

When you look at the stars in the sky, the history of the Universe is sending light signals to you from the depth of time. What is the direct experience of observing the night sky?

When you contemplate the night sky, some of those lights may be the only remains of stars that disappeared long ago.

How does it feel to investigate the past of the cosmos?

Is it possible that the movements of the stars influence you, your thoughts, and your mood?

To try a different approach, you can contemplate this question:
What is the reference point that you use to guide your thoughts, intentions, actions, and interactions?

3.30 Meditative integration (*samyama*) on the navel results in knowledge of the body.

This sutra begins a sequence of sutras listing some areas of the human body as focal points for *samyama*. Given the importance of the umbilical cord during pregnancy as a major conduit for blood, oxygen, and nutrients from the mother to the embryo, it seems to make sense that the navel can be used as a focal point to learn about the body. Although the navel does not seem to have much of a physiological function for humans after birth, it is often located at or very near your center of gravity. Is it possible that meditating on your navel can offer insight into your own body? You may also use the center of your body as a focal point to try to understand what your true center is at the physical, mental, and emotional level.

In recent years, researchers have found a complex system of neurons in the gastrointestinal tract called the Enteric Nervous System. The Enteric Nervous System seems to play an essential role in health, and it may also be an important factor in several diseases and neurological conditions.
Is it possible that ancient yogis had already found these critical connections between the systems in the abdominal area and the rest of the body?
Could it be that the common idea of gut feeling may be related to all of

this?

What can you discover if you meditate with the navel as your focal point?

3.31 Meditative integration (*samyama*) on the pit of the throat offers access to controlling hunger and thirst.

As you can see, this group of aphorisms seems very applied and practical. Most commentators do not elaborate much on this sutra. G. Maehle, in his contemporary comment, suggests that the focal point at the pit of the throat may be targeting the thyroid gland and its function in regulating metabolism. From the simplest perspective, you can try to explore if focusing your attention on the pit of your throat has any effect on your levels of hunger and thirst.

3.32 Meditative integration (*samyama*) on the tortoise channel (*kurma nadi*) gives steadiness.

In Sanskrit, a *nadi* is a vein, artery, nerve, or any other tubular organ in the body. Some people suggest that the *nadis* are indeed the channels throughout the body, including the circulatory system, lymphatic system and nervous system, as well as the more recently discovered primo-vascular system; other people state that the system of the *nadis* is not a physical system but a virtual system of patterns of life energy (*prana*) flowing through your body. According to Vyasa, the tortoise channel (*kurma nadi*) is below the pit of the throat. Other authors indicate that the tortoise channel extends from the lower abdomen to the throat underneath the *sushumna nadi* (mentioned in aphorism 3.27), while still others say that it is a tortoise like bundle of nerves in the chest area, the lotus of the heart. The result of *samyama* is translated here as steadiness. However, as it tends to happen with many Sanskrit words, the meaning of the word used here, *stharyam*, include solidity, hardness, constant, fixedness, stability, permanence, and steadfastness. A few other meanings useful in understanding this sutra include delight in, calmness, tranquility, perseverance and patience. To apply this sutra, you may inquire into the *kurma nadi*:

Does it exist?

Can you feel it slightly below the top of your sternum and a half inch in?

Or is the *kurma nadi* a channel connecting your lower abdomen to your throat?

Could it be at the center of your trachea?

Or is it perhaps at the center of your chest?

Is focusing on one of these areas more effective in creating an experience of solid tranquility and calm permanence without rigidity?

Does this practice enhance your capacity to persevere and be delightfully constant?

Is a deep meditation on any of these areas resulting in tranquil physical stillness?

3.33 On the light in the crown of the head (*murdha*), enables seeing those who are accomplished (*siddhas*).

The meanings of the Sanskrit word *murdha* include crown, top, and summit, as well as forehead, head, and skull. The other word to attend to in this sutra is *siddhas*. A *siddha* is an accomplished or perfected person, somebody who has reached liberation from suffering. It can also mean someone who has obtained *siddhis*, supernatural powers. This aphorism indicates that practicing *samyama* on the divine light that is the source of intelligence at the top of the head (or the midpoint where the top of the forehead and the hairline meet) enables you to see perfected beings. Some people call these perfected beings angels, guardians, guides, prophets, sages, or seers (*rishis*). As you prepare to put this aphorism into practice it is useful to notice how the space within your head feels. A simple way to explore this is by coming into a relaxed position, and then bringing your attention to the space behind your forehead. Next, think about something that makes you feel mildly worried, anxious, or upset and notice how those thoughts influence your experience of the space within your head. For the sake of comparison, think about something that you find uplifting and inspiring (1.39), and notice if and how your internal experience changes.

Would it be accurate to say that one of these two options feels more like radiance or light?

Is it possible that practicing each one of the limbs of yoga contributes to enhancing that feeling of clarity and lightness (*sattva*) throughout all aspects of your being?

Can that be a simple way to assess if your practice is effective?

If you feel light behind your forehead, can you stay with those sensations as you release the thoughts that triggered the clarity?

What happens when you stay with that radiance in your head?

Does that decrease your internal commentary and opinions?

Would that state be conducive to receiving guidance?

For instance, as you are pondering a decision you need to make, can you abide in the brightness in your head?

Does that make you more receptive and sensitive to subtle cues around and within you, like those cues suggesting viable and life-affirming paths of action?

In some cases, the gentle hints you receive come in the form of words that somebody says, or as a billboard on the side of the road. Sometimes that guidance appears as a message or phone call that comes in at a very precise moment. The teachers and guides are everywhere, especially if you are open to the possibility that life is an ocean of interconnectedness where everything articulates with grand precision and exquisite timing.

If it is the case that you notice some subtle hints providing options for you to make intelligent and conscious choices, can you cultivate a curiosity to know where that guidance originates? You may also engage in the inquiry:

Is it possible that there are perfected beings (*siddhas*) who live in harmony with the rhythms of life touching everything with kindness and compassion? Is this sutra echoing sutra 1.47 that says that the light of pure awareness shines through without being obscured by our ways of being?

3.34 Or, by intuitive insight everything becomes known.

Reiterating the message from aphorism 1.48, this sutra points out that with increasing internal clarity you can have access to wisdom through effortless intuition. Continuing the thread from application of the previous sutra, you can explore if, after developing a certain level of inner stillness and silence, you become more sensitive and receptive to intuition (*pratibha*). It is understood that your internal agendas and beliefs will likely interfere with the insight you receive, often opening the door for doubt and uncertainty. This is part of the process of learning to trust your intuition. One approach is to practice asking questions for guidance on small things during your day to notice how insight manifests. For instance, as you go to work, can you ask for guidance on the best route to take?
What happens as you try this regularly?
Does this listening invite you to be more aware?
Does guidance lead you to engaging in more useful actions?
Is it possible that the skill of being open to guidance from your intuition can be cultivated through consistent practice (*abhyasa*) and without expectations (*vairagya*)?

One of the potential challenges is not being able to distinguish the insight you are receiving from what some aspect of you desires. Honing your capacity to distinguish between what is and what you want is the path for developing discriminative awareness (*viveka* in sutras 2.26 and 2.28). On the path to full discernment, your internal environment may feel lighter and perhaps more luminous. This brightness is another way to interpret the Sanskrit word *pratibha*, and it is the same inner light suggested as an object of single-pointed focus mentioned in aphorism

1.36. That is also the same inner light revealed by practicing *pranayama* (2.52) as well as the light mentioned in sutra 3.36.

Notice also that this sutra is related to the practice of utmost humility (*ishvara pranidhana* in los sutras1.23 and 2.45). Relinquishing the illusion of control requires trusting that whatever you need to know and whatever you need access to will become available at the precise moment needed, neither before nor after. Moreover, consider that the more occupied you are with your ways of being (your beliefs, opinions and drama) the less likely it is for you to recognize insights. Once you quiet your mind, the insights become more evident in many of the experiences that you have during your day. When you notice a silent suggestion, beware of the potential interference of your tendencies and inclinations. Remember that you are in charge of making your choices, and the insights guiding you to transcend your current level of understanding will possibly ask you to step beyond the boundaries of your comfort zone. *This is what learning means.*

3.35 By meditative integration (*samyama*) on the heart, the mind is understood.

By practicing meditative integration on the center of the chest, the emotional heart, *citta* is understood. Remember that *citta* is one of the four words in the definition of yoga in Chapter One of the Yoga Sutra. *Citta* is also one of those Sanskrit words that has several meanings including intention, aim, attending, thinking, reflecting, wish, mind, memory, intelligence, and reason. In some of the ancient texts called the *Upanishads*, the space around the heart is said to be the dwelling of the light of awareness. Does it ever happen to you that you are trying to make a decision and that the logical reasons suggesting one choice are in conflict with your emotions and feelings? On the other hand, has it ever happened to you that you made a choice following your heart and then you found yourself in a difficult predicament? This sutra can be considered a pivotal aphorism for practice because it highlights the deep connection between your mind and your emotions. When mind and emotions align, the blockages created by doubt and fear disappear. Conflict between mind and emotions is a major source of pain and suffering for many people. Learning to integrate your mind with your emotions makes you more effective, decisive, and compassionate.

From the simplest perspective, you can start by exploring how your physical posture affects your state of mind and mood. Sitting in a hunched position with your shoulders raised, your chest collapsed, and your head down, try to think uplifting and inspiring thoughts. Then, explore what position would shift your internal environment towards feeling boastful and full of pride. Continue this inquiry by finding a posture conducive to feeling optimistic, hopeful, uplifted, and filled with kindness and compassion.

Does it seem that your posture, especially the space around your heart, can influence your mind and emotions?

Does one of these positions generate a feeling of lightness and clarity in heart and mind?

Can that lightness and spaciousness be the brightness mentioned in sutra 3.33?

Is it possible that, in addition to the relationship between your physical posture, your mind and your mood, there is a close connection between your mind and your heart?

Can you be curious to investigate this connection?

For instance, if your mind is open, does it cause your heart to feel more generous, caring and forgiving?

Does the connection work also in the opposite direction?

If your heart feels more open, generous, caring, kind and forgiving, does your mind feel more willing to be inclusive, cooperative, and understanding?

(As you inquire into the relationships between your heart and mind, remember that we are using the word mind as a stand-in for the concepts associated with the word *citta,* including intention, thinking, reflecting, wish, mind, memory, intelligence, and reason.)

One avenue for furthering this exploration is by linking this inquiry to the sutra immediately preceding this one, 3.34, where it says that intuitive insight provides access to all knowledge.

Can you become skilled at meditating on your heart when there is confusion or agitation in your mind?

As you become more practiced in receiving insight, might it be possible that intuitions arrive in your heart and from there are communicated to your mind?

Can it be the case that harmony between your mind and heart confirms your insights with your knowledge as mentioned in aphorism 1.6 (direct experience – *pratyaksha,* inference – *anumana*, and traditional wisdom coming from the past – *agama*)?

Does common sense resonate with both your mind and your emotions?

As you try to follow intuitive insight, check if it provides useful guidance for living your life with enthusiasm, intelligence and humility (*kriya yoga* 2.1).

3.36 Even a balanced and clear mind is different from pure awareness. When there is no distinction of this difference, individual awareness misidentifies with experiences, feelings, and perceptions. Meditative integration (*samyama*) on this distinction results in knowing pure awareness (*purusha*).

This sutra presents the core of the teachings of the Yoga Sutra. Once again, the major theme of the Yoga Sutra emerges restating the ideas presented in sutras 1.3 and 1.4 as well as in sutras 2.6 and 2.17. You can choose to see life and all that it offers as a playground for your senses, leading you to all kinds of experiences. If this is your viewpoint, you will likely pursue pleasurable experiences (*raga*) and push away whatever you dislike (*dvesha*). Yet, even if you are fortunate enough to have only pleasurable experiences, sooner or later, all the pleasurable experiences will come to an end – causing you pain and suffering (2.15). This aphorism is an invitation to investigate your essence and its relationship to your experiences. Hence, it invites you to engage deeply in the process of developing your discriminative awareness (*viveka*), just as aphorism 2.26 did before.

What do you notice when you observe yourself during your daily experiences?

What are your motivations?

What are your expectations?

How do you respond to the changing circumstances in the world around you?

Do you respond with kindness and grace?

Or do you react with defensiveness and aggression?

Can your internal environment become clear and free from cravings, opinions, and reactivity?

Can you accept your experiences and navigate them with grace and equanimity?

Remember the process invoked in the comment to sutra 2.10 and consider exploring the differences between who you think you are and who you actually are. Your thoughts and opinions about you and about life, are just comments that do not add anything to the quality of your experience. The direct experience of being is who you are.
When you release all your beliefs what is left?
Is there anything beyond the changeable aspects of your body, mind, and emotions?
Is it possible that once you are free from beliefs and grasping, you might be able to notice the distinction between who you think you are and who you are?
Then, can you focus your attention deeply and effortlessly (*samyama*) on the difference between the pure awareness that pervades all of existence and your individual awareness?
What do you discover?

3.37 As a result, intuition and extraordinary sense perception unfold.

Knowing the difference between your individual awareness and universal awareness removes the confusion that prevents you from seeing yourself as you are. And, according to the previous sutra, being clear on that distinction enables you to know pure awareness. This aphorism adds that the intuitive insight (*pratibha*) mentioned in sutra 3.34 results from being established in that clarity. As you consider the idea of deep intuition, consider whether it is possible that wild animals use their intuition to gain access to the wisdom guiding them to migrate, hibernate, and estivate. Some perspectives look for an explanation of these and other natural phenomena in the material make up of life. Other viewpoints suggest that there are multiple levels of embedded information orchestrating those processes. For instance, when you go to sleep, if you are not sleep deprived, and you know that you need to wake up at a certain time, does it ever happen that you wake up at the time you need, often before your alarm goes off? Is it possible that when you set your intention to wake up at a certain time you are setting that intention somewhere in between your internal processes and pure awareness?

Is it possible that it is your intuitive insight that wakes you up at the right time?

Could it be that uncluttering your inner world from wants, cravings, opinions, and beliefs may bolster your ability to tap into the wisdom that makes all processes in nature work?

Is your individual awareness embedded in universal awareness?

In addition to gaining deep intuition, knowing pure awareness results in heightened sensory perception. Aphorism 1.36 already offers subtle sensations as a productive object for single-pointed focus. Adding awareness to any of your senses is a way to enhance your perception, so that instead of staying with the gross level of sensory perception you access a richer, deeper, and more nuanced understanding of whatever you are perceiving. When you really want to determine what spices were used in preparing a delicious dish, you focus your awareness by not talking, by closing your eyes and by attending to the specific sensations in your mouth. As a result, you are better able to notice textures, moisture, softness, granularity and a wide range of sensations that make up the flavor you are tasting. A tea connoisseur may be able to distinguish very subtle flavors that differentiate one variety of tea from another, or even the subtle distinctions between the same variety of tea grown in different regions. This sutra suggests that even at this higher level of sensory awareness, these experiences do not access the deepest levels of subtlety. Remember that at the end of Chapter Two of the Yoga Sutra, in aphorisms 2.54 and 2.55, the fifth limb of yoga, *pratyahara*, consists of drawing your senses inward so that you can feel yourself from the inside and explore your inner world. In *pratyahara*, you invite your awareness into an internal journey of deep exploration leading you to the higher limbs of yoga, concentration (*dharana*), meditation (*dhyana*), and integration (*samadhi*). This sutra says that clarifying the distinction between your individual awareness and pure awareness grants you access to perceive the utmost essence of all sensory experiences. *As with every single sutra, rather than assuming this statement is true, remain open to the possibility that once you release all your beliefs, your perception may be enhanced beyond its current level.* Possibly this leads you to greater awareness of the perceptual process itself, so that instead of being aware of the object or experience you are perceiving, you tune into the process of perceiving which will, in turn, lead you to the clear experience of the perceiver. This aphorism reminds you, once again, that for most of us yoga is an incremental journey towards awareness. It is your choice to deepen your knowledge of yourself. Nobody else can do this for you.

Are you at the mercy of your senses, chasing after sensory experiences for fulfillment?

Or are your sensory experiences instruments for you to unveil the mystery of your existence?

May it be possible to access your primordial senses at the core of every sensory experience?

Can this lead you to feel with great clarity the perceptual process itself and its subtle ways of working?

If so, can this heightened sensitivity deepen your awe and appreciation for the indescribable miracle of life in its wondrous manifestations?

Which option is most conducive to living in joyful harmony with life?

Warning

3.38 These extraordinary powers can be seen as accomplishments or as obstacles.

Throughout this chapter, Patañjali follows the same structure as in the previous chapters: First, introducing definitions and a contextualization of the practices within the larger project of yoga; then, there is a list of applications of the techniques with their results. This sutra offers a clarification, like the one offered in sutra 2.18, where it said that whatever can be perceived manifests to the senses as experiences for enjoyment or as experiences leading to liberation. When you read about the many possible outcomes of meditative integration (*samyama*), it is not surprising that some of the meanings of the word yoga in Sanskrit include magical art, trick, and supernatural means. In fact, it was mentioned before that according to some sources, attaining extraordinary or magical powers is the sign of a yogin or yogini.

This aphorism serves as a reminder that you are in charge of your journey because you are the only person who can set a meaningful goal for your practice – that it enhances the quality of your participation in your life. For some of us it may mean that all the yogic tools are means to increase our sense of ourselves and our self-importance. If that is the case, then you will see any powers you acquire as a sign of your self-worth and success. You may even believe that it is you who have made all those things happen on your own. This will likely generate a sense of separation, isolating you from others and from the deep interconnectedness between life and awareness. Seeing these extraordinary accomplishments as ways to aggrandize yourself are obstacles not only to your progress but also to your ability to be of service. A different option is to see yoga as a way to grow in your capacity to open your mind and your heart to contribute your uniqueness to the world. Therefore, as you remove inefficiencies from your body, mind, emotions, and attitude, you can receive and transmit the wisdom of life through your actions and interactions more effectively. Then, all the practices lead you to see yourself as a humble conduit for love and awareness. This is the same message advanced in sutra 2.45, that practicing humility (*ishvara pranidhana*) confers extraordinary wisdom and powers (*siddhis*).

What are your goals for your practice?

What are you focusing your awareness and energy on?

What parameters are you using to measure the effectiveness of your practice?

Is your practice a way to build your self-importance, or a way to deepen your humanness?

These questions also prepare you to develop an appropriate mindset for the aphorisms that follow.

SUBTLE ENERGY FLOW

3.39 Releasing the causes of attachment to the physical body and by knowing the conduits through which the vital forces travel, the yogin can enter somebody else's body.

This is the first of a series of sutras dealing with more subtle aspects of life energy (*prana*) flow in the human body. The caution in the previous sutra acts as sound advice for practitioners interested in exploring these truly extraordinary attainments. Misidentification with your ways of being (1.4) leads you to confuse your sensations and experiences with your true nature (*avidya* 2.4). Sutra 2.17 underscores that the cause of all suffering is confusing awareness with what can be experienced. This confusion generates the afflictions (*kleshas*) listed in sutra 2.3, all of them resulting from not seeing clearly (*avidya*). *Avidya* manifests in thinking that you are your body, despite knowing that your body has been changing constantly from its conception. Identification with your body leads to fear of dying, an affliction endured even by the wise (2.9). Yogic action (*kriya yoga* 2.1) and the eight limbs of yoga (*ashtanga yoga* 2.28) remove this fundamental confusion. Attachment to your body is one of the most powerful instincts you have. The first part of this aphorism says that once that attachment to your physical body is released, if you know how life energy flows through the body, then you can find the gate through which life energy enters and exists in your body. If those conditions are met, you can detach from your body and enter somebody else's body. These two requirements offer already a complete program of internal inquiry.

Can you modulate your attachment to your physical body?

Can you release this attachment while remaining appreciative of the miracle that your human body is?

Are you only your body?
Can the *samyama* from 3.32 to achieve stillness contribute to such a deep stillness that it may be easier to release your attachment to bodily sensations?

To explore the second portion of this sutra you can investigate experientially how your life energy flows through your own body.

For instance, when you first wake up, is there a place where your energy seems to be more noticeable?
In the process of falling asleep, how do your vital energy patterns diminish? As your awake energy transitions towards the restfulness of sleep, does it move to a specific place?
When you fill emotionally drained do you notice any changes in your vital energy?
Is it different when you feel inspired?

3.40 Mastery over the *udana vayu* enables lightness, levitation and leaving the body at will.

Yoga studies life in all its aspects. The third limb of yoga, *pranayama,* presented in sutra 2.49, consists of developing an intimate knowledge of the flow of *prana*, the primordial force animating sensations and actions in all living beings. Their study of the life force led ancient yogis to classify the flow of *prana* into five major winds or vital airs (*vayu*). These five types of life energy are known as *prana*, *apana*, *samana*, *vyana* and *udana*. The first one, confusingly enough also named *prana*, is thought to be responsible for processes of bringing vitality into the body. Some sources suggest that *prana* is related to inhalation, whereas other sources maintain that *prana* is responsible for both inhalation and exhalation. This first form of *prana* is thought to sustain the organs of perception and to reside in the upper portion of the body, including the heart.

Apana animates the proccsses of elimination. Some authors associate *apana* with exhalation and with the lower section of the torso. *Samana* is connected to digestion and assimilation. *Samana* is thought to operate in the abdominal region. *Vyana* is the vital force pervading the whole body, including the limbs. Therefore, *vyana* sustains the organs of movement.

Udana is the ascending vital force, responsible for burping, speech, and elevated states of consciousness. *Udana* is in charge of sustaining the tissues of the body. This *udana* aspect of the life force is also thought to leave the body at will at the moment of death. Remember how in Chapter One of the Yoga Sutra aphorism 1.39 suggests directing your single-pointed focus to anything uplifting. In Chapter Two, sutras 2.33 and 2.34 encouraged the cultivation of uplifting thoughts and emotions (*pratipaksha bhavana*). This aphorism 3.40 says that meditative integration on the ascending life force, *udana*, will enable the practitioner to avoid sinking in water, mud, or stepping into thorns. Additionally, learning to regulate *udana* ensures ascending out of the body through the crown of the head at the time of death, which is believed to be the safe passage to escape the endless cycle of birth, death, and rebirth.

Is it possible to notice how the feeling of lightness operates in your being?

What thoughts and actions contribute to feeling light and buoyant?

Where do the sensations of lightness arise?
How do they travel?
Which of your choices and decisions support feeling light?
When you go to sleep, does focusing on the feeling of lightness influence the quality of your rest?
What happens if you choose to focus on lightness when you first notice that you are awake?
Does that choice influence your thoughts, attitude, actions, and interactions during your day?

3.41 Mastery over the *samana vayu* confers radiance.

As mentioned in the comment to the previous sutra, *samana* is the vital energy in the body related to digestion. When your digestion is less than optimal, you feel heavy, tired or with internal discomfort and agitation. When your appetites are adequate and your food intake appropriate, you will notice that your body will be able to digest your food effectively, contributing to efficient elimination, and giving you energy to accomplish whatever you need. This applies not only to your relationship to food but also to your intake of mental and emotional stimulation. Observing the ideas, emotions and food that you consume, how you handle each one of them and what effect they have on your overall state and mood will provide insight into your mental, emotional and physical digestive processes. Once this becomes clearer to you, you can enhance your capacity to regulate these ways of being to feel radiant.

The Tibetan practice known as *Tummo*[v], inner fire, has been mentioned often as the extraordinary power (*siddhi*) introduced in this aphorism. The *Tummo* practice is used at the closing ceremony of an extended period of meditative retreat, usually 3 years. During the ceremony, retreat participants engage in the *Tummo* meditation while walking or sitting in the cold Himalayan snow at below freezing temperatures with wet sheets draped over them. This type of meditation includes a specific breathing technique as well as a visualization. As a result of raising their body temperature, practitioners dry the wet sheets with their own body heat. Some authors argue that regulating one's temperature can contribute to enhanced immunity and neurocognitive function. You may begin an inquiry into your internal fire by enhancing your sensitivity in your abdominal area through the technique known as *Agni Sara*, which is best learned from a qualified teacher. You can further your exploration by using the following visualization technique: In a comfortable position, with your spine elongated, stable and relaxed, focus your attention on the area below your navel. Gradually, visualize a flame below your navel. Invite the flame to increase in size along the length of your spine. As you practice consistently, notice the effects of the practice on your body temperature and, perhaps more importantly, on your ability to infuse life energy into all your endeavors. What do you find?

3.42 Meditative integration (*samyama*) on the relationship between hearing and space (*akasha*) results in divine hearing.

The Sanskrit word *akasha* includes among its many definitions the concepts of space, sky, atmosphere, and the notion of the ethereal fluid that pervades the whole Universe. *Akasha* is also the vehicle of life and sound. One way to approach this meditative integration on the relationship between sound and space is to notice silence. Recognize that silence is the medium making sound possible. For example, when learning a language, you notice that there are different words when you can notice the silences that separate them.

Can you experience silence?

As you sit quietly, is there an ongoing internal commentary precluding you from having the direct experience of silence?

What happens when you invoke the deep silence you attain during dreamless deep sleep?

Then, can you investigate if developing an intimate relationship with silence influences how you perceive sounds?

When you are established in silence, are you better able to listen to others?

How does awareness of the relationship between silence and space affect your capacity to listen for the silent insights of wisdom?

3.43 Meditative integration (*samyama*) on the relationship between the body and space or meditation on lightness enables traveling through space (*akashagamana*).

Akashagamana is a Sanskrit word translated as traveling through space or traveling through the ether. Patañjali offers two ways of accomplishing this prodigious feat: by practicing *samyama* on the relationship between the body and space; or by practicing *samyama* on something that is very light, like cotton. When you observe highly proficient dancers, you can probably notice that they have developed a profound relationship with space that enables them to move gracefully and with extraordinary fluidity. It may seem that, somehow, they may not be subject to the same force of gravity as other people. The next time you take your shoes off and you walk, notice the relationship between your body and space.

What is the sound of your feet as they touch the ground?

Can your asana practice be a laboratory for exploring how to infuse lightness into your movements and actions?

Can you make yourself as light as cotton?

Might it be helpful to consider the fact that there is a lot of space between the electrons and the nuclei of each of the trillions of atoms that you are made of?

Could it be that the force that bonds electrons and nuclei may be one component of that elusive life force called *prana*?

Is it possible that *samyama* on the relationship between the body and space (*akasha*) may reveal dimensions other than the gross dimensions we are aware of through our senses, including mental, emotional, and spiritual dimensions?

3.44 Beyond the physical body and the ways of being (*vrtti*), the great disembodiment removes the veil over the inner light of awareness.

Similar to the section in Chapter One of the Yoga Sutra that talks about the highest levels of meditation and their characteristics, the previous sutras present increasing depth in exploring the subtlest aspects of existence. You may remember that sutra 1.19 mentioned two categories of existence beyond the physical plane: the disembodied (*videha*) and the merged in nature (*prakritilaya*). This sutra talks about the great disembodiment, or the ability to leave your physical body. Aphorism 3.39 indicated already that to enter somebody else's body the yogi needs to be able to release attachment to the physical body. In addition to releasing attachment to your physical body, you also need to release your ways of being (*vrtti*) to uncover your inner light of awareness.

As it was suggested in the "What is Yoga?" chapter, all of yoga is a lifelong process of noticing and regulating our ways of being (*vrtti*). Attachment to your ways of being and to your body results in confusing your body and ways of being with your true nature (1.2 to 1.4). The first five limbs of the yogic process lead you to decrease your ways of being and your attachment to your physical body. As you deepen your meditation practice, it becomes easier to remain focused effortlessly on a specific object of concentration. This sustained focused results from releasing your beliefs, worries, and fears, as well as from being so at ease in your body that you do not feel your body. This happens naturally any time you are absorbed in something that captures your attention and imagination, like when you are listening to your favorite music.

Would it be possible to explore this sutra by finding a very relaxed position that can be maintained for a good amount of time and then choosing to notice your body from the inside, starting at your bone marrow where your red blood cells and white blood cells are made? Then feel your bones and the continuous process of storage and release of minerals taking place in your bones. In your own time, feel the multiple layers of connective tissue and muscles intertwined with blood vessels and nerves into a living web that is adaptive and highly responsive. Feel also your organs and the exquisite connections and interrelations between them. Gradually move your attention towards your skin, the intelligent membrane regulating your molecular interaction with the world around you. Feel your skin as clearly and accurately as possible. Pay close attention to the outermost portion of your skin in its interaction with the world around you.

Can you increase your focus on the outside?

How far beyond the skin can you feel?

The object of your external focus is *akasha*, the notion of space mentioned in the sutras before this one.

How long can you remain with this external focus beyond your sense of the body and beyond your thoughts and emotions?

Can you remain anchored in awareness while letting go of any notions of me, myself and I?

What happens then?

Might it be possible that this practice can be taken even further?

HIGHEST ATTAINMENTS

3.45 Meditative integration (*samyama*) on the relationship between the physical, the generic nature, the subtle, the inherent qualities and the purpose of any element results in mastery over the constitutive elements of all natural phenomena.

Consistent with the rest of the Yoga Sutra, Patañjali continues describing the effects of these advanced practices, now at their highest levels. Already sutra 1.17 pointed out that meditation reveals increasing levels of subtlety in the object meditated upon. Remember also that aphorism 3.13 in this chapter already explained one perspective on how the world is organized as consisting of a substratum manifesting along the dimensions of characteristics, properties, and condition. These three dimensions are the field of interaction between the elements and your senses. In this sutra, the *samyama* practice is directed to the elements that make up everything in the universe. The elements mentioned here are the five elements listed by the *Samkhya* philosophical school. *Samkhya* is concerned with classifying existence according to its different categories of manifestation. According to *Samkhya,* the five fundamental elements are earth, water, fire, air and space or ether (*akasha*, mentioned in the previous aphorisms). This sutra states that practicing *samyama* on these elements and their different aspects of manifestation leads to mastery over the fundamental properties of all sensory phenomena.

Each element has five interrelated aspects: physical, generic, subtle, inherent qualities and purpose. The first level is what can be perceived by the senses. If you are tasting water, you taste its temperature, texture, and flavor. Each element has its own physical characteristics that change, they are not fixed. Increasing the level of subtlety requires practicing *samyama* on the generic aspect of the element. In the case of water, it would be its quality of being liquid. Deeper than the generic quality is the subtle aspect of the element, which is its indescribable most fundamental aspect, its essence. This is the indivisible essence beyond the level of the senses that can be perceived only in the state of integration (*samadhi*). The inherent qualities of that element are a combination of its interactive tendencies towards wholeness or clarity (*sattva*), inertia or darkness (*tamas*), and agitation or activity (*rajas*). These tendencies were mentioned previously in sutras 2.18 and 2.19. The final aspect of the element is its purpose as an object of experience: *Is it causing you to attach to your experiences, or is it a vehicle to liberation from your sense of self?* A complete experiential understanding of these five aspects of the five fundamental elements enables the practitioner to master anything that is made from these fundamental elements.

It is worth mentioning that according to the *Samkhya* philosophical perspective, consciousness (*purusha*) and the world (*prakriti*) are two fundamental and complementary aspects of existence. According to *Samkhya*, consciousness is the cause of all existence starting at the subtlest level and emerging into a sense of being that generates a sense of individuality that, in turn, generates the units of sensation and from there the senses, the elements and perception develop[vi]. Delving into this philosophical system is related to an ongoing debate in Indian philosophy over many centuries: Is there one pervading principle in the Universe that animates everything? Or are there more than one? Perhaps, is there only pervasive emptiness and impermanence? A similar debate exists in Western philosophy, and in some fields of science: does the physical universe give rise to consciousness? Or does consciousness exist before the material world and generate it? Of course, there are other possibilities including that consciousness and materiality emerge from their synergetic interaction that generates a more complex system than the sum of its parts. You may find these questions interesting enough to explore them and to use them as one filter for interpreting your experiences.

This can be a very dense sutra. How can it be put into practice? Would it be possible to start by moving all your practices (*yama, niyama, pratipaksha bhavana, asana, pranayama, pratyahara, dharana* and *dhyana*) from a gross level of experience to a subtler level? For instance, in present times the most popular aspect of yoga is the physical practice, *asana*. A yoga practice consisting only of *asana* will have results mostly in the physical realm, helping with fitness and health, when practiced consciously. When you expand your practice to have a strong foundation on the *yama* and *niyama*, your yoga practice will extend to your mind and emotions, helping you refine your attitude and perspective through love and contentment. Next, if you enrich your practice with *pranayama*, in addition to enhancing your respiratory function, you will directly experience its purifying effects, and you will prepare yourself for *pratyahara* and the meditative limbs. Each one of the limbs takes you into experiencing deeper levels of subtlety. Rather than isolating the different limbs of yoga, you can yoke them together to act synergistically on all aspects of your being. You may also choose to try the following questions to move towards application of this sutra:

What happens when you try to meditate on each one of the five elements?

Could it be possible to find out if the intricate levels of manifestation of each element can be experienced directly through meditation?

Might it be possible that such subtler levels of experience offer a different approach to your sensory experiences?

What is your purpose in experiencing the primordial elements that make up life?

Is it really possible to gain access to the most fundamental aspects of existence through meditative integration?

3.46 As a result, extraordinary powers, perfection of the body and immunity from the elements.

According to the traditional commentaries, the *samyama* technique presented in the previous sutra results in eight extraordinary powers (*siddhis*) including the abilities to become minute (*anima*), become light (*laghima*), become large (*mahima*), reach anything regardless of how far it may be (*prapti*), unrestrained will, like being able to merge into the earth or water (*prakamya*), control over the elements (*vashitva*), mastery of the elements to make them appear or disappear (*ishitrittva*), and omnipotence – the power to make anything happen according to whatever is desired (*yatrakamavasaitva*). In addition, the body of the practitioner becomes immune to the effects of the elements. This is a humbling aphorism for most practitioners as it puts into perspective what might be possible through advanced yoga practice. Moreover, the commentaries all indicate how, despite acquiring all of these powers, the yogi refrains from upsetting the cosmic order. This can be an excellent reminder that whatever powers may be obtained, they are all related to each individual's previous actions (*karma*) and life purpose (*dharma*). *As you reflect on your own practice and your life, can you see any changes indicating that you are growing in your humanity?*

3.47 The bodily perfections include beauty, grace, and the strength to withstand a thunderbolt.

Continuing with the effects of practicing *samyama* on the elements, this sutra lists the effects of mastering the elements. The fact that the traditional commentators have basically no commentary on this sutra reminds the student *that focus only on the physical misses the point of the practice.* This sutra points out that the body of the practitioner grows in beauty, grace and becomes unbreakable. These attributes are not a goal, but a side effect of the practice. At a basic level you may notice how when a person is loving, kind and emotionally balanced he or she seems to radiate joy. Also, a practitioner whose power comes from having an open mind, open heart, and deep integrity can navigate all aspects of life with ease and grace. No matter what happens, good or bad, the practitioner can withstand it all with equanimity. Even if you have not mastered the primordial elements of existence, is your practice keeping you vibrant, enthusiastic, and wholehearted?

Are you living your life with beauty, grace, and strength?

3.48 Meditative integration (*samyama*) on perception, essential character, sense of self, inherent qualities and purpose results in mastery of the senses.

This sutra presents the culmination of the *pratyahara* practice introduced at the end of Chapter Two of the Yoga Sutra (2.54 & 2.55). In this case, the single-pointed focus of *samyama* is directed to the senses themselves. It follows a similar approach to the focus on the elements presented in aphorism 3.45. Like the rest of yoga, this is a gradual progression from one level of experience into a subtler one. It begins with attention to the perceptual process. Every stimulus activates one sense organ causing it to receive the generic and specific qualities of whatever is perceived. Going deeper, attention rests on the essential character unique to the sense organ that is active. This leads to the sense of self ("I") manifesting through that sense. The tendencies of manifestation (activity-*rajas*, inertia-*tamas*, clarity-*sattva,* mentioned in sutras 2.18-2.19) inherent in that sense organ become more evident. Then, the process reveals the purpose of the sense as an instrument of experience for liberation from misidentification. True mastery of the senses liberates the practitioner from chasing after sensations. This sutra is an invitation to gain a profound experiential relationship with your senses as vehicles of freedom from sensory conditioning.

Is living in the world a never-ending journey of overloading your senses?

What are the sensory experiences you expose yourself to?

How in tune are you with your own perceptual systems and processes?

What is the purpose of your sensory experiences?

3.49 Consequently, a body as fast as the mind, independence from sense organs and mastery over the creative principle of nature (*pradhana*).

These highest attainments challenge everyday notions. As a result of mastery over the sense organs, the body can move as fast as the mind, regardless of distance or circumstance. Independence from the sense organs has been interpreted as the ability to perceive without using one's sense organs. Some commentators indicate that the practitioner has the capacity to generate an organ when needed. One of the sutras in Chapter Four of the Yoga Sutra, will refer to this ability to create a body at will. The final achievement is mastery over the essence of life (*pradhana*). Here again there are different opinions. Some commentaries say that this mastery means that the yogi has the power to control nature. A typical objection is that wanting to control nature shows that there is still attachment to the world. A different viewpoint suggests that the yogi can use this power to fulfill their purpose to be of service. This inquiry can be a useful point of inquiry:

What is your relationship to life's creative principle?

Do you try to control life?

Or do you embrace life in all its forms unconditionally?

3.50 Through discernment of the distinction between Pure Awareness and the transparently clear body-mind-heart, supremacy over existence and omniscience arise.

The recurrent theme in the Yoga Sutra emerges again: The problem humans face is suffering. Suffering results from forgetting one's own nature, or, more specifically, from believing that experiences and activities are our true nature (1.3, 1.4 and 2.5). The highest freedom is to be free from distractions caused by even the subtlest experiences (1.16). Freedom emerges from releasing this confusion between the power of witnessing, consciousness, and what can be experienced (2.17, 2.20, 2.24 and 2.25). This sutra reiterates that the whole yogic process is one of releasing one's ways of being at all levels to have the direct experience of unclouded awareness. Then, the distinction between one's immanent awareness and the primordial transcendental awareness that underlies all existence becomes clear. Since all identification has ceased and all agendas have been released, all experiences are perceived clearly in their impermanent nature. Having found undying consciousness, the practitioner is beyond all aspects of existence. Having access to primordial awareness results in omniscience, the simultaneous knowledge of all possible permutations of the essence of life at all times and in all places. Notice that these ideas echo the attributes of *ishvara* presented in sutras 1.24 to 1.29, as well as the statement in sutra 2.45 that being established in total surrender to the perfection of life results in *siddhis*.

As a present-day student of yoga, are you gaining some supremacy over your ways of being?

Is it becoming clearer to you that there is a vast body of knowledge yet to be discovered?

Is the internal tendency to comment on everything dwindling?

Does it seem like insight is more available to you?

Is your sense of "I" changing?

FREEDOM

3.51 Releasing even those attainments and removing the remaining seeds of afflictions delivers liberation.

The journey of yoga is a journey of releasing restrictions to the endless manifestation of life in its infinite diversity. By removing the focus on the limited realm of the sense of self, the sense of being an "I," the practitioner understands experientially the extraordinary richness of life and nature. The *siddhis* emerge when the practitioner releases her attachments to her opinions, beliefs, and other ways of being. Then, a profound understanding of the timeless interaction between consciousness and matter develops resulting in the extraordinary powers described in this chapter, the *siddhis*. This gradual process consists of returning persistently to presence (*abhyasa*) while releasing judgment and expectations (*vairagya*). Similarly, all limbs of yoga require a combination of this patient persistence. For instance, in meditation practice you learn to concentrate first, then you soften the amount of effort so that you can remain focused with minimal energy expenditure. The journey towards liberation is a progression towards the subtlest perception. After focusing on the distinction between pure awareness and one's individual awareness introduced in the previous sutra, all of nature in its grandeur is clearly recognized as a vehicle for awareness and not awareness itself. All the attainments presented in Chapter Three of the Yoga Sutra are only vehicles for liberation. This differentiation is the antidote to ignoring one's nature (*avidya* 2.3 to 2.5). In fact, it is the discriminative awareness (*viveka*) presented as the path to liberation in sutra 2.26. When the practitioner has reached this level, even the capacity to discern between pure awareness and individual awareness (*viveka*) is seen as one more way of being (*vrtti*). Once again, everything that is no longer needed, regardless of its previous usefulness, is released. By releasing all ways of being, the last impressions stored in one's awareness (*samskaras*) are effectively deactivated. There is nothing else to focus on. This is the transition from integration with a seed (*sabija samadhi*) and integration without a seed (*nirbija samadhi*) talked about in sutras 1.17, 1.18, and 1.47to 1.51; as well as at the beginning of this chapter in sutras 3.7 and 3.8. Only when everything is released (*vairagya*) is there liberation. This liberation emerges when there is no longer an illusion of separateness.

Where are you on your path towards liberation?
What ways of being are you holding on to?
Which ones have you identified as unhelpful and released?
Which ways of being are still serving a purpose?
Are there any moments when the notion of "I" becomes less established?

3.52 Self-importance and pride from contact with others, even with celestial beings, can result in undesirable consequences re-emerging.

Today the cult to personality is so widespread that it makes it easy to understand how being approached by the powerful and the famous may be a source of pride and self-importance. Moreover, it may also explain how pride and self-importance contribute to the undoing of some of those people who have reached positions of prominence. In this sutra, Patañjali states that even after the long process of releasing your identity, your exalted state may attract invitations from celestial beings that result in re-igniting the seeds of your ways of being in the form of self-importance and pride. There are countless examples of stories about temptation in all the wisdom traditions around the world. Temptation exposes lack of commitment to the path to freedom. As you may recall, one of the obstacles listed in sutra 1.30 was *anavasthitatvani*, instability or inability to maintain the level of progress reached. Remember also that at the beginning of Chapter Two of the Yoga Sutra, it says that not knowing your fundamental nature (*avidya*) becomes the field where other afflictions sprout, including misidentification with the sense of "I" (*asmita*), likes (*raga*), dislikes (*dvesha*), and a sense of self-importance (*abhinivesha*) (2.3-2.9). This almost seems like an invitation to be very well established in the practice of humility (*ishvara pranidhana*).

What are you tempted by?

When temptation emerges, what kind of imbalance does it reveal in you? How can you address that imbalance?

Are you following the teachings intelligently or are you following a charismatic teacher?

Are there traces of self-importance in you?

What are the triggers that activate your self-importance?

Do your thoughts, intentions and actions reveal pride?

How is your life purpose orienting you towards liberation?

Purpose

3.53 Meditative integration (*samyama*) on single moments and their sequence, results in wisdom born of discernment.

A moment is the smallest instant in which change can occur. Change is happening everywhere. Life is a continuous sequence of changes occurring simultaneously. As change takes place, a moment almost imperceptibly turns into another moment. However, changes only happen in the present moment. In the ancient commentary by Vyasa, he explains that time is a mental construct. Yesterday and tomorrow seem real in our minds, yet we have never been in yesterday or tomorrow. We can't go to either. We can only go to recollections in our mind to try to go back in time. Or, to think about the future, we have to speculate about what might happen. Time is a useful tool for practical purposes, such as choosing when to meet a friend for lunch. However, when you see time as something real, time can become a commodity, something that can be saved or wasted. Like with any other construct or tool, we can see time as helpful or unhelpful. *Is the expectation that there is a tomorrow waiting for you an excuse to postpone your wholehearted participation in your life? Or is the uncertainty about tomorrow a powerful motivation to engage meaningfully in your activities?* This sutra is a reminder to the call to action from sutra 1.1, the task of the yogi is to be present. If change happens only in the present moment, your actions can take place only in the present moment. *When you go*

beyond seeing time as something real, what happens? This aphorism says that meditative integration on moments and their succession, establishes wisdom out of discernment.
Can your meditation on the sequence of unique moments clarify the difference between the aspect of you that is changing constantly and the part that seems to be timeless?

For instance, in a comfortable position close your eyes and invite yourself to relax. Take some time to let everything, your body, breath, mind, and emotions settle. Focus on feeling the complete experience of being without adding any commentary.
Can you feel a timeless aspect of you?
Whatever the experience, it cannot be put into words accurately, but you may be able to feel it.
Can you stay with that and be curious about what happens when you focus fully on each moment and the changes that are taking place?

Can this practice offer you a useful vantage point for living your life?

3.54 Consequently, the essential difference between two otherwise seemingly identical objects (by species, characteristics, and location) can be discerned.

Continuing the idea in the previous sutra that the advanced yoga practitioner can notice the minute changes from one instant in time to the next, this sutra states that the practitioner can notice the minute changes that make an object unique, even when there are two otherwise identical objects. The typical example is that if there are two gold rings that are identical in all their characteristics, including their shape, color, weight and appearance, a yogi can tell if somebody switches the positions of the rings. This knowledge results from being able to discern the smallest changes taking place in an instant. Each identical ring has different atomic interactions with its surroundings, and the yogi can notice these infinitesimal differences. This is part of omniscience, the complete knowledge, awareness and understanding of the world mentioned in sutra 3.50. Another way of understanding this aphorism is that the yogi is completely attuned to whatever can be perceived.

To what extent are you able to notice the very subtle aspects of the phenomena that surround you?

How does that enable you to be uplifting and life affirming?

3.55 As a result of discernment (*viveka*), complete and all-encompassing transcendent knowledge that dissolves the illusion of time. Then, the yogi is free from conditioned existence.

The discernment (*viveka*) of the distinction between pure awareness and temporary experiences gives the practitioner the intuitional wisdom encompassing everything in existence, regardless of characteristics, properties, condition, realm, or sequence (time). This transcendent knowledge is *rtambhara* – mentioned in aphorisms 1.48 and 1.49 – a deep understanding, beyond inference, of the intricate synergy of everything in the cosmos. Free from all conditioning, the practitioner accepts unconditionally everything that exists.

To what extent are you still placing conditions on your participation in the endless flow of life?

What remaining ways of being pull you away from your natural state of

being?
What conditions keep you from saying yes to life?

3.56 Thus, when purity of the individual flawlessly mirrors the purity of Pure Awareness (*purusha*), liberation (as complete independence - *kaivalya*) comes into being.

Regardless of using meditative integration (*samyama*) and its results, or pure discernment (*viveka*) without any attainments (*siddhis*), reaching the utmost clarity leads into complete freedom (*kaivalya*). This utmost clarity is the final step in regulating one's ways of being (*vrtti*). First, the ways of being are noticed, then their helpfulness is assessed. The next step consists of regulating the ways of being and favoring the beneficial ones. Eventually, all the ways of being are released uncovering the natural state of complete awareness that mirrors absolute awareness. In the example of a movie projector, the lens, the film, the screen, and everything in the projection room is free from any blockages that might prevent the uninterrupted flow of light to animate the film. Similarly, at this stage in the journey, all misidentification (*avidya*) has been released. All past impressions (*samskaras*) have been resolved, with no new tendencies developing (*vasanas*). Consequently, actions are not attached to any expectation or consequences (*karma*). All participation in the flow of life happens according to the unimpeded flow of pure awareness through the practitioner's body, mind and emotions. This is abiding in one's natural state, one's true nature (1.3).
What is your natural state?
What is conducive for you to be in that natural state?

Summary of Chapter Three of the Yoga Sutra

With the first five limbs of yoga, the practitioner increases harmony between life and awareness, thereby reducing internal levels of reactivity. The final three limbs of yoga, concentration (*dharana*), meditation (*dhyana*) and integration (*samadhi*), complete the system of yoga. When applied together these three limbs are called *Samyama* and through gradual cultivation result in insight into the highest wisdom. *Samyama* is more internal than the first five limbs, yet it is still not as deep as the highest level of integration. *Samyama* is a process that continues the journey from *pratyahara*, inward sense orientation, to concentration that becomes effortless and invites growing inner silence. Since most of the obstacles to connecting to our true nature result from our misidentification, the release of erroneous beliefs about ourselves brings about a deep level of integration. This integration happens as a gradual transformation at the physical, physiological, mental, and emotional levels manifesting as growing inner peace and inward focus. As a result, a new tendency towards inner silence takes hold, becoming deeply rooted so that all distractions dissolve and single-pointed awareness gets established. Consequently, the illusion of separateness dissolves, and it is possible to notice the similarities between one instant and the next. Having released the limiting filters used to interpret all experiences, awareness attunes through the senses to the direct and unobstructed experience of life in its constitutive elements including their properties, characteristics, and states. Consequently, changes can be perceived with unparalleled clarity offering insight into all phenomena.

By directing meditative integration (*samyama*) into the dimensions of change, past and future become evident. Meditative integration can reveal languages and communication with all beings, knowledge of previous lives, a person's state of mind, and the time of one's death. *Samyama* can also confer imperceptibility. It can enhance qualities and strengths; offer perception of what is hidden as well as knowledge of the subtle realms of the universe, stars and constellations; understanding of the body; control of thirst and hunger; communication with perfected disembodied beings; access to the inner light of awareness; knowledge of one's mind; impartiality; extraordinary intuition; capability to enter somebody else's body; levitation; radiance; traveling through space; awareness beyond the body; extraordinary sense perception; extraordinary physical powers; bodily perfection; independence from sense organs; omniscience and omnipotence. However, only through detachment from these achievements can temptation be averted. By releasing all misidentification (*avidya*), the conditioning imposed by all the ways of being is finally removed. Only through discerning the distinction between one's true nature and one's ways of being can absolute liberation manifest. *The practitioner becomes an embodiment of true insight into all aspects of reality, absolutely free from conditioned existence.*

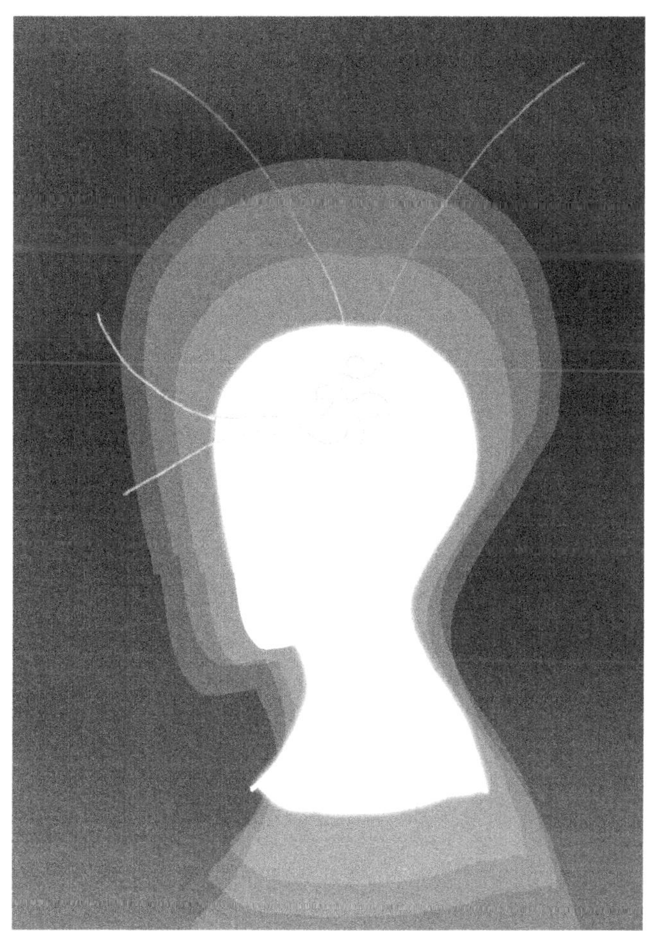

By abiding in your true nature, the constant struggles to make sense dissolve, freeing you up from your limited and limiting opinions, beliefs and misidentifications. Then your heart and mind open.

EMANCIPATION (*KAIVALYA*)

Kaivalya, the title of Chapter Four of the Yoga Sutra, has the following meanings in Sanskrit: *isolation, absolute unity, perfect isolation, abstraction, detachment from all other connections, detachment of the soul from matter or further transmigrations, beatitude, leading to eternal happiness* or *emancipation*. The aphorisms in this shortest chapter can be grouped as follows:

- Awareness & nature [4.1-4.5]
- Impressions, tendencies & consequences [4.6-4.11]
- Realm of experience [4.12-4.17]
- Consciousness and awareness [4.18-4.24]
- Emancipation [4.25-4.34]

Consciousness & Awareness

Consciousness is the aliveness, the presence or the beingness in everything that exists, everywhere.

Awareness is the individual sense of being alive; a manifestation of consciousness; the light that enables us to notice that we are conscious; the process of coming into presence; the active expression of consciousness; the key element in yoga.

Awareness and Nature

4.1 Optimal function and enhanced efficiency (*siddhis*) may result from birth, herbs, mantra, purification practices (*tapas*) and deep integration (*samadhi*).

After dedicating a major portion of Chapter Three to the yogic practices resulting in extraordinary attainments (*siddhis*), Patañjali begins Chapter Four by listing five possible ways of cultivating these faculties. The first is by birth, meaning that these powers are innate, with typical examples provided by prodigious children. The commentators explain that, in those cases, the person's merits in previous lives come into fruition as the person is born. The second way is by using herbs. All world traditions living in harmony with nature develop a profound understanding of their environment. Consequently, each tradition learns to use what nature provides for sustenance, health, and to fulfill all their needs, including entering states that give them access to a deeper understanding of the universe.

Mantra, the practice of reciting a series of words, is also a widespread practice in many traditional societies. They can be used for producing specific effects, such as bringing calmness to one's being, reaching heightened states of consciousness, and casting a spell. Extraordinary powers can also be obtained through intense purification practices, *tapas*. These types of practices are common in many traditional rituals throughout the world. The fifth way of enhancing function and efficiency is integration, *samadhi*. Remember that Patañjali already dedicated Chapter One of the Yoga Sutra to *samadhi*. This sutra reflects Patañjali's comprehensive perspective, by not claiming that only yoga can create these supernatural powers. Of course, it has already been said in aphorism 3.38 that these powers can be seen as accomplishments or as obstacles. It is the practitioner who decides how to apply these powers, either to generate more ways of being (*citta vrtti*) and entanglements or to move towards liberation.

Are you noticing changes in your ways of being and functioning?
Where do they come from?
Is your practice resulting in optimal function and enhanced efficiency?
How are your practices sustaining your vital energy?
How do they contribute to enhancing the quality of your participation in your life?
Are you increasing your entanglement in the world or are you living in harmony within and without?

4.2 Coming into being is a transformation that follows the flow of nature (*prakriti*).

The flow of life evolves according to the intrinsic tendencies in nature: movement (*rajas*), balance (*sattva*) and inertia (*tamas*) (2.18). These three tendencies manifest in nature (*prakriti*) in countless ways. In sutra 3.13 Patañjali talked about everything in nature changing along three dimensions: properties (*dharma*), characteristics (*lakshana*) and states (*avasthana*). At different times some of those features can be active, dormant, or latent (3.14). Changes in those features (properties, characteristics, or states) are not a fundamental change. For instance, water changing from liquid to vapor, or ice does not go through a fundamental transformation because its essence does not change. The changes caused through the five practices listed in sutra 4.1 do not represent a fundamental transformation because they do not change the fundamental essence of the object. In the case of birth, it was suggested that the cause of the supernatural faculties manifests at birth as a result of the accumulation of previous experiences of that being.

Remember that in the first half of Chapter Three of the Yoga Sutra Patañjali mentioned three significant changes accomplished through meditative integration (*samyama*): a change to increased inner stillness (*nirodha parinama* – 3.9), releasing all externalities (*samadhi parinama* – 3.11), and single-pointedness that removes all illusion of separation (*ekagrata parinama* – 3.9). Although these are not fundamental changes to your essence, they do have a powerful effect in transforming your body and mind. *Samadhi* seems to be preferable to the other options listed in 4.1 because it is more sustainable and within the control of the practitioner. In any case, being born is the unstoppable flow of life manifesting in nature.

To what extent are you conscious of the flow of life in you?

Are you aware of the constant changes as life unfolds all around you?

How do your movements influence the flow of life through you?

What are the effects of various ways of breathing into the aliveness in you?

Do your thoughts affect how alive you feel?

Is there a relationship between your emotions and the sense of aliveness in you?

What are the effects of your choices and actions on the flow of life in nature, including in your own being?

4.3 The flow of life in nature (*prakriti*) is not the result of incidental causes. When obstacles are removed, life flows organically according to its own potentiality.

Continuing the line of thought in the previous sutra, this aphorism acts as a reminder that nature has its own primordial tendencies. Your previous actions do not cause your life; your previous actions, however, will influence your birth, lifespan, and quality of experiences (2.13). When obstacles are removed, life flows according to its own potentiality, like when a farmer diverts the flow of water from one field to another to irrigate the field that needs it. The farmer does not actually cause the water to be absorbed by the plants that need it. Instead, the farmer creates the conditions conducive for water to be absorbed, which happens according to the nature of water, soil, ecosystem of bacteria in the soil, and plant root system. If you have ever tried to plant a garden, you may have noticed that you start by removing weeds, preparing the soil and planting the seeds appropriate to your geographic location, season, and sun exposure. Even when you prepare the whole section evenly and you use seeds from the same seed bank, you will notice that some seeds germinate, and some seeds don't. In other words, you orchestrate the incidental causes, creating propitious conditions for your plants to grow, but you have no control of how nature will manifest. These incidental causes that you manipulate are not the cause of life flowing into the seeds to germinate them.

The second half of this sutra presents the part that is within your control, removing the obstacles to the flow of life. You do this by amending the soil, removing weeds, ensuring that it is the right season and correct sun exposure. Although some seeds may have a chance to grow even when you do not prepare the ground, probabilities increase dramatically when you facilitate the process by removing the obstructions to the flow of life in nature.

Remember the definition and results of yoga in Chapter One of the Yoga Sutra, that yoga is regulating your ways of being (1.3). This regulation is precisely the removal of obstacles explained in this sutra. Because of regulating your ways of being, you embody your true nature (1.4). To embody your true nature is to live in what is often called the natural state. This point is reiterated here because it is crucial to yoga practice. The natural state is your birthright, it is the effortless joy and health you witness in a baby. You look at the baby and it looks back at you with a genuine smile and a carefree attitude. There is no effort on the baby's part to abide in the natural state; that is why it is called the natural state. *It happens often that we come to see yoga as a system to acquire, fitness, health, beauty, or extraordinary strength or flexibility. When that happens, we set up inaccurate goals for the practice.* At the same time, these goals generate expectations that will become the seeds of future frustrations, because even when you attain them, they will be temporary.

Yoga is a complete system to remove the obstacles that keep you from being in your natural state of effortless joy. That's why the first step is to become aware of what you are doing. Next, you decide how what you are doing is contributing to keep you in your natural state. You remove the unhelpful ways of being, the obstacles preventing you from living unconditionally.

Is there a difference between your normal state and your natural state?

How are you aligning with your natural state?

Are there any obstructions limiting your access to the joy and love permeating your being?

How many of those obstacles can you learn to regulate and, eventually, remove?

4.4 Created minds result from sense of self (*asmita*).

One fascinating aspect of the Yoga Sutra is that its terseness invites many different interpretations. One approach is to choose one perspective according to one tradition or belief and to interpret the sutra according to that tradition. Another approach is to consider that several interpretations may be correct at different times and for different levels of practice. This second approach was offered in the previous chapter, and in this whole book, to provide an accessible way to practice. For some commentators, this aphorism states that the practitioner creates other body-minds as vehicles of his consciousness that can all be active simultaneously without generating new impressions. The practitioner creates other body-minds to speed up burning his past impressions (*samskaras*) and *karma*. A slightly different perspective suggests that the practitioner creates many body-minds, out of compassion, to enhance the quality of life for all beings. Since the practitioner's being is free from thoughts, the actions accomplished through these bodies do not generate impressions causing future *karma*. These two complementary interpretations continue the thread of supernatural powers in Chapter Three, framed within the ideas in the past three aphorisms, that coming into being results from removing the obstacles to the flow of natural forces.

One further possible way of understanding this sutra is that the natural flow of life manifests as the sense of self (*asmita*). This sense of self is the very subtle sense of being. It is this sense of self that is at the core of all your experiences. In fact, it is this *asmita* that gives you the sense that you are a being, that you exist. Remember that at the very beginning of Chapter Two of the Yoga Sutra, the list of the five afflictions included not knowing your true nature (*avidya*) as the major obstacle enabling the other obstacles to emerge sequentially (2.3- to 2.9). The second obstacle to appear is the sense of self (*asmita* 2.6). When this very subtle obstacle is active, it can be neutral. However, it can also trigger the emergence of the other three afflictions, likes (*raga* 2.7), dislikes (*dvesha* 2.8), and sense of self-importance, also known as fear of dying (*abhinivesha* 2.9). According to sutra 4.4, this natural outcropping of nature, your sense of self, is the root of all your identifications. In other words, it is your basic sense of self that creates all the typical conflicting views of who you think you are, who you think you should be, and who you think others expect you to be. In the context of accomplishments, yogis at this level of mastery can connect to their sense of self and deactivate its tendencies towards identification to prevent generating other ways of being (*citta*).

One possible way of contemplating the message in this sutra is to experience how your sense of self is the point where nature and consciousness meet. Like any other point of interaction between two different principles, *asmita* is the field where friction between these two different principles will manifest. It may also be useful to remember that this sense of being (*asmita*) was one of the degrees of meditation mentioned in sutra 1.17. If you remember the idea that yoga is a process of refining your presence, you can approach this contemplation of your sense of being by considering the following two questions:
What are the different labels influencing who you think you are and your actions?

When you quiet down the level of internal activity and identification through meditation, what do you experience?

4.5 One singular awareness underlies all the many experiences in their wide variety.

When interpreting the previous aphorism as the capacity to generate a variety of body-minds, this sutra is thought to be a clarification of the fact that the yogi directs all the individual body-minds they've created. If the previous sutras are understood as dealing with the capacity to regulate the sense of self (*asmita*), this sutra can be thought of as confirmation that there is an underlying sense of self beneath all the individual experiences, regardless of how different they may be. As you observe yourself during your day, you'll probably notice that you adjust the way you interact with the world according to the context that you are in. If you are at a library and are talking to a friend, the tone of voice you use might be different from your tone of voice when meeting that same friend at a busy restaurant. Similarly, what you talk about and the level of emotion you display may be different at different times and with different people. *Is there a singular awareness underlying all the varied experiences you have? What is at the core of every one of your experiences?* This inquiry can be extended to consider that the sense of being is common to all humans and, quite likely, to all beings.

Could this be one way to facilitate developing a sense of compassion and interconnectedness?

Could this be put into practice in the common greeting at the beginning and/or end of many yoga asana group sessions when everybody says *namaste*?

What is at the core of your being?

Impressions (*Samskaras*), Tendencies (*Vasanas*) and Consequences (*Karma*)

4.6 The yogi's mind, stilled in meditation, does not generate or accumulate new subconscious impressions (*samskaras*), because its perception is not clouded by its ways of being.

Of the five paths to gain supernatural powers listed in sutra 4.1, only one path is established in meditation, that is the *samadhi* path. The other paths –birth, herbs, purification practices (*tapas*) and mantra – use external ways of gaining these attainments. Because these actions are external, they will generate echoes in the world, subconscious impressions (*samskaras*) that will result in future activities. According to this sutra, only the path that is based on meditation (*samadhi*) will not produce new impressions. In other words, the external paths are short-lived and therefore not sustainable, while the meditation path (*samadhi*) does not require the yogi to rely on external elements and is, thus, reliable and sustainable. Also, since *samadhi* brings the yogi into the natural state, the yogi's sense of self (*asmita*) is free from all identification and, thus, free from expectations and attachments to the results.

All actions have ramifications. The root of each action includes your intention and your attitude. When your actions are grounded in the natural state, free from the conflict between likes and dislikes, the ramifications of your actions do not become a burden or a source of future suffering as it was pointed out in aphorisms 2.15 and 2.16. Also, in Chapter Two of the Yoga Sutra, Patañjali indicated that the afflictions (*klesha*) dissolve when the sense of self dissolves into consciousness (2.10) and that meditation is a way to counteract the activities resulting from the afflictions (2.11).

Having reached this level of practice, although you still live in the world and participate in life through your actions and interactions, your actions spring from your emotional balance and unclouded awareness. As a result, your actions do not leave lasting emotional impressions (*samskaras*) that will otherwise generate future experiences gravitating around your sense of self, your likes, your dislikes, or your sense of self-importance.

Are any of your actions caused by your sense of self-importance?

To what extent are you free from the manipulations of your likes and dislikes? What motivates your actions?

How do you know if your actions result from your deep emotional balance?

Are you clear on your intentions?

4.7 The accomplished yogi, established in integration, is beyond dualities. Therefore, the yogi does not accumulate impressions that cause reactivity (*karma*). For everybody else, reactivity (*karma*) is of three kinds: positive, negative, and mixed.

The path of yoga is a lifelong journey. It starts with the desire to be present in our lives. That simple (yet profound) resolve motivates us to bring awareness into our thoughts, intentions, actions, and interactions. As we attempt to be present, we start noticing that we get distracted a lot of the time. When we observe ourselves systematically, we find some tendencies in all aspects of our being, our body, mind, emotions, and interactions (*cittta vrtti* – ways of being). *Knowing those patterns is the prerequisite for being able to modulate them*, increasing life-affirming tendencies and decreasing unhelpful ones. The unhelpful tendencies generate emotional impressions that will perpetuate a cycle of further painful or irritating actions. These are the seeds of negative reactivity, called black *karma* in this aphorism. The helpful, life-affirming patterns plant seeds of positive change, white *karma*. It is safe to say that out of most people, there are very few people who are completely virtuous all the time or completely non-virtuous all the time. Most of us show a combination of virtuous and not so virtuous intentions, thoughts, actions, and interactions. This is the third kind of *karma*, a mix of the results of virtuous and non-virtuous actions.

This sutra explains that yogis are in a different category altogether. A yogi, somebody who is established in integration (*samadhi*), is a person who has gone beyond regulating tendencies. He or she has extinguished all tendencies arising from a sense of self. As a result, all actions are completely detached from expectations (*vairagya*) because the yogi is fully aligned with pure consciousness. Being in the natural state, the yogi's actions are not driven by the afflictions listed in sutra 2.3, and thus, they do not accumulate unresolved emotional imprints (*sámskarás*), as pointed out in aphorisms 2.13 and 2.14. In other words, the yogi is not trying to be virtuous or non-virtuous, because he or she is participating in the everchanging flow of life without cravings or attachments. It is those attachments that create the illusion of separation.

To what extent are you aware of your tendencies?
How are you regulating your tendencies?
Is it possible that even tendencies that used to be beneficial may no

longer be serving a purpose and can be eliminated?

How many of your attitudes, intentions, actions and reactions are connected to unresolved emotional imprints from your past?

Can you notice how your present situation may be influenced by your previous intentions and actions?

Are you aware of the past impressions still active in you?

Do your actions reflect increasing evenness within you?

4.8 The subconscious impressions (*samskaras*) lie dormant until the conditions are appropriate for their manifestation. These impressions influence personality traits and tendencies (*vasanas*).

Remember that actions motivated by the five afflictions (*kleshas* 2.3) will influence your birth, lifespan, and quality of life (2.12), and will result in pleasant and unpleasant experiences (2.13). Recognize also that anything that you do, you get good at, including what you do with virtuous or selfish motives, and regardless of your actions being conscious or unconscious. Whatever you do, especially anything that is charged with emotion, leaves an impression that gets stored in your subconscious. If you think about something that caused you great joy or pain, it will bring forth memories and sensations that are stored in you but are timeless. The intensity of the sensations can move you, no matter how far back in time the event may have happened. Something that caused you emotional pain in your childhood may still be stored in you after many years, triggering responses and influencing how you perceive, interpret and behave in your life. In fact, all actions related to your sense of identity perpetuate further actions and reactions that will, in turn, influence your choices and preferences.

Is it possible that some events in your life manifest as the result of impressions left by your personal history?
If you notice some patterns repeating in your life, even when you have tried to change your behavior, is it possible that some unresolved previous impression may be influencing your decisions?
How are your motivations influencing your perspective and choices?

How are your past actions forming who you are or who you think you should be?
Is your personality a form of conditioning?

4.9 All actions result in accumulated impressions (*samskaras*) linked to memory in a unique configuration regardless of the time, place, or circumstances in which those impressions emerged.

Any activity you do has a beginning and an end. All activities leave impressions in your memory. The more meaningful the motivation for the activity and the stronger your emotional investment in it, the stronger its impression. These impressions include all kinds of emotions. Emotion is the glue that keeps all these impressions together and to yourself. As mentioned in the previous aphorism, these impressions are seeds that influence your actions and inclinations. When you tasted something sweet like ice cream or chocolate for the very first time, the experience left an impression in you. That impression is reinforced every time that you have a similar experience. The next time you eat that type of food, you will remember previous times, places, and circumstances when you had a similar experience, strengthening the hold of those impressions. Some of those impressions may be in your conscious awareness while others may be stored in your subconscious mind.

This sutra takes this idea further by saying that the impressions from all your actions, thoughts and intentions are linked to your memory in a unique way. This aggregate of impressions becomes part of your ways of being. As long as the impression generates some level of emotional reactivity, it will remain and, as it was pointed out in aphorism 4.8, the impressions remain dormant until a propitious time for them to emerge. Over time, these impressions accumulate subconsciously and create a feedback loop of associations that generates tendencies and recurring experiences. The resulting experiences offer potential lessons that have not been fully assimilated and thus will need to emerge again until they do not generate any emotional reactivity. When these impressions remain active, they perpetuate your process of living through your *karma*, as mentioned in sutras 4.7, 2.12, 2.13 and 2.14.

As you become familiar with your ways of being, can you notice if these ways of being tend to appear again and again?
Do your ways of being seem to overlap?
Are those ways of being related to your beliefs and opinions?
If your ways of being seem to repeat, is it possible that the external circumstances of their manifestation might differ, but their emotional content and agitation may be the same?
For instance, if you keep getting frustrated by a diverse set of circumstances and people, could it be that there is an unresolved previous emotional experience common to these irritations, like a deeply ingrained feeling of scarcity, or a deeply seated need for approval?
Might it be possible that this collection of impressions, when unresolved, remains in your individual space of awareness offering you ways to overcome your identification with these experiences?
If you trace the irritants that bother you, can they be trying to show you

what needs to be released so that these experiences do not become another source of misidentification?

For instance, the person who finds it difficult to voice his needs will find himself in situation after situation prompting him to assert his voice until he can finally do it. Consider if the unique configuration of impressions and emerging circumstances for their resolution are perfectly calibrated for you to decrease or remove some of your ways of being.

One traditional interpretation of this sutra indicates that the conglomerate of impressions and memory continues from one lifetime to the next in a potentially endless cycle of life, death, and rebirth (*samsara*). This unique collection of memories and impressions is what some people call the individual soul. There is a controversial idea about recipients of organ donation experiencing new cravings and predilections matching those of the organ donor. Other recipients of organ donation have reported unusual dreams that seem to coincide with traumatic experiences lived by the organ donors close to the time of their demise. These stories are controversial because there are no ways to prove or disprove them. However, if these reports are true, would it be possible for the impressions of previous actions to be stored in our organs through some mechanism that we do not understand yet? Furthermore, decades of rigorous research on children who remember their previous lives suggests that consciousness survives death, remaining even when the bond to the physical body has been severed.[vii] Can these stories about transfer of some personal traits from one person to another point to how awareness infuses our embodied existence? Also, if some personal tendencies (*vasanas*) can survive after death, might this suggest that the journey of learning extends beyond this lifetime?

Is it possible then that your unique configuration of memories, impressions and tendencies continues from one life to the next?

4.10 It is unknown when these subconscious impressions (*samskaras*) originated, and since they are powered by desire, they will remain for as long as desire remains.

This sutra says that there is no clear explanation of when or why desire started. Desire is a powerful force compelling us to act. The will to live is an expression of a primordial desire in all living beings. Desire is an emotional charge causing impressions to stick to your awareness. These latent impressions emerge when the conditions are ripe for them generating more impressions in an endless cycle (4.8). Then, is it possible or necessary to eliminate all desire? At the beginning of this book we suggested harnessing the power of desire to move toward presence.

Can desire be like all experiences, either a vehicle for enjoyment or for liberation?

What desires are prevalent in you?

To what extent are those desires perpetuating some of your existing tendencies and inclinations?

Can you modulate your desire?

Is your desire a way to deepen your identification with temporary phenomena?

Is it possible to orient your desire towards liberation from conditioning?

As you cultivate presence, are you more aware of your own impressions emerging?

For instance, when you set your mind to focus on an idea or object during meditation, can you notice that the seemingly random thoughts distracting you emerge from your subconscious mind?

Can those distracting thoughts suggest viable paths for releasing them?

4.11 These impressions are caused by the afflictions (*klesha*) and result in birth, lifespan, as well as pleasant and unpleasant experiences. The impressions are supported by ways of being (*citta vrtti*), tendencies (*vasanas*) and by the objects that can be experienced. When the causes, effects, support and objects are removed, the impressions disappear.

This aphorism weaves together the major themes from the Yoga Sutra. Related to sutras 2.12 to 2.14, this sutra explains how the five afflictions –not knowing your true nature (*avidya*), your sense of self (*asmita*), your likes (*raga*), your dislikes (*dvesha*) and your sense of self-importance (*abhinivesha*) –keep generating impressions that manifest as ways of being through your actions and interactions. The objects and circumstances in which they appear will facilitate the emergence of some of your ways of being, which will leave new imprints in your memory. These impressions will create new potential conditioning that will influence your future perceptions, intentions, actions, circumstances, and experiences. *How can you make these impressions, and their effects disappear*? As in other sections of the Yoga Sutra, Patañjali in this aphorism states the problem and its solution. If the impressions are caused by the afflictions (2.3 to 2.9) and all the afflictions sprout in the field of not knowing one's true nature (*avidya*), then being established in discernment (*viveka*) will help remove the misidentification and its consequences. Notice that aphorism 1.16 already explained that being aligned with Truth was the sign of success in freedom from attachments (*vairagya*). The patient persistence of practice (*abhyasa*) and detachment (*vairagya*) is the method for regulating your ways of being (1.12), which are the support of the impressions. Eventually, the ways of being are turned off.

The objects that can be experienced include both sensory objects that draw our senses as well as situations and circumstances leading to storage of new impressions. Notice how the eight limbs of yoga provide a complete program for the removal of causes, effects, support, and objects that generate more internal reactivity. The *Yamas* provide ways to create mental, physical, and emotional harmony around you. The *Niyamas* lead you to establish contentment through creating inner mental and emotional harmony. *Asana* practice optimizes body function. *Pranayama* enhances the flow of vital energy by purifying and modulating your respiratory processes. *Pratyahara* draws your senses inwardly to delve deeply into the subtler aspects of yourself. *Dharana* and *Dhyana* establish the focus of your mind for accurate perception free from interference from beliefs and preferences. Then you abide in your natural state, in deep harmony with the flow of life and established in true wisdom (*Samadhi*).

To what extent are you able to notice the causes of your deep-seated emotional interferences?
What ways of being support your emotional imbalances?
What circumstances are conducive to their survival?
How are you removing your deeply ingrained subconscious impressions? When you choose to be still, is there inner silence or endless internal commentary?

How are you creating effortless peaceful impressions (3.10) through your practice and life?

The Realm of Experience

4.12 Past and future, in subtle form, latent or potential, exist in the present.

The previous sutra already indicated that since active impressions are constantly triggering actions and reactivity, removing their causes, effects, support and objects removes the impressions. With less active impressions, the practitioner's reactivity decreases. Although every action leaves impressions in memory, some of the impressions are beyond conscious access; in other words, they are not manifesting in the present, they are only latent. Because those impressions are not active but latent, those impressions will manifest in the future, when circumstances are propitious (4.8). Remember that sutra 3.14, stated that there is an underlying essence to everything that can be perceived. What varies is the degree of manifestation. Impressions exist in every moment: in a latent state when they remain only in memory, in potential state awaiting the adequate conditions for its future manifestation, or in manifest state when they are active. Just like an acorn carries with it the essence of the whole lineage of oak trees from where it came, it also carries the potential of one oak tree and all its possible descendants. Yet, currently, the acorn is the present manifestation.

Sutra 4.10 already indicated that the origin of impressions is not known, which may lead to inferring that impressions do not actually disappear. If you know your impressions, discernment can clarify how to prevent the future manifestation of the impressions that you have (2.15 and 2.16). For example, if you fill a bottle with water and just place the lid on top of the bottle without securing it because you are preoccupied with something else, you might forget that the bottle is not fully closed, and it may spill all over when you place it in your lunch bag. If you do not know your tendencies, when everything in your lunch bag is soaked in water, you may think to yourself *"Why does this always happen to me?"* When this happens enough times, it can cause you to pause and examine your actions. Then, you may notice your tendency to be preoccupied with many things at once, causing you not to attend fully to some of your actions. Perhaps you can choose to avoid future spillage by bringing your presence into packing your lunch. In this case, the impression may remain in potential state but a new impression of attending to all steps of packing your lunch may block that impression of distractedness, as suggested in sutra 1.50.

Can you notice recurring circumstances leading you to suffering and agitation?
Is there an impression coming into manifestation in those cases?
What impressions lead you to harmony with your natural state?
What impressions foster misidentification with temporary phenomena?
To what extent are you aware of the impressions left by your past experiences?
Are some of your actions the effect of a distant impression in the past?

4.13 Manifest or subtle, characteristics change due to the primordial tendencies (*gunas*) of nature.

This sutra relates to the ideas presented in aphorisms 2.18 and 3.14. Anything that can be perceived will be influenced by a combination of the three fundamental tendencies in nature. These tendencies, the *gunas* are inertia (*tamas)*, activity (*rajas*), and harmony (*sattva*). When internal activity and reactivity are stilled through meditation, it is possible to notice the underlying essence of what is perceived along with its characteristics. Meditating on the changes of its characteristics reveals the past and future of the object meditated upon (3.14-3.16 & 4.12). The process is related to subconscious impressions. As part of nature, subconscious impressions are influenced by these primordial tendencies. Nature follows its course. In other words, *your impressions result in inclinations and tendencies according to the intentions motivating your thoughts, actions, and interactions.* You do have a choice, especially when you become aware of your tendencies and their effects on your ways of being. In some cases, you are influenced by your own inertia (*tamas*), like when you have decided to ride your bike more often because it is enjoyable and a good way to exercise, but when it is time to go to a place nearby you override that previous decision because it is more convenient to drive your car. Other times, your own excitement may lead you to overreach beyond your capacities, leading you to exhaust your energy (*rajas*). Other times, you make choices that feel balanced, require an appropriate amount of energy and have balancing effects (*sattva*). So, even when you are not aware of your own inclinations, just living your life you may notice that every time a situation manifests you have choices for your actions. Your choices and actions will be influenced by your past impressions as well as by the three fundamental tendencies in nature. The sensations, emotions, and thoughts that you perceive at any point may indicate the presence of some of your conscious and unconscious impressions, in tandem with the primordial tendencies of nature.

When your choices are entangled in your sense of identity, they will tend to bring up more agitation. For instance, when you have an interaction with a colleague and you are trying to impose your idea or perspective because you want to impress or you want to feel superior, it will be challenging for you to stand outside your own identity. Thus, it will be harder for you to witness the situation from your own presence in order to make a balanced choice. Similarly, the way you interact with others is influenced by the primordial tendencies of nature. When you feel agitated or anxious, your ways of moving and speaking are different from when you feel tired or lethargic. These ways of expressing yourself also change when you feel at peace and satisfied.

How can you become aware of the effects of the basic tendencies of nature in your own inner world?
To what extent are some of your thoughts, emotions, and actions influenced by inertia, agitation and harmony?
Do your activities influence your own levels of energy?
Are you able to regulate your own levels of energy?
Can the eight limbs of yoga (from Chapter Two of the Yoga Sutra) offer you ways to fine tune your ways of participating?
When you do something, can you notice your own habitual patterns?
Do you engage superficially or with too much intensity?
What feedback offers you cues to modulate your actions?
Is it possible that your tendencies are constantly offering you lessons to learn? In fact, is it possible that everything in nature can be seen either as pure sensual enjoyment or as a way to connect to your true nature as

intimated in sutra 2.19?

What would happen if you contemplate this idea: Is life a foe trying to set you up to suffer or a compassionate teacher helping you move towards greater integration?

Can every single action and every single interaction be an opportunity for presence?

4.14 Although undergoing constant change, each unique object is real.

This and the following sutras ascertain one perspective on the world, existence, and perception according to Yoga from Patañjali's perspective. There have always been competing ideas about the world and how it works.

Is the world real, or is it a figment of your imagination?

Just like the seemingly real scenes from a dream disappear when you wake up, is it possible that the experiences you have during your awake state are imaginary because they seem to disappear while you are dreaming?

Is being awake more real than dreaming?

Some people have argued that only that which can be experienced through the senses is real, while others argue that everything that exists is an illusion. These ideas regarding the world and its perception will influence what you focus on. *No matter how thorough your way of thinking about the world, it is by necessity incomplete, because life in its diverse complexity cannot be encompassed fully in the mind.* However, the framework you choose to interpret the world is a useful tool to try to make sense of your experiences, of yourself and of your life. Even with a well-established theory about the world and how it works, there are many aspects that may not be explained satisfactorily for everybody.

In this group of sutras Patañjali offers a yogic explanation of reality, according to which everything in nature is subject to the constant interaction between the three different tendencies mentioned in aphorisms 2.15, 2.19, and 4.13. These qualities are interpreted sometimes as steadiness (*tamas*), activity (*rajas*) and illumination (*sattva*), and other times as inertia (*tamas*), energy (*rajas*) and harmony (*sattva*). They can also be thought of as delusion (*tamas*), passion (*rajas*) and intelligence (*sattva*). These three tendencies are responsible for the changes that characterize all of life. Life is the field where these qualities interrelate. Although these tendencies interact causing constant change, there is something in each object that remains, as it was suggested in sutra 3.14. For instance, some days you feel energized and others you feel tired. Even when your activities are quite similar, it is highly likely that there are variations in your attitude, mood, and level of energy. However, is there something in you that remains the same? In the cycle between birth and death, your body is in constant change, yet there is some thread of continuity in you. No matter how much your body ages, when you look at yourself in a mirror you can still recognize that it's you.

Regardless of how real or unreal your dreams seem to be, or how real or unreal your awake life seems to be, can you feel that you exist? Despite all the constant changes in your sensations, emotions, and thoughts, is there some continuity in you?
What makes you aware of that continuity?
Is it possible that the continuity in you may also be changing?
Another possible avenue of exploration can be accessed through these

questions:
Can you recognize that you are a unique being in the world?
Is that uniqueness what remains consistent in your experience?
Is there uniqueness in everything you can perceive?

4.15 The object remains consistent regardless of being observed by different minds or by one mind in different states. In other words, the object exists independently of individual perception.

This group of sutras offers arguments to counteract other philosophical positions active at the time that the Yoga Sutra was compiled. This is part of a tradition of debate as a healthy exchange of ideas to clarify one's own perspective and understanding of the world. This sutra states that rather than the world being created by perception, the world is real, it exists even when it is not being perceived. Since different people can all perceive the same object and compare their perceptions, the object must exist. Of course, each person's perception will be influenced by that person's ways of being.

How do your ways of being influence your perception?
Are there some aspects of your life that remain constant?
Are there some aspects of you that remain constant?
More importantly, as you deepen in the exploration of this sutra consider, what is real in your life?
How many stories are you willing to believe?
To what extent are your stories real?
Do your stories enable you to experience your presence?
Or are your stories ways to move away from being present?

Are your thoughts, intentions, actions, and interactions charged by your conscious and deliberate presence?
Is your commitment to participating in your life real?
How are you putting your commitment into concrete actions?

4.16 The object does not depend on being perceived. Otherwise, what would happen when the object is not being perceived by a mind?

Continuing the same thread of thought, this sutra says that objects in the world are not created by your imagination. Since objects remain in existence even when you are not perceiving them, objects exist independent from perception. Remember that Patañjali makes a clear distinction between knowledge and imagination in aphorisms 1.7 and 1.9. This distinction is relevant particularly for applying this sutra.
If you believe that everything that exists is only an illusion, would you be less inclined to participate in your life?
Is it possible that everything in the universe exists instead of being just a figment of your imagination?
What is your attitude towards the world?
What is it that makes it possible for you to perceive anything?
What is the relationship between your awareness and the world that can be perceived?
If there is a relationship between your individual awareness and what can be experienced, is that an integrative, adversarial, or neutral relationship?

If you wish, you may contemplate further questions: What is the purpose of everything that exists?
What is your purpose as a person in the world?
To what extent do your intentions, actions and interactions align with your purpose?
Are your purpose and the purpose of the world in alignment or in conflict?

4.17 An object becomes known or unknown depending on the coloring of perception.

Nature is real. It exists even when it is not perceived. In addition, nature changes continuously. Although nature and everything that can be experienced exist independently from the perceiver, sutra 2.21 suggests that everything that exists has the purpose of being experienced by the perceiver. Awareness, the active expression of consciousness, enables perceptions, actions, and interactions. However, experiences are influenced by your level of awareness and by the coloring of your awareness. For instance, if you are having a conversation with one of your friends but you keep thinking about another place or time, you will not come to know or understand whatever your friend is saying, because you are not orienting your presence to the interaction with your friend. In addition, even when you are paying attention to your friend's words and gestures, the content of your friend's talk will be influenced by your personal, social, and cultural biases. The stronger your beliefs and opinions on the topic your friend is talking about, the more they will influence your perception. Both lack of presence and interference of your ways of being will affect the quality of your participation and interactions. Besides, everyone perceives uniquely according to personal history.

This sutra serves as a reminder that becoming aware of one's tendencies, opinions and habits will influence perception. When you do any type of yoga practice, the practice itself will help you notice some of the colorings of your own perception. For instance, it is quite common for the person who overreaches in life to find themselves overreaching in yoga.

To what extent are you present in your daily activities?

Can you inquire into the sources of distractions keeping you away from doing what you are doing fully?

How do those distractions influence your perception?

Are there other ways of being interfering with your perception and participation in your life?

Remember sutras 1.6 and 1.7 about knowledge, how do you know what you know?

Is what you know just information that you repeat?

Is what you know, true knowledge, the result of your direct experience?

Is there a difference between what you know and your opinions?

What is the relationship between what you know and timeless pure common sense?

Consciousness & Awareness

4.18 Unchanging, Consciousness is the substratum pervading all existence. Ways of being are always known to Consciousness.

After explaining in the previous aphorisms that the world is real and that ways of being influence perception of the world, in this and the next two sutras, Patañjali focuses on the relationship between consciousness and the world that can be experienced. Remember that this topic was explored already in sutras 2.17 to 2.23 where it says that suffering results from conflating awareness and experiences. When you identify with your passing experiences, you are bound to ride an emotional rollercoaster. Experiences offer you the opportunity to recognize the fundamental difference between unchanging consciousness and the world of change.

Consciousness is what is often called the seer, witness, source or the absolute (all words used to try to help our minds understand something that is beyond our minds.) Western philosophy has tried to understand and explain consciousness for centuries without reaching a conclusive resolution. In recent years, consciousness has emerged as a new field of scientific study including areas such as psychology, cognitive science, neuroscience, physics, mathematics, and philosophy. Contemporary science has tried to explain consciousness by formulating competing theories that still cannot explain adequately what it is that gives us the feeling of being alive. *Perhaps no word or theory can ever encompass the complete sense of what it means to be alive.* And even if it could, the pervasive aliveness throughout all of existence is certainly beyond the mind, so it cannot be fully apprehended by the mind. You certainly experience the sense of being alive as you are reading this, while at the same time you're noticing the sensations in your body offering information about the space you are in, including temperature, humidity, noises and sounds, textures, scents and visual information. The aliveness in all of life does not change but our relationship to that aliveness does. This explains how some days you wake up feeling out of sorts and other days you wake up feeling energized.

We are using the word Consciousness as the aliveness or the life in everything that exists everywhere. In contrast, we are using the word awareness to refer to your individual sense of being alive. Sometimes you feel more alive, that is, more vibrant and with more vitality than at other times. **The major theme in the Yoga Sutra is that you can connect to your natural state, a state when your aliveness flows harmoniously with the flow of life.** When you allocate your attentional energy to the experiences that you are having and become emotionally entangled in the play of opposites inherent in all experiences, you will likely misidentify and end up believing that you are the experiences that you have. In other words, you will confuse your aliveness with the vehicles that enable that aliveness to experience the world. This is the major theme in the Yoga Sutra, mentioned thus far in sutras 1.3 and 1.4, 2.20 to 2.25, and 3.36.

Experiences are not intrinsically good or bad. In fact, being alive offers you the option of experiencing a complete range of sensations and emotions. If you believe that you are those experiences or emotions, you are setting yourself up to suffer, because you will long for something that appears better than what you are currently feeling, or you will fear the end of the experience that you are enjoying. In either case, you are not present because you are distracted by the "shoulds," "coulds," "woulds" and "what ifs" related to your perspective on your experience.

This process of misidentification consists of all the ways of being that you inherit, learn, and cultivate in your life. These ways of being exist in your internal space and, according to this sutra, they exist in the space of universal aliveness with Consciousness (universal awareness) witnessing all ways of being.

What are your thoughts on Consciousness, awareness, experiences, and the relationships between them?

How do those ideas relate to your direct experience of your own aliveness?

Does your feeling of aliveness fluctuate?

Is what fluctuates your awareness or your ability to connect to your awareness?

Are there ways to regulate your connection to your own aliveness?

4.19 Individual awareness is not independent or autonomous. However, individual awareness can serve as a transparent window between consciousness and the world of experience.

This sutra continues exploring the ideas of universal aliveness (Consciousness), individual aliveness (awareness) and the manifestation of life as the world of experience. Individual awareness is not independent. In other words, you did not create yourself or your sense of aliveness. However, once you are alive, when you manifest in the world of experience, you are endowed with the gift of awareness. Awareness of being alive is a thread of connection between your individual self and the universal aliveness (Consciousness). Once again, it is impossible to put into words the ineffable nature of Consciousness.

Nevertheless, as part of the yoga tradition, there is an idea that the nature of Consciousness consists of three components often presented in the compound word *saccidananda (sat-chit-ananda)*: *sat* meaning existence, presence or being; *cit* meaning awareness or spirit; and *ananda* meaning joy, happiness or bliss. Throughout the Yoga Sutra all the practices are intended to remove obstacles that prevent individual awareness from experiencing the world accurately in order to serve as an interference-free conduit between the world of experience and universal aliveness. The sense of aliveness is founded on presence, which is another word for awareness. This aliveness or awareness is only accessible in the present moment. Every time that your awareness gets distracted by your internal activities the quality of your connection to presence decreases.

What is the relationship between individual awareness, your own sense that you are alive, and universal aliveness?
To what extent are your ways of being – including your activities, tendencies, beliefs, and personal history – illuminating or obscuring the connection between aliveness and the world of experience?
Is it possible that the fluctuations in your aliveness may be related to your ways of being?
Does the relationship between universal aliveness and your individual aliveness change when you modulate your ways of being?

4.20 Both pure awareness and the world of experience cannot be apprehended simultaneously.

This sutra offers one perspective on the process of attending. You can either focus your awareness on the world of experience or on the universal awareness, but you cannot do both simultaneously. This aphorism echoes the dichotomy presented by sutras 1.3 and 1.4: Either you direct your attention to your natural state of awareness and wholeness, or you focus on your doings and becomings. Sutras 1.20 and 1.23 offer a similar two-pronged approach to reaching integration, either by directing your attentional resources with trust, vitality and memory towards stillness and wisdom, or by directing your awareness towards pure aliveness with complete surrender. The first approach focuses on the world of experience, while the second emphasizes pure awareness as the focal point. This is reiterated in sutra 2.18, by saying that the world of experiences can be used as a system for enjoyment when the focal point is the experiences themselves. The second approach is to understand that the world of experiences can be used as a way towards liberation by noticing how the temporal nature of all experiences highlights the all-encompassing permanence of pure aliveness. Chapter Three of the Yoga Sutra also offers a similar idea in sutras 3.50 and 3.51, by saying that discernment of the difference between pure consciousness and individual awareness brings about liberation. *You make a choice to focus on pure aliveness.* This message is reinforced by inviting a release of the focus on the world of experience by letting go of the attainments listed in the third chapter of the Yoga Sutra.

What is your intention when you direct your awareness to the world of experience?

What happens?
Do you notice a difference when you focus on aliveness itself? If the process of focusing on aliveness itself uncovers distractedness, there may still be a need to empty yourself from whatever imprints that may be triggering distractions. What happens when you try to focus on both experience and pure aliveness?

4.21 One part of the individual awareness cannot observe another portion of itself, or an endless succession would confuse memory.

As you explore the relationship between your awareness, universal consciousness and the world of experience, questions may emerge:
Can there be more than one instance of your individual awareness?
Can one aspect of your awareness watch another aspect of itself?
If that were the case, argues this sutra, several instances of your awareness could watch one another creating an endless loop resulting in confusion. One way to explore this idea is to assume that you can observe different aspects of your awareness at the same time. If that were the case, you could direct your attention to noticing the sounds and noises in your surroundings. Simultaneously, you can start another process where you direct awareness to your list of things to do. If both processes can take place at the same time, can yet a different part of your awareness focus on noticing the sounds and the other on the process of thinking about your to-do list? If that is possible, can another portion of your awareness pay attention to the simultaneous process of observing each thread of your awareness?

Another very simple way to explore this notion is by bringing the tip of your thumb and the tip of your index finger in one hand to touch (*jñana mudra*) as lightly as you can. Feel the sensations at the point of contact as clearly as possible. Then try the same hand gesture with the other hand as well. Notice the sensations at the points of contact in each hand and notice if the sensory streams are perceived simultaneously or if your awareness keeps switching from one side to the other almost imperceptibly. What do you find? If it seems like you can feel both streams of tactile sensation coming in simultaneously, can you also observe yourself while you notice the tactile sensations from both hands? You can conduct a similar experiment during your daily activities. Notice the mental processes you are engaged in at any time. Notice if they are taking place at the same time. What aspect of you is keeping track of each one of these processes?

4.22 When the ways of being are stilled, individual awareness experiences its fundamental nature as embodied consciousness.

Deepening the exploration of the nature of existence, awareness and their relationship, this sutra indicates the core idea in the Yoga Sutra presented in sutras 1.3 and 1.4. Your individual sense of being can identify with your ways of being or with its natural state (the state of yoga), consciousness. There are many models of the relationship between nature and Consciousness. One predominant perspective states that there is a fundamental split between Consciousness and nature or between spirit and body. Other viewpoints maintain that the world is just materiality, and thus, only what can be explained in terms of observable phenomena is real. Examining your own perspective on the nature of the relationship between your sense of aliveness and your experiences provides a concrete way to delve into the meaning of this sutra. Becoming aware of your assumptions can help you identify how your assumptions may be influencing your perspective and understanding.

If you think that all that exists is only what can be experienced through your senses, how will that assumption influence your understanding and your actions?
How do your thoughts, which have no materiality, influence your physical body and physiological processes?
To what extent are your experiences only about your senses?
How can your experiences of friendship, kindness, compassion, and love be explained by your current assumptions?
Is it possible that you are embodied consciousness?
In other words, can your physical manifestation be a vehicle for conscious awareness to experience the world?
If you are embodied consciousness, are your ways of being contributing to enhancing your experience of Universal Consciousness?
Are your ways of being detracting from your experience of universal aliveness?
Another idea you may consider is that everything in existence is one organism manifesting in a myriad of forms conducive to recognizing the interconnectedness between everything that exists.
Could that perspective illuminate how what appears to be coincidences may be synchronicities of countless elements coming together for a purpose?

4.23 When free of identification and reactivity, individual awareness can reflect everything, Consciousness (the seer) and the objects/experiences (the seen), with complete neutrality and all-inclusiveness.

This sutra describes the natural state of individual awareness. This is the state presented as the state of yoga in aphorism1.3. It is also the state described in sutra 1.41 as *samapatti*, when the mind and heart are completely open and clear, like a pure crystal reflecting whatever is near without any distortion. This is the state of harmonious integration between individual awareness and the world of experience. Rather than a state of becoming inert, this is a state of joyful participation in the world to enhance the flow of aliveness everywhere. Notice that anything you identify with will potentially become something to explain, justify, perpetuate, or defend.

For instance, if you choose to alter your diet, you probably have good reasons to make that decision. This new choice may generate a label to use to identify yourself as a raw foodist, vegan, fruitarian, vegetarian, lacto-ovo vegetarian, pescatarian, flexitarian, paleo, omnivore. As a result, you may come to see differing options as something that competes with, undermines or challenges your perspective. These can lead you to invest time and energy in ensuring that your choice is the best for your life experiment. Noticing this process and your previous views on diet may indicate how your beliefs and ways of thinking and identification have changed over time. It will also show you how those beliefs may have influenced your thoughts, intentions, choices, actions, and interactions. They may even have caused you to become more judgmental of your own actions and of other people's choices and lifestyles. Notice also that as your preferences and choices change, you internally find ways to create a coherent narrative about you and your life experiment. Holding on to your own identifications requires lots of energy and effort. In addition to reactivity, your investment in your opinions creates an obstacle to opening your heart and mind.

Is there a relationship between your reactivity and your identification with a set of ideas and beliefs?
Is it possible that your reactivity originates in your deeply held opinions?
Are your opinions contributing to open or to close your mind and heart?
To what extent is your heart open?
Is your mind clear and still like the surface of a lake without any ripples?
Are you neutral and inclusive or partial and limiting?
Which of these two attitudes is more conducive to enhancing your aliveness?

4.24 In spite of its many latent impressions, the individual awareness can serve its higher purpose as a vehicle for liberation by offering a distortion-free reflective surface for universal Consciousness.

Remember that sutra 1.50 says that meditation creates peaceful impressions that keep the distracting impressions at bay. In fact, the seven preparatory limbs of yoga (*yama*, *niyama*, *asana*, *pranayama*, *pratyahara*, *dharana* and *dhyana*) offer an effective progression for removing distractions, obstacles and inefficiencies so that your wisdom grows and your ability to discern your true nature (2.28) increases. Yoga is a process of transformation that increases inner awareness (3.9) and establishes peaceful impressions (3.10). Only latent impressions remain (1.18). Then the yogi's awareness, when free from distractions, becomes as a clear crystal (1.41) so that it can serve its purpose: to become an open conduit between universal awareness and the world of experience to facilitate liberation from the shackles of the ways of being (2.18). The progression towards liberation is a lifelong journey of discovering the obstacles, first by making them evident and then by noticing them in all aspects of its manifestation from gross to subtle. Eventually, individual awareness releases its ways of being. In other words, *yoga unravels the fabric of the identity woven from the threads of beliefs, opinions, stories, as well as from the external narratives in movies, books, songs, and media.* Yoga practice decreases the tendencies to misidentify with all external and internal temporary phenomena.

Have you noticed a change in your ways of being because of your practice?

Can you notice that, even though there are still some distractions, they are becoming more sporadic?

To what extent are you participating in your life with neutrality and all-inclusiveness instead of allowing your assumptions to cloud your perception, intentions, actions, and interactions?

In your daily activities, are you becoming more effective by setting aside your agendas and allowing awareness to become your guide?

Is it possible that you are acting in the world with clarity, kindness, and compassion?

EMANCIPATION

4.25 Realizing through direct experience the distinction between pure consciousness and experiences dissolves the notion of individual self.

These last sutras in Chapter Four of the Yoga Sutra are weaving together the threads that appear throughout the whole treatise. Some scholars argue that Chapter Four of the Yoga Sutra is a later addition, while others maintain that it's part of the original compilation done by Patañjali. Regardless, continuity with the themes and topics in the previous chapters is evident. From the beginning of Chapter One, the problem faced by humans has been stated in terms of the dichotomy between the natural state of being grounded in the spacious peace of awareness and misidentifying with the world of temporary experiences. Remember that the first aphorisms in Chapter Two introduced the idea of not knowing one's own true nature (*avidya*) as the major field where all afflictions sprout, including the notion of the individual self (*asmita*). Sutra 2.10 stated that subtle afflictions dissolve when the sense of identity dissolves. Discernment (*viveka*) of the fundamental difference between awareness and experiences is the means to liberation (2.26).

All mental processes are, by their own nature, temporary. This is evident in the impermanence of thoughts and all mental constructs. Emotions are similarly momentary. However, despite being impermanent, sensations, thoughts and emotions effectively attract attention to lead you to experience life in its richness. As sutra 2.18 indicated, your experiences are a vehicle for liberation from misidentification with what is temporary. When misidentification dissolves, the yogi returns to the natural state. With no wants, no needs and no agendas, the yogi experiences directly the difference between the world of experience and pure awareness. As explained in sutra 1.7, experiential knowledge is the highest form of knowledge. Rather than just thinking about this distinction, the yogi becomes established in the discriminative awareness formulated as the solution to suffering (in 2.25 and 2.26). That distinction, which is the foundation of freedom from attachment (1.16), the vehicle for liberation (2.26) and the threshold of omniscience (3.50) finally comes into being. **The notion of an individual self who is isolated from the ongoing flow of life dissolves.**

What are the remaining obstacles on your path?
Are thoughts, sensations and emotions drawing you away from presence? What beliefs and opinions lead you to forget that every single day you are alive is an extraordinary gift?
How can you clarify your true nature?

4.26 As a result, free from the sense of identity, the discriminating individual awareness gravitates towards liberation.

Having left behind all attachments to the limited and limiting notions that used to trigger all kinds of reactivity, the call of the natural state predominates. The yogi is firmly established in knowing the fundamental distinction between Consciousness and temporary experiences.
What is liberation for you?
Is it isolating yourself from the ever-changing flow of life in its newness?
Or is liberation freeing yourself from your limiting concepts and

perceptions? Is liberation letting go of the boundaries keeping you to feel at one with all of existence?

4.27 Some latent impressions may still generate internal activity.

The last remaining impressions are the last obstacle to complete liberation. In other words, if you notice yourself returning to "me," "mine" and "I," you may be getting entangled again in your sense of identity with its beliefs and preferences. *What are the impressions still lingering? Are there still some subtle sources of agitation, reactivity, and drama?*

4.28 Those impressions may be removed in the same way as the other obstacles (*kleshas*).

These latent impressions can be removed by using the same approach presented before, through meditation and discernment of the fundamental distinction between who you are and who you think you are (2.10 and 2.11). The path remains the same, releasing assumptions and embodying presence by recognizing the uniqueness of every single moment. *How do you keep returning to presence?*

4.29 Having released all investments (goals, attachments, and expectations), the deepest degree of integrated harmony arises as complete absorption in serving the ongoing flow of life (*dharma megha samadhi*).

This is the culmination of the process of transformation mentioned in sutras 3.9-3.12. Removing the last remaining impressions results in the deepest degree of integrated harmony (*asamprajñata samadhi*) when there is complete and unconditional acceptance of existence as it is. This highest kind of integration is known as the integrated cloud of virtue or the integrated cloud of characteristics (*dharma megha samadhi).* Being established in discriminative awareness brings about the complete release of any traces of individuality, so that attention is directed to serving the flow of aliveness. The mind is completely open and so is the heart. At this level there are no practices to be done or achievements to accomplish. **All doing is at the service of existence, being.**

4.30 Thus, previous impurities are cleansed, and no new impressions accumulate.

Living in harmony with the ongoing flow of awareness in every changing moment cleanses any remaining obstacles and prevents the accumulation of new impressions related to an individual sense of identity. Then, the yogi is fully unconditioned and unconditional in intention, thought, action and interaction.

4.31 As a result, free from ignorance (*avidya*) and with all impurities (*klesha*) removed, endless wisdom arises with little that remains to be known.

There are no longer any goals. All the desire to achieve and to know is now extinguished because the yogi lives in a state of harmony through wisdom. The wisdom of the yogi manifests as embodied pure common sense. This is what Patañjali describes in aphorism 1.3 as the state of yoga, when there are no longer any ways of being to regulate so the yogi abides in the natural state, simply living in the deep peace of an unencumbered heart. Then, all that is left to know is to participate in every moment with utmost clarity, free from all struggle and agitation. There is no longer the need to choose something as either an experience or an opportunity for liberation. Every situation and all circumstances are met by the yogi with wisdom, accepting the perfection of life in its continuous changes.

4.32 After having fulfilled their purpose, to provide experiences for liberation, the tendencies towards change in nature (*gunas*) come into balance and inactivity.

These last aphorisms of the Yoga Sutra present the scenario at the end of the yogic journey. This sutra relates to sutras 2.18 and 2.22: the world is real, and although for the yogi established fully in discernment the world is no longer a source of distractedness, for others, the world of experience remains to serve its purpose as a vehicle leading to liberation. A literal interpretation of this sutra might suggest that once one yogi reaches the highest point of integration, *dharma megha samadhi*, the world would cease to exist. This would mean that everything in existence would dissolve also. A different perspective is that since all change results from the constant interaction between the tendencies of nature (*gunas*: *rajas*, *sattva* and *tamas*), for the yogi, the *gunas* come into balance and recede into inactivity. The yogi steps outside of the cycle of cause and effect (as it was stated in 4.6), abiding in awareness and without generating *karma*.

4.33 The imperceptible succession of instants in which change takes place ceases.

Abiding in awareness, the yogi is no longer chasing after the world of experience. Thus, the yogi clearly witnesses the otherwise imperceptible succession of instants along the three dimensions mentioned in sutra 3.13, properties (*dharma*), characteristics (*lakshana*) and state (*avastha*). When most of us see a tangerine, we usually do not recognize the flower where it originated or the continuous process of transformation that converted the pollinated flower into a ripe fruit with specific characteristics. Changes along those three dimensions create the idea of time – what was, what is and what might be. Time is only a mental construct, a convention used by humans to keep track of the constant changes from one instant to the next. For the yogi, since the agents of change (*gunas*) recede into inactivity, time also ceases. According to the previous sutra, the yogi steps out of the cycle of causality. This sutra states that the yogi steps out of the cycle of time as well. *The yogi abides in the natural state in the beginningless and endless ever-changing present moment.*

4.34 Having fulfilled their purpose, the tendencies of nature (*gunas*) return to their original state, and awareness, no longer being veiled by the activities of the *gunas*, abides in its own essential nature, the power of consciousness.

The yogi is liberated from the flow of causality, time, and experiences. The sense of I, with its limiting perspective, no longer colors existence, so there are no longer any personal agendas, opinions or drama. The yogi continues to exist with heart and mind fully open, abiding in the bottomless wisdom of ever-present consciousness until the body of the yogi reaches its death.

Summary of Chapter Four of the Yoga Sutra

The yogic process is a continual journey consisting of removing inefficiencies, restrictions and restraints impeding the optimal flow of awareness through all life processes. In the previous chapters, Patañjali presented yogic paths towards integration (*samadhi*), transformational yoga practice (*sadhana*), and the results of the highest yogic practices (*vibhuti*). This chapter explores the fundamental aspects of nature, awareness, and the manifestation and effects of different kinds of impressions. Chapter Four also explains perception, objects, notions of time, and individual awareness and its purpose. Eradicating misperception delivers lasting freedom from afflictions and integrated harmony with the ongoing flow of life as we fulfill our purpose – to be of service in creating connections with others.

Emancipation (Kaivalya)

Chapter Four of the Yoga Sutra begins by listing different approaches to cultivating extraordinary powers, a continuation of the major theme in Chapter Three. Subsequently, Patañjali explains the nature of existence and the mutability of nature where primordial energy manifests according to its potential, especially when obstacles to its organic development are removed. The individual sense of self results from its identification with changing phenomena. Through meditation, the impressions of those activities are neutralized so that they stop generating tendencies (*vasanas*) and potentialities (*karma*). Those tendencies and potentialities, although they may have been collected at different times and places, will emerge when the conditions are ripe for their fruition. Patañjali continues by formulating a model of mental perception, where the objects perceived are real, not imaginary. The whole process of perception is animated by pure awareness. Eventually, individual awareness releases its ways of being and turns from focusing on the world of experiences to reflecting pure awareness without distortion. With this extraordinary clarity, and without any further distractions, all afflictions and impressions cease. Having released all the binds to temporary experiences, the deepest degree of integrated harmony emerges as complete absorption in serving the ongoing flow of life. Thus, the qualities of nature, having fulfilled their purpose, can merge into consciousness.

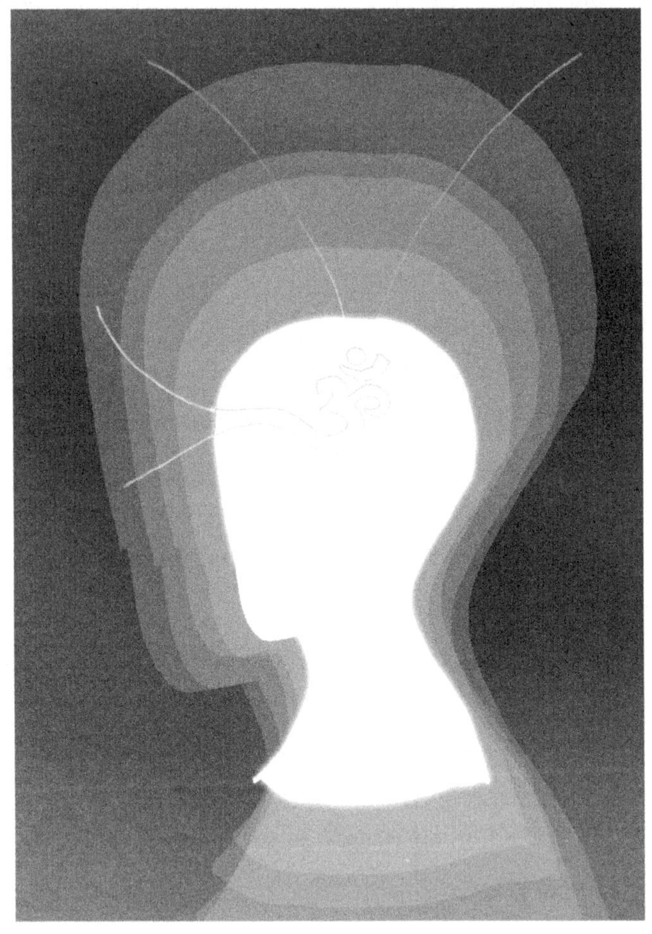

Participate in your life with heart and mind open.

WEAVING THE THREAD OF YOGA INTO LIFE

This book was born of a simple question: *Is it possible to apply the wisdom of the Yoga Sutra into everyday life?* Indeed, practical application of the Yoga Sutra is the major directive in every section of this book. In the Presence chapter, recall, we discussed life as an experiment. Consciously or unconsciously, each of us is running that experiment. Yoga offers you a systematic approach for making your life experiment conscious and deliberate. As it is the case with every part of your life journey, you are in charge. You control the exploration of your options; you choose the decisions that are most conducive to living a vibrant, meaningful, and joyful life. Although it can be tempting to attach to and stick with what we prefer or like, life is constant change. Your circumstances, options and choices will be different at different times... what remains the same is that you are fully present, for all of it.

Y.O.G.A.: You, Organically Growing Aware

Yoga is Presence. Presence is attending to every unique here and now moment of your life. Being present is a choice that only you can make. When you decide to pay attention to your life, you have already started on the journey (1.1). Yoga offers you a path to grow your awareness organically. Awareness is what makes presence possible. Organically means that you do the best that you can do comfortably.

When you explore your options for thoughts, feelings, movements, breathing, and interactions with deliberate and heartfelt consistency (1.12-1.14), you will notice limitations, obstacles, and restrictions as well as strengths, abilities, and virtues. Knowing what enhances your presence and what detracts from being present (1.5-1.11) enables you to make adjustments that help your awareness grow. This requires releasing your attachments to your current ways of being that obstruct the flow of your awareness (1.4 & 1.15-1.16). Instead of trying to make yourself into somebody different, you are trying to let go of the misperceptions distorting who you really are.

One of the biggest obstacles in Yoga is impatience, combined with the misperception that trying to do more than you can will get you to your destination faster (1.30). In fact, pushing yourself harder than you can handle is the fastest way to regress. **If you consistently try to do what you can do comfortably, you will notice that what you can do comfortably expands at the natural level that you can handle.** It's like wanting to start a program of exercise by walking. Just walk for as long as you can comfortably. If you walk regularly, you will notice that the distance you can walk increases gradually without exhausting yourself and without causing you unnecessary strain or pain. Besides, you grow in awareness by expanding your understanding, your kindness, your compassion, and your humility. When you use this approach, which combines persistence (*abhyasa*) with patience (*vairagya*) (1.12), you can enjoy the journey and its fruits. As a result, your yoga practice becomes a combination of Self-Awareness, Self-Care, and Self-Regulation. This perspective enhances the quality of your participation in your life so that you live with enthusiasm, wisdom, and humility (2.1).

S.I.M.P.L.E.: Self-Inquiry to Modulate Predilections for Life Enrichment

In all endeavors it is tempting to keep making things more complex. Keep your yoga practice SIMPLE.

Self-Inquiry. Know your tendencies. Pay attention to your ways of being (*citta vrttis*) in the form of attitudes, thoughts, emotions, beliefs, posture, movements, breathing, intentions, and interactions. Clarify what you know and what you don't know.

Modulate Predilections. Notice restrictions and inefficiencies that hinder your ability to participate consciously, deliberately, and wholeheartedly in your life. Also notice the tendencies and inclinations that are life-affirming. *Knowing your tendencies is the first step to regulating them.* Clarify what is within and beyond your control. Set aside whatever is beyond your control and focus on what you can regulate. Develop your skill for mastering your ways of being instead of allowing your ways of being to determine your attitude, choices, actions, and goals.

Life Enrichment. Direct all your attention and energy to enhancing the quality of your participation in your life through your intentions, actions and interactions. Keep attending to the quality of your participation in whatever you do.

Range of Action

Believing that more is automatically better is a current tendency in many societies. A related common mistake is to confuse range of motion and range of action. Range of motion is often misperceived as the most movement possible instead of the potential range of healthy movement. Rather than thinking in terms of doing the most, cultivating your complete range of natural action is most beneficial in yoga. Range of Action encompasses the complete range of natural possibilities available to you. When you are learning to play the piano, you may not start using the complete set of 88 keys. It is more appropriate to learn to play using a smaller section of the keyboard that would be more manageable while also enabling you to play a variety of pieces. As you develop your playing skills, your hands will adapt and will be able to reach more keys without strain. You will eventually expand your repertoire to include the full keyboard. Since you are not overextending your hands, you will be able to develop nuance in your touch so that you can adjust how soft or hard you press the keys to make your playing more expressive and with a wide dynamic range.

As a human being, your body, mind, and emotions are your instrument. Yoga enables you to access your complete repertoire of attitudes, feelings, thoughts, intentions, breathing, and movements. Whenever possible, attend to your range of action at each level, emotional, psychological, mental, respiratory and physical and get skilled at articulating all your systems seamlessly depending on your context, needs and intentions. *As a result, yoga becomes a balanced and balancing system empowering you to show up fully to your life every day, at every moment.* From this perspective, your yoga practice is at the service of your conscious participation in your life. Knowing your full range of healthy action enables you to decide the practice, duration, and level of intensity most appropriate for you at every time. If you are practicing at the end of your day, the practice will likely be different from a practice that you do at the beginning of your day or during your lunch break at work. As a result, you can show up to life with an open heart and open mind and ready to participate with graceful harmony (2.1).

Guidelines for Yoga Practice

Please remember that the Yoga Sutra has been a practical workbook offering reminders to teachers and dedicated students in their yogic endeavors. The guidelines below intend to assist you in your journey towards open-hearted, open-minded, unconditional presence.

- Meet yourself where you are and just as you are.
- Release strain, struggle, and self-judgment.
- Bring a smile into whatever you do.
- Explore everything with playful curiosity to learn about all aspects of yourself.
- Clarify your intentions.
- Make your own decisions.
- Act consciously and deliberately.
- Pause, Feel, Notice, Validate, Clarify, Choose and Respond.
- Do the best that you can do.

YOUR FOUNDATION

Every person intending to be present will sooner or later run into countless distractions. Distractions will probably happen very often. Remember, noticing distractions is not a sign of failure. On the contrary, when you notice your distractions you can witness how some tendency or preference is hijacking your intention. This enables you to drop the distraction and patiently return to your meaningful intention.

Start from your baseline.

- What is your nature? (1.3, 1.17, 1.41 to 1.51)
- Is there a difference between your nature and your activities (internal and external)? (1.4)
- Is it possible that you are complete, whole, and enough? (1.3)
- Do you know yourself thoroughly? (1.5 to 1.11)
- What do you know?
- How do you know what you know? (1.7)
- Is it knowledge or information? (1.7)
- What are your blind spots? (1.8)
- Are you doing what you think you are doing? (1.8)
- Are you aware of your assumptions and pre-conceived ideas? (1.9)
- How is what you think related to reality? (1.9)
- What are the stories you use to entertain yourself? (1.9)
- What are you learning from you dreams, sleep, and sleeping patterns? (1.10)

- How are the quality of your sleep and of your dreams influenced by your daily thoughts, emotions, and activities? (1.10)
- What do you store in your memory? (1.11)
- To what extent is what you remember accurate? (1.11)
- How are you arranging, editing, and modifying your memories? (1.11)
- Is your memory filled with shrines to previous moments of your life? (1.11)
- Are you aware of your habits and their effects? (1.5 to 1.11)
    - Mental
    - Emotional
    - Postural
    - Kinesthetic-Movement
    - Respiratory
- Are you your best friend or your worst enemy? (1.5)
- How are you addressing your habits? (1.12 to 1.16)
- Are you consistent in addressing your habits? (1.13 & 1.14)
- Are you patient in regulating your ways of being? (1.15 & 1.16)
- How dedicated are you to aligning with presence? (1.20 to 1.22)
- Are you in control or is control an illusion? (1.23 to 1.29)
- What obstacles distract you from your natural state? (1.30)
- How are you addressing those obstacles? (1.31 to 1.39)
- How do you know that your practice is working? (1.41 to 1.51)
- Do your actions indicate a balance of enthusiasm, wisdom, and humility? (2.1)

Limbs of Yoga

The *Yamas, Niyamas,* and *Pratipaksha bhavana* are practical ways of optimizing your energy and creating harmony internally and all around you. These yogic tools help you fine-tune your attitude to enhance the quality of your internal experience. Verify that these guidelines do not go against your own common sense. They may create friction with some of your beliefs. Notice that friction and try to explore it mindfully. The friction may generate internal agitation (*tapas*) that acts as feedback enabling you to modulate your actions. The test of these guidelines is in how you feel as you put them into practice. When you put these ideas into practice do you feel your aliveness and well-being growing?

YAMAS

- Cultivate your capacity for kindness and compassion until, eventually, you learn to love life unconditionally. This does not mean that you are passive or indifferent.
- What is your fundamental assumption? Is the world a place for cooperation or competition?
- Cultivate gratitude, compassion, and your capacity to love (*ahimsa* 2.31& 2.35).
- Think, talk, and act with integrity (*satya* 2.31 & 2.36).
- Live in abundance. Be fair and generous (*asteya* 2.31& 2.37).
- Ignite the spark for curiosity and reverence for life (*brahmacharya* 2.31 & 2.38).
- Thrive in simplicity (*aparigraha* 2.31 & 2.39).

Niyamas

Cultivate your gratitude and inspiration until you live in contentment. This does not mean that you become complacent.

- Is your attitude inspired by gratitude or entitlement?
- Grow in clarity (*shaucha* 2.32, 2.40 & 2.41).
- Abide in contentment (*santosha* 2.32 & 2.42).
- Participate with passion and enthusiasm (*tapas* 2.32 & 2.43).
- Know yourself thoroughly (*svadhyaya* 2.32 & 2.44).
- Touch the world with humility (*ishvara pranidhana* 2.32 & 2.45).

Pratipaksha Bhavana

Make a conscious choice to be an uplifting presence in the world (2.33 & 2.34).

Choose uplifting:

- Emotions
- Thoughts
- Intentions
- Words
- Actions
- Interactions
- Relationships
- Occupations
- Hobbies

- Entertainment

Asana

Embody fully your kinesthetic intelligence to enhance your innate harmony, grace, and overall well-being. In your *asana* practice (2.46-2.48):

- Act with clear intention.
- Do what you can consciously and deliberately.
- Clarify your steady foundation to facilitate upward actions.
- Engage your body with gentle firmness to enhance circulation of blood, nutrients, and information.
- Breathe with natural, smooth, and continuous inhalations and exhalations.
- Make your joints comfortably stable.
- Avoid pinching, forcing, or squashing, especially at your joints.
- Distinguish clearly between tolerable discomfort and pain.
- Distribute your movement evenly throughout all participating joints.
- Stabilize and strengthen unstable and weak areas.
- Enhance flexibility and mobility in tense, tight and rigid areas.
- Beware of tendencies to over-stretch, favor comfortable lengthening instead.
- Beware of tendencies to over-contract, choose 50% of muscular contraction instead.
- Can your posture and movements be a whole-body event?

- Smile and enjoy.
- Your practice relaxes and energizes you.

PRANAYAMA

Fall in love with your breath and become exquisitely familiar with your breathing processes (1.34 & 2.49 to 2.53). In your *pranayama* practice:

- For inhalation and exhalation explore:
    - Qualities (texture, taste, moisture, temperature, pace)
    - Location (abdomen, ribcage, upper torso, combinations)
    - Duration (full range from shortest to longest without any agitation)
    - Breathing options that improve
    - Energy
    - Relaxation
    - Calm attentiveness
- What connections between physical body, intellect and emotions can be explored through variations in breathing?
- Become familiar with the variety of options available for pausing your breathing.

PRATYAHARA

Direct your senses masterfully (1.35, 2.54, 2.55 & 3.48).

- What do you feed your senses?
- Is your mind chasing after sensory experience?
- What happens when you follow a sensation from the outside in?
- What does it feel like to be you from the inside?

DHARANA

Direct your attention to a focal object steadily (3.1, 1.32 to 1.39).

- Relax.
- What is interesting enough and important enough to deserve your time, energy, and attention?
- Contemplate ideas that engage your curiosity.
- Focus on sensations.
- Remember that feeling is different from thinking about.
- Distractions will happen.
- Get good at returning to your focal point, again and again without strain, struggle, or self-judgment and with a gentle smile.

Dhyana

Learn to remain effortlessly focused (3.2).

- Remove the distractions offered by:
    - Your sense of self importance (2.9).
    - Likes (2.7) and dislikes (2.8).
    - Your sense of identity including your opinions and beliefs (2.6).
- Develop your meditation gradually (3.6 & 1.17).
- Cultivate
    - Single pointed focus (1.32 & 3.12).
    - Internal harmony (1.33, 3.9, 3.10 & 3.11).
    - Insight and wisdom (1.20, 3.35).
- Clarify difference between
    - Who you are and who you think you are (1.3 & 1.4).
    - Being and experiences (2.20 to 2.22 & 4.18 to 4.24).

Samadhi

Integrate all your systems by releasing attachment to who you think you are or should be (1.17, 1.18).

- Get very good at relaxing.
- Soften your grip on everything.
- What does it take to let go of your stories?
- Be established in kindness and compassion.
- Accept each moment unconditionally.

Verify that your practice is working

You are the most interested participant in your life experiment because you cannot escape your life or the effects of your actions. Everything that is happening in your life is offering you lessons to grow beyond your current level of understanding. When your intention is clear it is easier to assess that your actions have the desired effects. Some of the potential effects of your practice are listed below.

Internal and external harmony flourish

- *Yamas*
  - Peace (2.35).
  - Effectiveness (2.36).
  - Prosperity (2.37).
  - Vitality (2.38).
  - Simplicity (2.39).
- *Niyamas*
  - Evenness of mind and heart (2.40).
  - Focus (2.41).
  - Joy (2.42).
  - Heightened senses and abilities (2.43).
  - Communion with Supreme Being (2.44).
  - Insight (2.45).
- *Asana*
  - Optimal body function.
  - Evenness beyond opposites (2.48).
- *Pranayama*
  - Long and subtle breath (2.50).
  - Inner radiance (2.52).

- *Pratyahara*
    - Senses within control (2.55).
- You gravitate towards your natural state (1.3).
- Ways of being decrease (1.5 to 1.11).
- Inner silence and inner peace increase (1.18, 2.2, 3.9 to 3.11).
- Distractions, disturbances, and obstacles diminish (1.29 to 1.31).
- You perceive with greater clarity and less assumptions (1.41 to 1.51, 3.12 & 3.12).
- Suffering becomes optional (2.15 & 2.16).
- Confusion is removed (2.25 to 2.27).
- Removal of impurities, increased wisdom and discernment (2.28).
- Release of limitations and beliefs (3.56).
- Enhanced intuition (3.34).
- Impressions do not accumulate (4.6 & 4.30).
- Embodied awareness serving the flow of life (4.22, 4.23 & 4.29).

ॐ शान्तिः शान्तिः शान्तिः

OM Shantih Shantih

May there be peace within, without and everywhere

APPENDICES

YOGA SUTRA CONTINUOUS INTERPRETATION

Chapter One - Integration (Samadhi)

1.1 Now, yoga practice.

1.2 Yoga: regulating ways of being.

1.3 As a result, embodied presence.

1.4 Instead of identifying with ways of being.

1.5 Ways of being manifest in five different ways, sometimes helpful, sometimes unhelpful.

1.6 They are knowledge, misperception, imagination, deep dreamless sleep, and memory.

1.7 Knowledge (*pramana*) results from direct experience (*pratyaksha*), inference (*anumana*), and transmitted wisdom (*agama*).

1.8 Error (*viparyaya*) results from inaccurate perception.

1.9 Imagination (*vikalpa*) is the activity of the mind not based on direct experience.

1.10 Dreamless deep sleep (*nidra*) is when the mind is empty of content.

1.11 Memory (*smriti*) is retaining experiences.

1.12 Integration (*samadhi*) results from practice (*abhyasa*) AND freedom from attachments (*vairagya*).

1.13 Practice (*abhyasa*) is established through deliberate intention.

1.14 And is firmly rooted over a long time of continuous, wholehearted, and sincere action.

1.15 Freedom from attachment (*vairagya*) develops with an attitude of evenness that releases all cravings for external stimuli and internal dialogue.

1.16 Awareness established in Truth does not become distracted, even by the subtlest fluctuations in nature

1.17 A gradual progression towards deep inner integration (*samprajñata samadhi*) develops through subtle refinement of attention from reasoning (*vitarka*), to contemplation (*vichara*), to joy (*ananda*) and then to the sense of being (*asmita*)

1.18 Resulting from practice, a higher state of integration (*asamprajñata samadhi*), with no thoughts remaining, only subconscious impressions (*samskaras*).

1.19 Higher integration results from objective existence for disembodied beings (*videhas*) and for those merged in nature (*prakritilayas*).

1.20 Others, rooted on trust and confidence (*shraddha*), that ignites vitality (*virya*); and on remembrance (*smrti*), that steadies their focus; grow into evenness of mind (*samadhi*) that leads to insight and wisdom (*prajña*).

1.21 It is near for those who apply themselves with intensity.

1.22 There are three degrees of intensity within each level: mild, moderate, and excessive.

1.23 Or, by wholeheartedly relinquishing the illusion of control (*ishvara pranidhana*).

1.24 Supreme Being (*ishvara*) is a special kind of being untouched by afflictions (*kleshas*), actions (*karma*), consequences (*vipaka*) or their impressions.

1.25 In Supreme Being the seed of omniscience is unsurpassed.

1.26 Not conditioned by time, Supreme Being is the unequaled teacher of all times.

1.27 OM is the sound that designates Supreme Being.

1.28 Chanting OM and contemplating its meaning.

1.29 Awareness turns inward, and all disturbances are removed.

1.30 The distractions (*vikshepa*) and obstacles (*antaraya*) on the path to deeper inner stillness and inner silence are disease (*vyadhi*), dullness (*styana*), doubt (*samshaya*), carelessness (*pramada*), laziness (*alasya*), indulgence (*avirati*), confused perception (*bhranti darshana*), inability to be grounded (*alabdha bhumikatva*), inconsistency (*anavasthitatvani*).

1.31 The symptoms of the distractions include: distress (*duhkha*), despair, suffering, trembling, and abruptness in breathing.

1.32 Practicing single pointed focus eliminates the distractions and disturbances.

1.33 Cultivating the habits of friendliness (*maitri*), compassion (*karuna*), inspiration (*mudita*) and equanimity (*upeksha*) purifies mind, body, and heart.

1.34 By exhalations and breath retentions.

1.35 Focusing steadily on subtle sense perceptions.

1.36 Cultivating the inner light.

1.37 Concentrating on serenity beyond desire or on the mind of someone who is beyond likes and dislikes.

1.38 Gaining insight from dreams and cultivating deep sleep.

1.39 Or, by focusing on anything uplifting.

1.40 Steady and focused awareness reveals insight on all aspects of the universe from the smallest to the largest.

1.41 Free from distractions, the mind and heart of the yogi become pure, like a crystal reflecting completely and without distortion whatever is in front of it (*samapatti*).

1.42 When awareness is colored by the focal object, its name and its meaning, integration with reasoning (*savitarka samadhi*).

1.43 When the object of meditation stands out without any thoughts or memories associated to it, integration beyond conceptualization (*nirvitarka samadhi*).

1.44 When the object of meditation is experienced in its subtle constitutive essence, contemplative integration (*savichara samadhi*). Even subtler, integration beyond contemplation (*nirvichara samadhi*) brings the yogi to experience directly the focal object.

1.45 Deepening levels of subtlety reveal the undifferentiated substratum of existence.

1.46 These previous states of deep meditation (integration- *samadhi*) are called with seed (*sabija*), because they use either a gross or subtle focal point.

1.47 Integration beyond contemplation (*nirvichara*) purifies the inner self.

1.48 Then awareness dwells in absolute true wisdom (*rtambhara*).

1.49 Absolute true wisdom, arising from pure insight and discernment, differs from knowledge gained through inference and testimony.

1.50 The impressions created by absolute true wisdom prevent other impressions (*samskaras*) from sprouting, also deactivating dormant, as well as unmanifested impressions or karma.

1.51 When all impressions dissolve, the highest level of integration emerges (*nirbija samadhi*) when all identification ceases and only consciousness, self-contained, pure, and liberated remains.

Chapter Two - Practice (Sadhana)

2.1 Yogic action (*kriya yoga*) combines enthusiasm (*tapas*), intelligence (*svadhyaya*) and humility (*ishvara pranidhana*).

2.2 Yogic actions minimize afflictions (*klesha*) and bring about integration (*samadhi*).

2.3 The afflictions include not knowing who I am (*avidya*), misidentification (*asmita*), likes (*raga*), dislikes (*dvesha*) and fear of death (*abhinivesa*).

2.4 Ignorance of my nature (*avidya*) is the field where the other afflictions sprout. The afflictions can be dormant, weak, intermittent, or fully active.

2.5 To mistake what is impermanent as permanent, impure as pure, painful as blissful, and the non-self as the Self is ignorance (*avidya*).

2.6 Confusing awareness with my body, mind and emotions results in self-centeredness (*asmita*).

2.7 Craving enjoyment is desire (*raga*).

2.8 Rejecting pain is aversion (*dvesha*).

2.9 Even the wise develop a sense of self-importance that causes attachment to living and fear of dying.

2.10 Subtle afflictions dissolve when the sense of being merges into pure awareness.

2.11 When the afflictions manifest as ways of being (*vrttis*), they are counteracted through meditation.

2.12 These afflictions (*kleshas*) are the source of an accumulation of impressions (*samskaras*) that influence present and future experiences (*karma*).

2.13 Determining birth, lifespan, and quality of life experiences.

2.14 Producing pleasant and unpleasant experiences according to virtues and defects.

2.15 The discerning person knows that all internal activities and experiences resulting from the mutability of nature (*gunas*) will eventually cause pain and suffering.

2.16 Future suffering can be avoided.

2.17 The cause of the suffering that can be avoided is the tendency to conflate awareness with what is experienced.

2.18 What can be perceived has three attributes: activity (*kriya*), steadiness (*sthiti*) and illumination (*prakasha*). It manifests in the elements and sense organs in order to provide experiences leading to liberation.

2.19 The states of the three attributes (*gunas*) change from unmanifest to manifest to subtle to apparent.

2.20 The Seer is pure. It is only the power of seeing that witnesses the activities of the body-mind-emotions without being affected by them.

2.21 Everything that can be experienced exists for the benefit of the Seer.

2.22 Although worldly experiences do not exist any longer for the yogi who has reached liberation, the world remains. The world is real.

2.23 The reason for awareness and experiences to come together is to recognize what is permanent and what isn't.

2.24 Identifying with experiences is confusion (*avidya*).

2.25 Freedom arises from removing confusion.

2.26 The means to liberation is uninterrupted discriminative awareness (*viveka khyati*)

2.27 Liberation unfolds in seven stages.

2.28 Practicing the eight limbs of yoga removes impurities, increases wisdom (*jñana*) and establishes discriminative awareness (*viveka*).

2.29 The eight limbs of yoga are: opening your mind (*yama*), opening your heart (*niyama*), optimizing body function (*asana*), enhancing vital energy flow (*pranayama*), clarifying the senses (*pratyahara*), focusing the mind (*dharana*), effortless awareness (*dhyana*) and integration (*samadhi*)

2.30 The *yamas*, wise ways for removing strain, are: Love (*ahimsa*), Integrity (*satya*), Fairness and Generosity (*asteya*), Curiosity and Reverence for Life (*brahmacharya*) and Abundance and Simplicity (*aparigraha*).

2.31 The *yamas* are a great universal vow to appreciate and honor the interdependent nature of life in all forms and manifestations.

2.32 The *niyamas*, wise ways for releasing struggle, are: Clarity (*shaucha*), Contentment (*santosha*), Enthusiasm (*tapas*), Wisdom (*svadhyaya*) and Humility (*ishvara pranidhana*).

2.33 When unhelpful thoughts and emotions arise cultivate uplifting thoughts and emotions (*pratipaksha bhavana*).

2.34 Choosing not to engage in negative and violent thoughts, emotions or actions at any level prevents never ending pain, imbalance, and suffering. (*pratipaksha bhavana*).

2.35 The person established in love and compassion (*ahimsa*), becomes a positive peaceful influence everywhere she or he goes.

2.36 The person established in integrity (*satya*), acts effectively and efficiently.

2.37 For the person established in fairness and generosity (*asteya*), prosperity unfolds effortlessly.

2.38 For the person established in nurturing curiosity and reverence for life (*brahmacharya*), great vitality and enthusiasm develop.

2.39 The person anchored in freedom from cravings and appreciation of abundance (*aparigraha*) recognizes impermanence, clarifies her purpose in life and gains insight into past and future.

2.40 Developing and refining mental, physical, and emotional clarity (*shaucha*), results in releasing blockages that inhibit optimal function, including habits and attitudes towards yourself and interactions with others.

2.41 [As a result of *shaucha*] increased evenness of mind and heart, joyful attitude, focused one-pointedness, mastery over the senses and insight into one's true nature.

2.42 By cultivating contentment and inner peace (*santosha*), supreme joy unfolds.

2.43 Cultivating enthusiasm through removing inefficient patterns in body, mind, and emotion (*tapas*) heightens all senses and abilities.

2.44 Deepening your understanding of yourself and embodying wisdom (*svadhyaya*) results in communion with Supreme Being.

2.45 Humility, relinquishing the illusion of control (*ishvara pranidhana*), enables integration into deep inner stillness and silence (*samadhi*) that facilitates extraordinary insight and effectiveness.

2.46 Steady and joyful posture.

2.47 Releasing struggle and endlessly integrated.

2.48 As a result, evenness beyond dualities.

2.49 Once unified and free from struggle, *pranayama*, regulating inhalation, exhalation, air flow and retention.

2.50 The breath becomes long and subtle when inflow (*puraka*), outflow (*rechaka*) and retentions (*kumbhaka*) are observed precisely according to location, count and duration.

2.51 The fourth type of breath is beyond internal and external regulation.

2.52 As a result, the inner light of awareness becomes brighter.

2.53 Subsequently, the mind is fit for concentration.

2.54 *Pratyahara*, cultivating inner sensitivity to bring awareness into its own form.

2.55 Then, the senses are mastered and at the service of the highest goal.

Chapter Three - Magnificence (Vibhuti)

3.1 Concentration (*dharana*) is directing the mind to a specific point.

3.2 Meditation (*dhyana*) is to maintain the focus effortlessly.

3.3 *Samadhi* is the ensuing dynamic integration empty of separateness.

3.4 *Samyama* (meditative integration) combines concentration (*dharana*), meditation (*dhyana*) and integration (*samadhi*).

3.5 Meditative integration (*samyama*) results in direct insight into higher wisdom.

3.6 Meditative integration (*samyama*) unfolds gradually.

3.7 *Dharana, Dhyana* and *Samadhi* are more internal than the previous five limbs.

3.8 Yet, *Dharana, Dhyana* and *Samadhi* are still external to the subtlest state of pure awareness (*nirbija samadhi*).

3.9 Increased tendency to inner stillness and away from outward attention. Growing inner awareness transforms the body, mind, and senses (*nirodha parinama*).

3.10 Effortless inner silence is established through peaceful impressions

3.11 Releasing internal commentary and identification with externalities brings about a transformation toward integration (*samadhi parinama*).

3.12 Single pointedness (*ekagrata parinama*) is the transformation that enables noticing similarities between arising and subsiding perceptions from one moment to the next. Then the illusion of fragmentation and separateness subsides.

3.13 Consequently, awareness attunes to changes in the senses and in the natural world. These changes manifest as variations of properties (*dharma*), characteristics (*lakshana*) and states (*avastha*) and include changes in one's own being.

3.14 The characteristics of an object can be dormant, active, or potential, yet there is an essence underlying the object.

3.15 Awareness of the sequence of manifestation of these states causes the perception of change.

3.16 Meditative integration (*samyama*) on the three dimensions of change (properties, characteristics, and condition) reveals past and future.

3.17 Meditative integration (*samyama*) on the difference between word, object and concept offers insight into the language of all beings, enabling deep communication with all beings.

3.18 Meditative integration (*samyama*) on impressions (*samskaras*) offers insight into previous births.

3.19 Meditative integration (*samyama*) on somebody's gestures, actions and demeanor indicates his/her state of mind.

3.20. However, the cause of that state of mind is not revealed.

3.21 Meditative integration (*samyama*) on the relationship between form, light and the eyes enables the yogi to become invisible.

3.22* Similarly with sound and other stimuli.

3.23 Meditative integration (*samyama*) on active (*prarabdha*) and dormant (*sanchita*) karma, or on the omens of death, discloses the time of death.

3.24 Meditative integration (*samyama*) on friendliness (*maitri*) and the other qualities (compassion-*karuna*, inspiration-*mudita*, and equanimity-*upeksha*) brings about their powers and effects.

3.25 Meditative integration (*samyama*) on the strength of an elephant and similar qualities, delivers them.

3.26 Meditative integration (*samyama*) on the inner light reveals the subtle, hidden, and distant.

3.27 Meditative integration (*samyama*) on the sun results in knowledge of the universe (the 7 realms).

3.28 Meditative integration (*samyama*) on the moon results in knowledge of the constellations.

3.29 Meditative integration (*samyama*) on the polestar unveils the movements of the stars.

3.30 Meditative integration (*samyama*) on the navel results in knowledge of the body.

3.31 Meditative integration (*samyama*) on the pit of the throat offers access to controlling hunger and thirst.

3.32 Meditative integration (*samyama*) on the tortoise channel (*kurma nadi*) gives steadiness

3.33 On the light in the crown of the head (*murdha*), enables seeing those who are accomplished (*siddhas*).

3.34 Or, by intuitive insight everything becomes known.

3.35 By meditative integration (*samyama*) on the heart, the mind is understood.

3.36 Even a balanced and clear mind is different from pure awareness. When there is no distinction of this difference, individual awareness misidentifies with experiences, feelings, and perceptions. Meditative integration (*samyama*) on this distinction results in knowing pure awareness (*purusha*).

3.37 As a result, intuition and extraordinary sense perception unfold.

3.38 These extraordinary powers can be seen as accomplishments or as obstacles.

3.39 Releasing the causes of attachment to the physical body and by knowing the conduits through which the vital forces travel, the yogin can enter somebody else's body.

3.40 Mastery over the *udana vayu* enables lightness, levitation and leaving the body at will.

3.41 Mastery over the *samana vayu* confers radiance.

3.42 Meditative integration (*samyama*) on the relationship between hearing and space (*akasha*) results in divine hearing.

3.43 Meditative integration (*samyama*) on the relationship between the body and space or meditation on lightness enables traveling through space (*akashagamana*).

3.44 Beyond the physical body and the ways of being (*vrtti*), the great disembodiment removes the veil over the inner light of awareness.

3.45 Meditative integration (*samyama*) on the relationship between the physical, the generic nature, the subtle, the inherent qualities and the purpose of any element results in mastery over the constitutive elements of all natural phenomena.

3.46 As a result, extraordinary powers, perfection of the body and immunity from the elements.

3.47 The bodily perfections include beauty, grace, and the strength to withstand a thunderbolt.

3.48 Meditative integration (*samyama*) on perception, essential character, sense of self, inherent qualities, and purpose results in mastery of the senses.

3.49 Consequently, a body as fast as the mind, independence from sense organs and mastery over the creative principle of nature (*pradhana*).

3.50 Through discernment of the distinction between Pure Awareness and the transparently clear body-mind-heart, supremacy over existence and omniscience arise.

3.51 Releasing even those attainments and removing the remaining seeds of afflictions delivers liberation.

3.52 Self-importance and pride from contact with others, even with celestial beings, can result in undesirable consequences re-emerging.

3.53 Meditative integration (*samyama*) on single moments and their sequence, results in wisdom born of discernment.

3.54 Consequently, the essential difference between two otherwise seemingly identical objects (by species, characteristics, and location) can be discerned.

3.55 As a result of discernment (*viveka*), complete and all-encompassing transcendent knowledge that dissolves the illusion of time. Then, the yogi is free from conditioned existence.

3.56 Thus, when purity of the individual flawlessly mirrors the purity of Pure Awareness (*purusha*), liberation (as complete independence - *kaivalya*) comes into being.

Chapter Four - Emancipation (Kaivalya)

4.1 Optimal function and enhanced efficiency (*siddhis*) may result from birth, herbs, mantra, purification practices (*tapas*) and deep integration (*samadhi*).

4.2 Coming into being is a transformation that follows the flow of nature (*prakriti*).

4.3 The flow of life in nature (*prakriti*) is not the result of incidental causes. When obstacles are removed, life flows organically according to its own potentiality.

4.4 Created minds result from sense of self (*asmita*).

4.5 One singular awareness underlies all the many experiences in their wide variety.

4.6 The yogi's mind, stilled in meditation, does not generate or accumulate new subconscious impressions (*samskaras*), because its perception is not clouded by its ways of being.

4.7 The accomplished yogi, established in integration, is beyond dualities. Therefore, the yogi does not accumulate impressions that cause reactivity (*karma*). For everybody else, reactivity (*karma*) is of 3 kinds: positive, negative, and mixed.

4.8 The subconscious impressions (*samskaras*) lie dormant until the conditions are appropriate for their manifestation. These impressions influence personality traits and tendencies (*vasanas*).

4.9 All actions result in accumulated impressions (*samskaras*) linked to memory in a unique configuration regardless of the time, place, or circumstances in which those impressions emerged.

4.10 It is unknown when these subconscious impressions (*samskaras*) originated, and since they are powered by desire, they will remain for as long as desire remains.

4.11 These impressions are caused by the afflictions (*klesha*) and result in birth, lifespan, as well as pleasant and unpleasant experiences. The impressions are supported by ways of being (*citta vrtti*), tendencies (*vasanas*) and by the objects that can be experienced. When the causes, effects, support, and objects are removed, the impressions disappear.

4.12 Past and future, in subtle form, latent or potential, exist in the present.

4.13 Manifest or subtle, characteristics change due to the primordial tendencies (*gunas*) of nature.

4.14 Although undergoing constant change, each unique object is real.

4.15 The object remains consistent regardless of being observed by different minds or by one mind in different states. In other words, the object exists independently of individual perception.

4.16 The object does not depend on being perceived. Otherwise, what would happen when the object is not being perceived by a mind?

4.17 An object becomes known or unknown depending on the coloring of perception.

4.18 Unchanging, consciousness is the substratum pervading all existence. Ways of being are always known to consciousness.

4.19 Individual awareness is not independent or autonomous. However, individual awareness can serve as a transparent window between consciousness and the world of experience.

4.20 Both pure awareness and the world of experience cannot be apprehended simultaneously.

4.21 One part of the individual awareness cannot observe another portion of itself, or an endless succession would confuse memory.

4.22 When the ways of being are stilled, individual awareness experiences its fundamental nature as embodied consciousness.

4.23 When free of identification and reactivity, individual awareness can reflect everything, consciousness (the seer) and the objects/experiences (the seen), with complete neutrality and all-inclusiveness.

4.24 In spite of its many latent impressions, the individual awareness can serve its higher purpose as a vehicle for liberation by offering a distortion-free reflective surface for universal Consciousness.

4.25 Realizing through direct experience the distinction between pure consciousness and experiences dissolves the notion of individual self.

4.26 As a result, free from the sense of identity, the discriminating individual awareness gravitates towards liberation.

4.27 Some latent impressions may still generate internal activity.

4.28 Those impressions may be removed in the same way as the other obstacles (*kleshas*).

4.29 Having released all investments (goals, attachments, and expectations), the deepest degree of integrated harmony arises as complete absorption in serving the ongoing flow of life (*dharma megha samadhi*).

4.30 Thus, previous impurities are cleansed, and no new impressions accumulate.

4.31 As a result, free from ignorance (*avidya*) and with all impurities (*klesha*) removed, endless wisdom arises with little that remains to be known.

4.32 After having fulfilled their purpose, to provide experiences for liberation, the tendencies towards change in nature (*gunas*) come into balance and inactivity.

4.33 The imperceptible succession of instants in which change takes place ceases.

4.34 Having fulfilled their purpose, the tendencies of nature (*gunas*) return to their original state, and awareness, no longer being veiled by the activities of the *gunas*, abides in its own essential nature, the power of consciousness.

YOGA SUTRA AS INQUIRY

At the beginning of the book, it was suggested that yoga philosophy has always been an applied endeavor. This list can serve as a quick reference of questions related to each specific sutra so that you can use the questions to guide your inquiry. Contemplating the questions, that is learning to live with the questions and love the questions themselves is more conducive to your growth than rushing in search of answers. Staying with the questions will invite you to sharpen your awareness. And it is your sharp awareness that will find teachers and lessons leading you beyond the confines of your current understanding. The main question you may ask at any point during your day is: **What is the quality of my participation?**

Chapter One - Integration (Samadhi)

1.1 Am I present?
1.2 Can I regulate my internal activities?
1.3 What is my true nature? Who Am I?
1.4 Who do I think I am?
1.5 Which tendencies are helpful? Which tendencies are unhelpful?
1.6 Can I notice the differences between what I know, what I don't know, my imagination, my dreams and my memories and their influences on my attitude, choices, and actions?
1.7 What do I know? How do I know it?
1.8 Am I aware of what I think I know but don't really know?

1.9 What stories do I imagine?

1.10 What is in my dreams?

1.11 What is my relationship to my memories?

1.12 What do I dedicate time and energy to and with what kind of an attitude?

1.13 What intentions motivate me to practice presence?

1.14 What do I do with continuous, wholehearted, and sincere dedication?

1.15 How am I releasing my attachments to external stimuli and internal dialog?

1.16 What do I attend to with no distractions whatsoever?

1.17 Am I noticing a gradual progression in my ability to stay focused? Can I be absorbed in reasoning that leads to contemplation and transforms into joyfulness and eventually into pure sense of being?

1.18 Can I be in stillness, silently witnessing the subtle subconscious impressions at the edge of my awareness?

1.19 Have I released all my beliefs?

1.20 How am I cultivating my trust and confidence, vitality, remembrance, evenness of mind, insight, and wisdom?

1.21 Am I committed to my own process of growth?

1.22 How is my commitment: mild, moderate, or excessive?

1.23 Can I relinquish the illusion of control?

1.24 Is there anything unaffected by obstacles, actions, their results, or their impressions?

1.25 Is omniscience possible?

1.26 Am I noticing the lessons custom tailored to me everywhere I go?

1.27 Is there anything that can symbolize pure being?

1.28 Can I chant OM while contemplating its meaning?

1.29 What do I discover when I chant OM?

1.30 Am I noticing any distractions and obstacles such disease, dullness, doubt, carelessness, laziness, indulgence, confused perception, inability to be grounded and inconsistency?

1.31 Am I feeling distress, despair, suffering, trembling and abruptness in breathing?

1.32 Am I practicing single pointed focus to eliminate distractions and disturbances?

1.33 What happens when I cultivate the habits of friendliness, compassion, inspiration, and equanimity?

1.34 What happens when I concentrate on my exhalations and breath retentions?

1.35 What happens when I concentrate on my subtle sense perceptions?

1.36 What happens when I concentrate on cultivating the inner light?

1.37 What happens when I concentrate on serenity beyond desire or on the mind of someone who is beyond likes and dislikes?

1.38 What happens when I concentrate on gaining insight from my dreams and on cultivating deep sleep?

1.39 What happens when I concentrate on something that is meaningful and uplifting to me?

1.40 When my awareness is steady and focused am I more sensitive to insights?

1.41 Is my mind becoming pure, like a crystal reflecting completely and without distortion whatever is in front of it?

1.42 Can I focus on something and be absorbed in the focal object, its name, and its meaning?

1.43 Can I focus on something without any thoughts or memories associated to it?

1.44 Can I focus on something and experience its subtle constitutive essence? Can I focused deeper to experience the focal object directly?

1.45 Am I gaining a growing awareness of the underlying nature of existence?

1.46 Am I aware, that even those deep levels of meditation gravitate towards a gross or subtle focal point?

1.47 Can I be deeply absorbed in just being?

1.48 Can I experience absolute true wisdom?

1.49 Can I discern the difference between knowledge gained through inference and testimony and absolute true wisdom?

1.50 Am I noticing a new tendency to dwell effortlessly in absolute true wisdom?

1.51 Have I released all identification?

Chapter Two - Practice (Sadhana)

2.1 Do my actions combine enthusiasm, intelligence, and humility?

2.2 Are my actions minimizing afflictions and bringing about integration?

2.3 What obstacles keep me from feeling whole and complete?

2.4 Am I aligning with my essence?

2.5 Am I confusing what is impermanent as permanent, impure as pure, painful as blissful, and the non-self as the Self?

2.6 Am I confusing awareness with my body, mind, and emotions?

2.7 Am I driven by my cravings for enjoyment?

2.8 Am I driven by avoiding pain?

2.9 Am I ruled by my sense of self-importance? Is my fear of dying an obstacle to living my life consciously?

2.10 Do these obstacles dissolve when my sense of being merges into pure awareness?

2.11 Is meditation helping me curb my internal activities?

2.12 Am I aware of how these afflictions are influencing my current situation and experiences?

2.13 How is my lack of awareness determining my future options and life experiences?

2.14 To what extent can I notice the connection between pleasant and unpleasant experiences and my actions?

2.15 Are there any internal activities and experiences that never cause pain and suffering?

2.16 Am I planting seeds of future suffering?

2.17 Is suffering caused by conflating awareness with what is experienced?

2.18 How can my experiences lead me to liberation?

2.19 Can I notice the sequence of subtle states of anything that can be experienced from unmanifest to manifest to subtle to apparent?

2.20 Is there anything witnessing the activities of the body-mind-emotions without being affected by them?

2.21 What is the purpose of everything that can be experienced?

2.22 Is the world of experience real?

2.23 Can I recognize the differences between what is permanent and what isn't?

2.24 Am I identifying with my experiences?

2.25 What happens when I stop identifying with my experiences?

2.26 Am I established in discriminative awareness?

2.27 Am I noticing a gradual process of personal growth? What are the stages I am going through?

2.28 Is my yoga practice removing impurities, increasing wisdom and establishing discriminative awareness?

2.29 Does my yoga practice include all eight limbs of yoga?

2.30 How do I define the *yamas*?

2.31 Am I practicing consistently and wholeheartedly?

2.32 How do I define the *niyamas*?

2.33 How am I cultivating uplifting thoughts and emotions?

2.34 How am I effectively removing negative and violent thoughts, emotions, and actions at all levels?

2.35 How am I established in love and compassion? What am I noticing as a result?

2.36 How am I established in integrity? What am I noticing as a result?

2.37 How am I established in fairness and generosity? What am I noticing as a result?

2.38 How am I established in nurturing curiosity and reverence for life? What am I noticing as a result?

2.39 How am I anchored in freedom from cravings and appreciation of abundance? What am I noticing as a result?

2.40 How am I developing and refining mental, physical, and emotional clarity? What am I noticing as a result?

2.41 Am I experiencing increased evenness of mind and heart, joyful attitude, focused one-pointedness, mastery over the senses and insight into my true nature?

2.42 How am I cultivating contentment and inner peace? What am I noticing as a result?

2.43 How am I cultivating enthusiasm through removing inefficient patterns in body, mind, and emotion? What am I noticing as a result?

2.44 How am I deepening my understanding of myself and embodying wisdom? What am I noticing as a result?

2.45 How am I practicing humility and relinquishing the illusion of control? What am I noticing as a result?

2.46 Is my posture steady and joyful?

2.47 Am I releasing struggle and becoming endlessly integrated?

2.48 Am I beyond dualities?

2.49 How am I growing in my ability to regulate my inhalations, exhalations, air flow and retention?

2.50 Am I observing my inhalations, exhalations and retentions according to location, count, and duration? Is my breath becoming long and subtle?

2.51 Am I noticing an even subtler spontaneous way of breathing?

2.52 Is my inner light of awareness becoming brighter?

2.53 Is my mind fit for concentration?

2.54 How am I cultivating inner sensitivity? What am I noticing as a result?

2.55 Am I increasing my ability to direct my senses purposefully?

Chapter Three - Magnificence (Vibhuti)

3.1 How am I practicing concentration?

3.2 Am I growing in my ability to maintain my focus effortlessly?

3.3 Is my ability to remain integrated and without internal commentary growing?

3.4 Can I progress from concentration to meditation and then into integration?

3.5 Are insights growing from my meditative integration practice?

3.6 How is the process of meditative integration developing for me?

3.7 Can I feel how the meditative practices are more internal than the previous five limbs?

3.8 Is there even a more internal and subtle state of awareness?

3.9 Is a tendency towards greater inner stillness and away from outward attention growing in me?

3.10 What are the dominant impressions in my inner realm?

3.11 Am I releasing internal commentary and identification with externalities?

3.12 Can I remain in single pointedness? Does single pointedness enable me to notice similarities between arising and subsiding perceptions from one moment to the next? Am I feeling less fragmented?

3.13 Is my capacity to notice subtle changes in the natural world and in my own being increasing?

3.14 Can I apprehend the characteristics of an object as well as its essence?

3.15 Am I able to notice change as the sequence of manifestation of the characteristics of an object?

3.16 What happens when I focus my meditative integration on the three dimensions of change (properties, characteristics, and condition)?

3.17 What happens when I focus my meditative integration on the difference between word, object, and concept?

3.18 What happens when I focus my meditative integration on subconscious impressions?

3.19 What happens when I focus my meditative integration on somebody's gestures, actions, and demeanor?

3.20. If I focus my meditative integration on somebody's gestures, actions and demeanor can I discover the cause of their state of mind?

3.21 What happens when I focus my meditative integration on the relationship between form, light, and the eyes?

3.22* What happens when I focus my meditative integration on the relationship between sound and the ears and other stimuli?

3.23 What happens when I focus my meditative integration on active and dormant karma?

3.24 What happens when I focus my meditative integration on friendliness, compassion, inspiration, and equanimity?

3.25 What happens when I focus my meditative integration on the strength of an elephant and similar qualities?

3.26 What happens when I focus my meditative integration on the inner light?

3.27 What happens when I focus my meditative integration on the sun?

3.28 What happens when I focus my meditative integration on the moon?

3.29 What happens when I focus my meditative integration on the polestar?

3.30 What happens when I focus my meditative integration on the navel?

3.31 What happens when I focus my meditative integration on the pit of the throat?

3.32 What happens when I focus my meditative integration on the tortoise channel?

3.33 What happens when I focus my meditative integration on the light in the crown of the head?

3.34 What is intuitive insight revealing to me?

3.35 What happens when I focus my meditative integration on the heart?

3.36 Can I notice the differences between my awareness and pure awareness?

3.37 What happens when I focus my meditative integration on this distinction between my awareness and pure awareness?

3.38 How do I view the improvements brought about by my practice?

3.39 Is it possible to release the causes of attachment to the physical body? Can I know the conduits through which my vital forces travel?

3.40 What happens when I focus my meditative integration on the ascending vital force?

3.41 What happens when I focus my meditative integration on the abdominal vital force?

3.42 What happens when I focus my meditative integration on the relationship between hearing and space?

3.43 What happens when I focus my meditative integration on the relationship between the body and space?

3.44 What happens when I focus my meditative integration beyond my physical body?

3.45 What happens when I focus my meditative integration on the relationship between the physical, the generic nature, the subtle, the inherent qualities and the purpose of any element?

3.46 To what extent is my body becoming stronger and immune to the elements?

3.47 To what extent am I familiar with all the levels of subtlety in my own organism?

3.48 Do I have a profound experiential understanding of my own senses?

3.49 What is my relationship to life's creative principle?

3.50 To what extent can I discern the distinction between Pure Awareness and my own unblemished awareness?

3.51 Can I release all attainments and remove the remaining seeds of my afflictions?

3.52 Am I free of self-importance and pride from contact with others?

3.53 What happens when I focus my meditative integration on single moments and their sequence?

3.54 Can I discern he essential difference between two otherwise seemingly identical objects?

3.55 How do I know if I am free from conditioned existence?

3.56 Am I participating in the constant newness of life without blocking the permanent flow of Pure Awareness?

Chapter Four - Emancipation (Kaivalya)

4.1 Am I noticing optimal function and enhanced efficiency in my life?

4.2 How does life manifest into being?

4.3 What are the obstacles keeping life from flowing organically according to its own potentiality?

4.4 What are the by-products of my sense of self?

4.5 Is it possible that there is one singular awareness underlying all the many experiences in their wide variety?

4.6 When my mind is stilled does it generate or accumulate new subconscious impressions?

4.7 Am I beyond dualities? What causes reactivity in me?

4.8 What causes my subconscious impressions to manifest? How do they influence my perspective and decisions?

4.9 Is it possible that my unique configuration of memories, impressions and tendencies continues from one life to the next?

4.10 When did these subconscious impressions originate?

4.11 What are the causes of my impressions? What are their results? What perpetuates the existence of these impressions in my own awareness? Can the causes, effects and support for these impressions be removed?

4.12 What is the relationship between past, present and future?

4.13 What causes the changes in characteristics for all phenomena?

4.14 Are the objects I experience real?

4.15 Does the object experienced remain consistent or is it affected by the different minds that perceive it?

4.16 Does an object I perceive depend on being perceived? What is the purpose of everything that exists?

4.17 How does an object become known?

4.18 What is my direct experience of consciousness, awareness, experiences, and the relationships between them?

4.19 What is the relationship between my individual awareness, my own sense that I am alive, and universal aliveness?

4.20 What happens when I try to focus on both experience and pure aliveness?

4.21 Can one part of my individual awareness observe another portion of itself?

4.22 What happens when my ways of being are stilled?

4.23 What happens when I am completely free of identification and reactivity? Can I witness life with complete neutrality and all-inclusiveness?

4.24 Is my individual awareness serving its higher purpose as a vehicle for liberation?

4.25 What happens when I realize through my direct experience the distinction between pure consciousness and experiences?

4.26 What is my experience when I am free from the sense of identity?

4.27 Are there some latent impressions still generating internal activity?

4.28 Can I modulate the subtle latent impressions remaining in me in the same way that I have deactivate active impressions?

4.29 Have I released all goals, attachments, and expectations?

4.30 Am I becoming less conditioned and more unconditional?

4.31 Am I free from all misidentification and all impurities?

4.32 What happens once the tendencies of nature fulfill their purpose?

4.33 Is it possible to step outside the flow of time?

4.34 Can my individual awareness be free from the activities of nature?

GLOSSARY

abhyasa: Study, practice, repetition, use, habit.

agama: What is known from tradition, testimony of trustworthy sources.

agami karma: Consequences of previous actions yet to manifest, future karma.

ahimsa: Do no harm. The *yama* practice of seeing through the eyes of love and compassion.

akasha: Open space, ether, sky, the ethereal fluid pervading the universe, the vehicle of life and sound.

akashagamana: Going through the atmosphere, going through space.

alasya: Idleness, sloth, laziness. One of the disturbances listed in sutra 1.30.

ananda: Joy, Delight, Pleasure.

anima: Ability to become minute, one of the siddhis listed in sutra 3.46.

anumana: Inference, logical deduction.

aparigraha: Renounce or not accept. The *yama* practice of living in abundance and simplicity.

asana: abiding, stool, dwelling, place, seat, stopping, sitting, sitting down
and posture. Living in knowledge and meditation, empty of distractions, likes and dislikes.

asmita: Sense of I, sense of being.

asteya: Not-stealing. The *yama* practice of living in fairness and generosity.

atha: An auspicious particle, then, moreover, rather, certainly, but.

avidya: Foolish, unwise, not educated, ignorance, spiritual ignorance, the fundamental obstacle that causes confusion and misidentification.

avirati: Lack of self-restraint, excessive indulgence, incontinence, intemperance. One of the disturbances listed in sutra 1.30.

bhasya: Remark, note, comment, commentary, explanation.

bhavana: Causing to be, producing, manifesting, producing welfare.

bhrantidarshana: Confusion, wavering and vacillating perspective. One of the disturbances listed in sutra 1.30.

bija: Seed, source, origin, truth.

brahmacharya: Student or follower of Brahma, the absolute. Celibacy. The *yama* practice of honoring the absolute and following supreme wisdom.

citta: Intention, aim, attending, observing, thinking, reflecting, wish, heart, mind, memory, intelligence, reason.

devanagari: Literally divine city script. The script in which Sanskrit is usually written.

dharma: Duty, life purpose and living according to one's conscience.

duhkha: Unpleasant, disagreeable, suffering, pain, distress, sorrow.

gunas: The qualities and attributes in nature and all that exists, activity-rajas, inertia-tamas, balance-sattva.

ishitrittva: Mastery over the elements to make them appear or disappear, one of the *siddhis* listed in sutra 3.46.

ishvara: Queen, prince, god, king, lord, ruler, god of love, Supreme Being, supreme soul, master.

ishvara pranidhana: Honoring Supreme Being, contemplating Supreme Being with wholehearted devotion. The niyama practice of living with humility and relinquishing the illusion of control.

japa: Muttering, whispering, the practice of whispering or silently repeating a mantra.

kaivalya: Freedom, Liberation.

karma: Action.

karmashaya: The repository of all impressions accumulated throughout life.

laghima: Ability to become light, one of the *siddhis* listed in sutra 3.46.

mahima: Ability to become large, one of the *siddhis* listed in sutra 3.46.

mantra: Instrument of thought, speech, sacred text or speech, a prayer or song of praise, a sacred formula addressed to an individual deity, a mystical verse or magical formula, incantation, charm, spell.

nadi: A vein, artery, nerve or any other tubular organ in the body.

nidra: Sleep, deep sleep.

nirodha: Confinement, restraint, check, control, suppression.

pada: Foot, quarter, chapter of a book consisting of four parts, a ray or beam of light.

pradhana : The creative principle of nature.

prakamya: Unrestrained will, like the ability to merge with the earth or a rock, one of the *siddhis* listed in sutra 3.46.

pramada: Negligence, carelessness. One of the disturbances listed in sutra 1.30.

pramana: Correct perception.

prana: Vital energy, breath of life.

pranava: The mystical syllable ॐ, transliterated as OM and AUM.

pranidhana: Attention, vehement desire, profound religious meditation, great effort, prayer, endeavor, abstract contemplation of, assiduousness, vow, access, entrance.

prapti: Obtaining, acquisition, gain. Ability to reach anything regardless of distance, one of the *siddhis* listed in sutra 3.46.

prarabdha karma: Consequences of previous actions that are manifesting at this time, currently active karma.

pratibha: Light, intelligence, presence of mind, understanding, wit, genius, thought, idea.

pratiprasava: Involution, return to original state. *Prati* means against and *prasava* means product, fruit, generation. *Pratiprasava* is often translated as return to the original state or counter order.

pratyaksha: Direct experience.

rishi: Sage, prophet, seer.

sadhana: Furthering, guiding well, leading straight to a goal, effective, efficient, propitiation, accomplishment, fulfilment, completion.

sama: Even, level, equable, complete, and whole.

samadhi: Joining, whole, accomplishment, trance, concentration, union.

samapatti: Giving way, completion, coming together, yielding, coalescence.

samshaya: Doubt, hesitation, uncertainty. One of the disturbances listed in 1.30.

samskara: Mental impression or recollection.

samyama: Neutrality, being equable, whole self-control. Meditative integration, the articulation of the three internal limbs of yoga, *Dharana*, *Dhyana* and *Samadhi*.

sanchita karma: Dormant karma, consequences of previous actions awaiting the appropriate circumstances to manifest in one's life.

santosha: Delight, contentment, pleasure, joy, satisfaction. The niyama practice of living in contentment.

satya: True, truth, sincere, valid, authentic, pure. The yama practice of living with integrity.

shaucha: Cleanliness, clarity, cleanness, purification, purity of mind. The niyama practice of cultivating clarity in mind, body, emotions, and intentions.

shraddha: Faith, belief, trust.

siddha: An accomplished or perfected person, somebody who has reached liberation from suffering; someone who has obtained siddhis, supernatural powers.

siddhi: Accomplishment, performance, fulfilment, complete attainment (of any object), success, solution of a problem, readiness, prosperity, personal success, fortune, good luck, advantage, bliss, perfection, acquisition of supernatural powers by magical means.

smriti: Memory, reminiscence, remembering.

stharyam: Solidity, hardness, constant, fixedness, stability, permanence, and steadfastness.

styana: To grow dense, coagulated, stiffness, rigidity, apathy. One of the disturbances listed in sutra 1.30.

sushumna: The gracious and kind channel. The conduit of life energy (nadi) at the central axis of the body.

sutra: Formula, string, thread, twain, cord, short sentence.

svadhyaya: Read, study, recite, study true wisdom, self-study. The niyama practice of knowing yourself thoroughly.

tapas: Fire, heat, austerities, self-inflicted torture, pain, deep meditation.

vairagya: Disinclination, dislike, freedom from worldly desires, asceticism, apathy.

vasana: Inclination, tendencies, proclivities, propensities.

vashitva: Control over the elements, one of the *siddhis* listed in sutra 3.46.

vayu: Wind of the body, vital air. There are five major vital airs in the body, *prana*, *apana*, *samana*, *udana*, and *vyana*.

vibhuti: Penetrating, abundance, welfare, wealth, magnificence, great power, prosperity, splendor, greatness, and fortune.

vichara: Contemplation, thought, consideration, reflection.

vidya: Knowledge, learning, science, philosophy.

vikalpa: Imagination.

viparyaya: Misperception, incorrect knowledge.

virya: Vitality, energy, vigor, splendor, luster.

vitarka: Argument, imagination, opinion.

vrtti: Way of behaving, course of action, tendency, nature, comment, explanation, maintenance, activity, mode of being, character, disposition.

vyadi: Ailment, illness, sickness, disease, disorder. One of the disturbances listed in sutra 1.30.

yatrakamavasaitva: Power to make anything happen according to one's desire, omnipotence, one of the *siddhis* listed in sutra 3.46.

FURTHER READING

Books

Aranya, Hariharananda Swami. *Yoga Philosophy of Patañjali.* Albany: State University of New York Press 1983.

Bryant, Edwin F. *The Yoga Sutras of Patanjali.* New York: North Point 2009.

Carrera, Jaganath. *Inside the Yoga Sutras.* Yogaville, Va.: Integral Yoga Publications, 2006.

Deshpande, Purushottam Yashwant. *The Authentic Yoga: Patanjali's Yoga Sutras.* London: Rider and Company, 1978.

Desikachar, T.K.V. *The Heart of Yoga: Developing a Personal Practice.* Rochester, Vermont: Inner Traditions International 1995.

Devi, Nischala Joy. *The Secret Power of Yoga: a Woman's Guide to the Heart and Spirit of the Yoga Sutras.* New York: Three Rivers Press, 2007.

Feuerstein, Georg. *The Yoga-Sutra of Patañjali: a New Translation and Commentary.* Folkestone, Eng.: Dawson, 1979.

Hartranft, Chip. *The Yoga-Sutra of Patanjali.* Shambhala Publications, 2003.

Further reading

Iyengar, B.K.S. *Light on the Yoga Sutras of Patañjali*. London: Thorsons 2002.

Maehle, Gregor. *Ashtanga Yoga: Practice and Philosophy*. Novato, Ca.: New World Library, 2007.

Prabhavananda, Swami and Christopher Isherwood. *How to Know God: The Yoga Aphorisms of Patanjali*. Hollywood, Ca.: Vedanta Press, 1983.

Prasada, Rama. *Patañjali's Yoga Sutras*. New Delhi, India: Munshiram Manoharlal Publishers, 2002.

Satchidananda, Swami. *The Yoga Sutras of Patanjali*. Yogaville, Va.: Integral Yoga Publications, 1990.

Satyananada Saraswati, Swami. *Four Chapters on Freedom: Commentary on the Yoga Sutras of Patañjali*. Munger, Bihar, India: Yoga Publications Trust, 2013.

Stoler Miller, Barbara. *Yoga: Discipline of Freedom: the Yoga Sutra Attributed to Patanjali*. Berkeley, Calif.: University of California Press, c1996.

Taimni, I.K. The Science of Yoga. Adyar, Chennai, India: The Theosophical Publishing House, 2007.

White, David Gordon. *The Yoga Sutra of Patanjali: A Biography*. Princeton, NJ: Princeton University Press, 2014.

Woods, James Haughton. *The Yoga System of Patañjali*. Cambridge, Mass.: The Harvard University Press, 1914.

Online Sources

YOGA SUTRA

Unravel the Thread podcast and chanting of the Yoga Sutra https://simple-yoga.org/yoga-philosophy/

Patanjali's Yoga-Sutra – the Guide of Yoga, with translation and commentary by Dr. Ronald Steiner https://www.ashtangayoga.info/source-texts/yoga-sutra-patanjali/

Yoga Sutras of Patanjali - Raja Yoga - Ashtanga Yoga by Swami Jnaneshvara Bharati (SwamiJ) http://www.swamij.com/yoga-sutras.htm

SANSKRIT

Spoken Sanskrit dictionary http://spokensanskrit.org/

Monier-Williams dictionary https://www.sanskrit-lexicon.uni-koeln.de/scans/MWScan/2014/web/webtc/indexcaller.php

Sanskrit dictionary http://sanskritdictionary.com/

ABOUT THE AUTHOR

Rubén started practicing meditation in 1993 and established a daily yoga practice in 1996. He committed himself to studying, practicing and teaching yoga full-time in 2005. Rubén approaches yoga as a complete lifestyle grounded in traditional yoga philosophy, which is applied with common sense and without dogmatism. Focused on practicing all aspects of yoga with playful curiosity, Rubén continues exploring, refining, and adapting yoga techniques to integrate an open mind with a heart filled with gratitude and love in a body that functions efficiently. With thousands of hours of experience teaching all aspects of yoga in group classes, individual sessions, workshops, study groups, international retreats and teacher training, Rubén enjoys teaching yoga to a wide variety of students including absolute beginners, seasoned practitioners and yoga teachers. Rubén lives in sunny St Petersburg, Florida.

More information is available at https://simple-yoga.org/

REFERENCES

Feuerstein, G. (2001). The Yoga Tradition. In G. Feuerstein, *The Yoga Tradition* (p. 123). Prescott, AZ: Hohm Press.

Krauss, L. M. (n.d.). Atom: An Odyssey from the Big Bang to Life on Earth...and Beyond.

Lutz, A., Brefczynski-Lewis, J., Johnstone, T., & Davidson, R. J. (2008). Regulation of the Neural Circuitry of Emotion by Compassion Meditation: Effects of Meditative Expertise. *PLOS One.*

Maehle, G. (2012). *Pranayama, the breath of yoga.* Innaloo, WA, Australia: Kaivalya Publications.

Monier-Williams, M. S. (1899). A Sanskrit-English dictionary, etymologically and philologically arranged, with special reference to cognate Indo-European languages. London.

Narayanan, C. R. (n.d.). Yoga Sutras Lessons 1.

Satchidananda, S. (1990). The yoga sutras of Patanjali. In S. Satchidananda, *The yoga sutras of Patanjali.* (p. 93). Yogaville, Va.: Integral Yoga Publications.

Sharma, C. (2000). The Vedas and The Upanishads. In C. Sharma, *A Critical Survey of Indian Philosophy* (p. 13). Delhi: Motilal Banarsidass Publ.

White, D. G. (2014). The Yoga Sutra of Patanjali. A Biography. In D. G. White, *The Yoga Sutra of Patanjali. A Biography* (p. xvi). Princeton, NJ: Princeton University Press.

Wolkin, J. (2015, September 15). Cultivating multiple aspects of attention through mindfulness meditation accounts for psychological well-being through decreased rumination. *Psychology*

Research and Behavior Management , 8:171-180 https://doi.org/10.2147/PRBM.S31458. Retrieved 06 06, 2018

ENDNOTES

[i] These variations in internal activity seem to be corroborated by current scientific research https://www.nationalgeographic.com/magazine/2018/08/science-of-sleep/

[ii] Recent research also indicates that the tongue, because of its direct connection to the brain stem, may serve as a suitable point of access for rehabilitation of a variety of body functions including balance and other symptoms of neurological disorders as featured in Norman Doidge's book The Brain's way of healing and in an article by Esther Hsieh https://www.scientificamerican.com/article/tongue-shocks-hasten-healing/

[iii]The growing number of research on meditation and its effects include a study suggesting that meditation may produce more folds in the cerebral cortex http://newsroom.ucla.edu/releases/evidence-builds-that-meditation-230237, another study also indicating that meditation changes the physical structure of the brain with effects on sensory, cognitive and emotional processing https://www.ncbi.nlm.nih.gov/pmc/articles/PMC1361002/, while another study suggests that long-term meditation practice changes pain sensitivity https://www.ncbi.nlm.nih.gov/pubmed/20141301; another study looked at changes in brain activity and structure conducive to the capacity to choose between automatic thoughts and habits and mindful behavior as well as enhanced feelings of wellness, deep pleasure and oneness https://www.ncbi.nlm.nih.gov/pmc/articles/PMC3184843/

[iv] Some researchers have found that it is possible to gain strength from exercising mentally even without physically performing the exercise https://www.sciencedirect.com/science/article/pii/S0028393203003257

while other studies have also found that the nervous system can influence muscular strength or weakness https://www.physiology.org/doi/abs/10.1152/jn.00386.2014

[v] An article examining the Tummo meditation technique including its physical and meditative components, variations and their results https://doi.org/10.1371/journal.pone.0058244 . You may be aware also of Wim Hof who has offered numerous demonstrations and who has participated in many research studies related to regulating the autonomic nervous system with specific beneficial effects on the immune system through breathing and meditation techniques.

[vi] *Samkhya* is a complete philosophical school. One of the commentaries that provides a detailed explanation of the Yoga Sutra from the *Samkhya* perspective is the ninth or tenth century commentary, *Tattva-Vaisharadi* by Vachaspati Mishra, a commentator famous for writing complete commentaries on the six orthodox systems of ancient Indian philosophy.

[vii] For more than 50 years, the Division of Perceptual Studies at the University of Virginia has systematically documented the experiences of children remembering their past lives, with extensive questionnaires, cross-checking and triangulating different sources, and creating a comprehensive record of thousands of cases that are documented in numerous academic articles and books. https://med.virginia.edu/perceptual-studies/publications/academic-publications/children-who-remember-previous-lives-academic-publications/

Made in United States
Orlando, FL
23 October 2025

71302640R00312